7 Steps to Health and The Big Diabetes Lie

By: Max Sidorov

In cooperation with the doctors at the ICTM

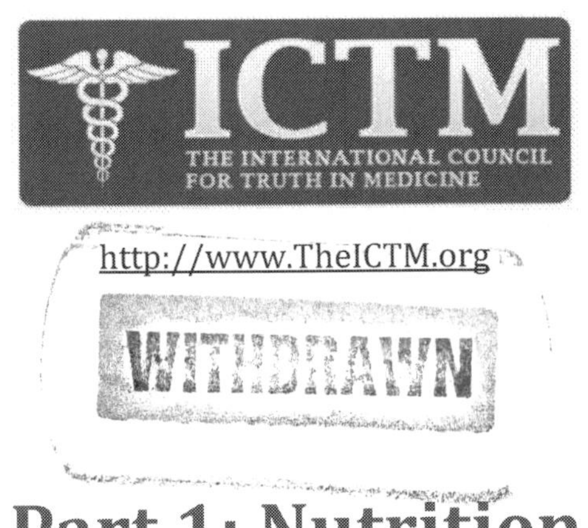

Part 1: Nutrition

Disclaimer

Due to the laws and rules regarding health and wellness, the medical establishment has made it very difficult for anyone to even mention the word "cure" next to a disease or illness. Even though what you are about to read has been studied for decades, proven and researched as fact by medical doctors, scientists, researchers, dieticians, nutritionists, and may just as well "cure" you and restore your full health, by law we are not allowed to do so or say so. Thus, the law requires us to state the following:

This book is not in any way offered as prescription, diagnosis nor treatment for any disease, illness, infirmity or physical condition. Any form of self-treatment or alternative health program necessarily must involve an individual's acceptance of some risk, and no one should assume otherwise. Persons needing medical care should obtain it from a physician. Consult your doctor or health practitioner before making any health decision.

All material in this book is provided for your information only and may not be construed as medical advice or instruction. No action or inaction should be taken based solely on the contents of this information; instead, readers should consult appropriate health professionals on any matter relating to their health and well-being.

The information and opinions expressed here are believed to be accurate, based on the best judgment available to the authors; and readers who fail to consult with appropriate health authorities assume the risk of any injuries. No warranty or guarantee of a cure is expressed or implied with any information in this book. In no event shall the author, 7 Steps to Health, The ICTM, its employees or associates be liable to any person or individual for any loss or damage whatsoever which may arise from the use of the information in this book. To put it simply; before doing anything, make sure to consult your doctor.

Introduction

Before you begin, the most important point we need to stress is the power of proper nutrition. The food you eat; or better yet, not eat plays a much more essential role in reversing your diabetes than any drugs or fancy diets your doctor may prescribe you.

There are no shortcuts, no magic pills and no magic powders. The only thing you need to do to is change the things you eat.

What many doctors and other health specialists practicing mainstream medicine don't realize is how important nutrition is to good health. How could they? Doctors barely get 6 hours of nutrition education for every year they are in medical school.

Doctors aren't being trained to help you; they are trained to become glorified prescription drug dispensers. And since the multibillion dollar pharmaceutical companies are the ones sponsoring and writing curriculum for medical schools, nothing is going to change anytime soon.

And this big pharma influence doesn't stop in medical school; pharmaceutical companies legally bribe doctors to prescribe you more drugs. Many doctors get kickbacks from drug companies for every drug they prescribe or certain brand of insulin meter they recommend to you.

The entire medical system is made to keep you hooked on drugs for life while lining the greedy pockets of pharmaceutical companies. Nobody wants to cure you or make you get better. Everything is made to keep you as sick as possible, thereby guaranteeing profits to them for life.

Sounds grim? Well it is. Think about it. If your diabetes goes away, they lose a customer. They can't sell you any more insulin pumps, glucose meters or monthly drug refills. That's tens of thousands of dollars lost from every patient. This is why they have absolutely no intention of helping you get better. If they were actually in the health business, they'd be putting themselves out of business.

We couldn't just sit there and watch so many diabetics suffer and struggle their entire lives, which is why we wrote this book. In this book we cover the many aspects of proper nutrition and how it relates to perfect health. Countless scientific studies over the years have shown that proper nutrition is many times **more effective** than most drugs and pills at reversing, curing and eliminating disease.

We think you deserve to know the truth regarding our medical system, food and drug system, and health policy.We think you deserve to know what is being done and not being done to keep you sick and unhappy, and we want to shed some light on what is *actually* important and what *actually* matters. You deserve to know that the most common notions you have been told about the food you eat, and about health and disease are wrong:

- Hoping that drug manufacturers or genetic research is eventually going to discover the miracle pill to "cure" any disease is ignoring the decades of scientific studies and research that already proves how disease can be reversed and prevented with diet alone.
- Chemicals in the environment, as bad as they might be, as well as your "predisposition" to disease are not the main causes of most illnesses.
- The genes that you inherit from your parents are not the most important factors that will determine whether you will suffer from any illnesses or diseases.
- Controlling any one aspect of your diet, for example carbohydrates, fats, protein, or any one nutrient is not going to lead to any strong improvement in your health.
- Drugs and surgery DO NOT cure the diseases that kill most people today.
- Most likely, you doctor has absolutely no idea what you need to do to be the healthiest that you can be.

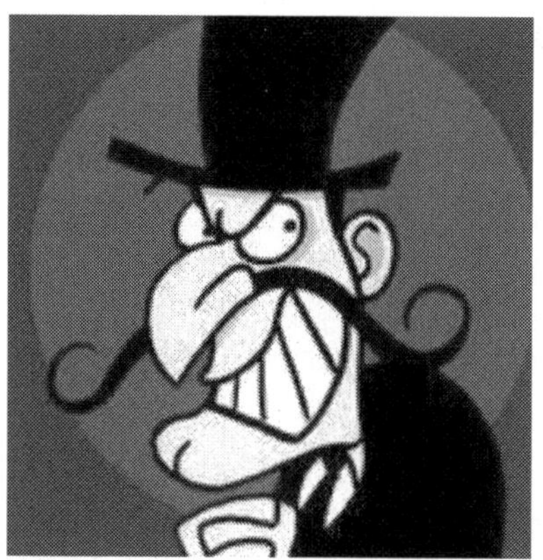

The health industry, just like any other industry, is just that; an industry. And the sole purpose of any giant mainstream industry is to increase profits. How does the health industry make money? They need **more and more** unhealthy people each year who will buy their products. What would happen if people became healthy, and happy? That's right, the whole industry would collapse overnight, and all their billion dollar profits would disappear.

Drugs and pills are not made to cure you. Their goal is to relieve your symptoms to make you FEEL better and trick you into believing they worked. They run an industry to increase their profits, they do not want you to become health, their billions of dollars **depend** on you staying sick and unhealthy.

We want to dispel the mystery and confusion and bring you to the foundation of your **TRUE** health and wellbeing.

Countless scientific studies (which we will get to later on) over the years have proven that simple dietary and lifestyle changes work much better than conventional methods involving drugs and surgery - and without the side-effects. When you take drugs, you still LIVE with the disease you are treating. You still LIVE with the side-effects from the disease while throwing away your money on pointless pills. When you start eating right, when you eliminate the harmful oils, fats, and chemicals, your diabetes goes into remission and overtime even disappears - and with it disappear all the horrible side-effects. Without the use of drugs, pills, surgery or injections.

And trust me, you are going to be quite angry when you see for yourself what the drugs and pills that you might be taking really do to you - and why you never even had to take them in the first place.

Tomorrow's Medicine

"Let thy food be thy medicine and thy medicine be thy food"
-Hippocrates

2500 years ago, Hippocrates, the "Father of Medicine", said to his students, "Let thy food be thy medicine and thy medicine be thy food". Moses Maimonides, the great 12th century physician, repeated the Hippocratic statement when he said, "No illness which can be treated by diet should be treated by any other means". In essence, Hippocrates and Maimonides were insisting that their students practice nutrition therapy, healing the body not by pills, drugs, or surgery, but by changing the things you eat. This type of medical therapy is being used by doctors today, but only by a very small minority.

If you went to your mechanic because there was a loud noise coming from the car and instead of fixing the problem he gave you some ear plugs, would you be satisfied? If a red warning light started blinking and all your mechanic would do is remove the light, would you be happy? This is the same problem with doctors. When you go to a doctor, many of them don't tell you how to cure your disease or ailment but prescribe pills to fight the SIDE EFFECTS of this problem. The drugs simply turn off the warning lights that your body is frantically flashing.

High cholesterol? They tell you to take some cholesterol lowering drugs without analyzing you body to find out WHY you have high cholesterol. High cholesterol is a warning sign of something much worse.

Have heart disease? Blocked arteries? They say you need heart bypass surgery or blood thinning drugs. They never tell you how to clear up your arteries or reverse your heart disease.

Do you have diabetes? The doctor puts you on drugs, and makes you measure your blood sugar daily. None of these things will ever cure diabetes, they are just treatments.

Have you ever wondered why some people have diabetes, heart disease, high cholesterol and other illnesses while others don't? It's all very simple - they eat different foods.

Doctors are not trained in nutrition; they are trained to prescribe drugs and other medicines. They are not allowed by law to even mention natural ways to cure illness or disease using anything other than prescription drugs.

Toximolecular medicine, used by the majority of doctors (especially in the past 50 years) is the administration of drugs at sub-lethal levels to cover up diseases or ailments. Drugs, of course, are alien chemicals which serve to cover-up the disease - to mask it, help relieve symptoms, but never to eliminate the real cause. They offer symptomatic relief but often at the cost of severe and dangerous side effects (if you read the side effect list on some of the most popular drugs, they actually cause much more problems than they solve).

Drugs create dependence on the part of the patient and often complicate the doctor's job by masking or alleviating the symptoms, which are valuable clues as to the real source of the disease or illness.

Of course drugs can save the life of an ill patient, as can surgery and the other techniques at which doctors are very good at. But the paradigm is changing. The common practice of using drugs or surgery to treat what is caused by nutritional deficiencies is slowly on its way out the door. As a doctor in Dublin recently said, "The evidence for nutritional therapy is becoming so strong that if the doctors of today don't become nutritionists, the nutritionists will become the doctors of tomorrow."

Patrick Holford, Director of the Institute for Optimum Nutrition in London which is at the forefront of research and education in this field, makes this very clear: "Tomorrow's medicine will not be about using nutrients instead of drugs. It will be about looking through a new pair of glasses which reveal the true causes of disease. In most cases these lie in faulty nutrition, pollution, stress, negativity, addiction and lack of exercise - the greatest cause of all being ignorance. The original meaning of the word 'doctor' is "teacher or learned man" and that is perhaps the most important role a health professional can perform."

Let's figure out the basics first. We do not have a headache because of a lack of Tylenol, and we don't develop diabetes because of a lack of Metformin. Our stomachs don't get upset because of a lack of Pepto-Bismol, and I'm sure we don't get high cholesterol because of a lack of cholesterol lowering drugs. Do you see where I'm going?

Tylenol does not cure your headache, it just stops you from feeling it, Metformin does not cure diabetes, it just makes your liver release less glucose, and Aspirin thins the blood which "seems" to help with heart disease, but why was the blood thick anyway? Why did you have a headache? Why is there so much glucose in your blood? What is the CAUSE of all those diseases? Has anyone ever asked what the real cause of their disease was instead of just taking a pill to make the symptoms go away?

The entire approach and foundation of Orthodox Medicine is based on Luis Pasteur's *Germ Theory*, a flawed concept. A disease condition is viewed by the orthodoxy as an isolated event, confined to the area in which it manifests itself (E.g. an ear infection, eye infection, gum infection, lung cancer, skin cancer, diabetes, heart disease, etc.). Under this theory, *for unknown reasons*, microbes or tumors indiscriminately grow in the patient and must be cut (surgery), burned (radiation), or poisoned (drugs) out of the body. In the orthodox model, the solution is sought through **mechanical** and **chemical** means. Seeking to understand WHY the infection or disease condition appeared in the first place, is not explored. The quick fix with a prescription for drugs to smother the symptoms is the typical orthodox 'answer'.

A contemporary of Pasteur, **Antoine Bechamp**, had a different opinion as to why disease conditions 'took hold'. Bechamp felt that the ENVIRONMENT, or the ECOLOGY of the blood played the critical role in deciding whether disease conditions would manifest or not.

It is important to discover the **stressors** (environmental, biological, chemical, psychological, and emotional) in a patient's life that cause a *weakening* of a particular bodily system; which in turn allows the manifestation of a disease condition in a weakened area. In order to maintain a state of health, all systems within the body need to exist in a state of **balance** or **equilibrium**. Imbalance leads to conditions of discomfort (dis-ease) which eventually spirals into ill health if not corrected. The Chinese and Indians (Ayurvedic medicine) had worked all of this out **thousands of years** ago.

Orthodox or Allopathic Medicine utilizes poisonous substances (drugs) in non-lethal dosages in order to suppress symptoms in an affected area. ***This approach neither addresses the cause of the disease condition, nor is it responsible for healing the patient.*** Rather, the use of drugs often will **temporarily mask** the outer manifestations of the malady, while at the same time, drive the disease deeper into the body...**only to reappear at a later date, as a more serious, and chronic health threat**. One of the many flaws of the orthodox approach is that it focuses on the disease condition itself, *rather than the patient*. The term **holistic** (or holistic) originally sprang up to distinguish those physicians whose diagnostic methods consider all of the physical and emotional factors interacting with the patient.

Why is medicine these days so concerned about the symptoms, why do we have so many drugs for so many diseases? Every year there is a thousand new diseases added to the list. It's because treating the symptom is much more profitable for the billion dollar drug companies than curing the cause.

There are a few principles guiding the pharmaceutical "business of diseases," and none of them have anything to do with your health. The financial interests of the pharmaceutical industry do not lie in the cure or prevention of the common disease - the maintenance and expansion of diseases is the only way for the financial growth of this industry. A key strategy to accomplish this goal is the development of drugs that merely mask symptoms while avoiding the curing or elimination of diseases. This explains why most prescription drugs marketed today have no proven efficacy and merely target symptoms.

Medical doctors are not trained in nutrition; they are trained in drugs, drugs, and more drugs. Asking a doctor about nutrition is like asking a train conductor about brick laying. This is why you need to educate yourself on the science of nutrition.

Processed Junk

Acids, anticaking agents, bulking agents, food coloring, emulsifiers, thickeners, stabilizers, flavors, humectants, preservatives, sweeteners.

Science in the field of food and agriculture has become very advanced, we are able to preserve things longer, cook things faster, and make things taste better. All these things require a heavy route of processing transforming otherwise healthy ingredients into Frankenstein like concoctions.

It is only the last few hundred years scientists began experimenting with chemicals on food, and only in the past 50 years we have really amped up the process with strong additives for preservation, color, or taste enhancement. Before that, people used to eat things completely unprocessed, and in its natural state. All the "Western" diseases like cancer, diabetes and heart disease as well as obesity were almost non-existent. Nowadays, millions of people die every year because of these illnesses.

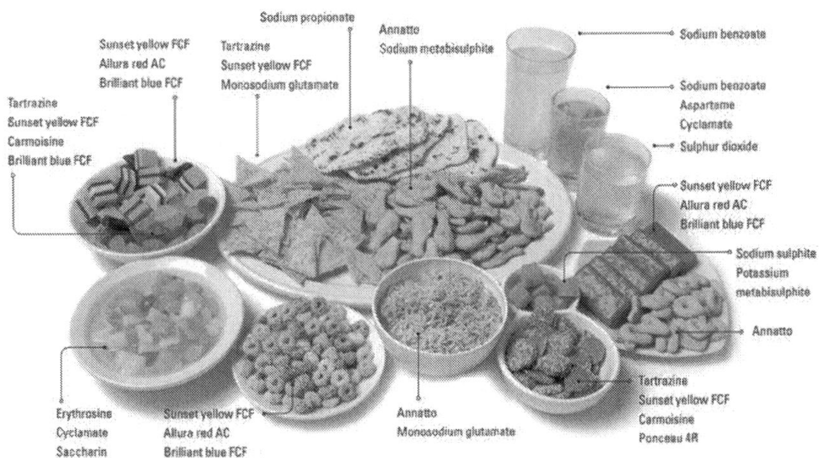

Our bodies are meant to run on natural, unprocessed, whole, organic foods, good quality proteins, healthy fats, fruits, vegetables, nuts and seeds. The chemical soup that comprises most grocery store and fast foods that so many people ingest every day wreaks absolute havoc on our immune, hormone, nervous, vascular, and all other systems in our body creating chemical and hormone imbalances, and just like a computer virus, messing around with our body's processing until everything begins to self destruct.

Forget the low carb, low fat or fat free (loaded with sugar and starch), sugar-free (chemical poison and fat storing fuel). Forget the fast foods and the microwave foods (loaded with a mixture of chemicals and toxic ingredients taking years off your life by stimulating inflammation, immune/hormone/metabolism imbalances, heart disease, diabetes, cancer, just to name a few). Let's go back to REAL food and REAL water and allow our bodies to clean up, detox, and loose the weight once and for all!

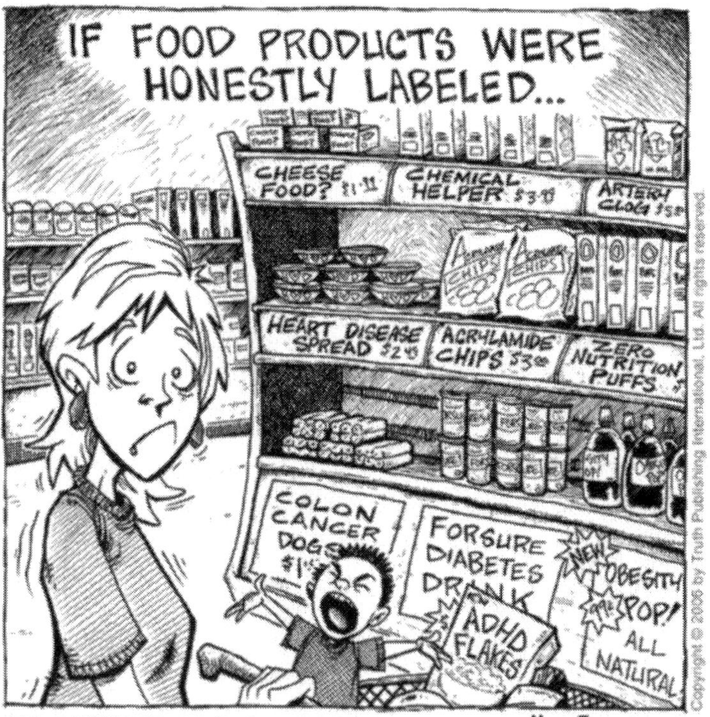

www.NaturalNews.com

Where to look for food additives on a product label?

When buying groceries, these additives are listed (if it's given by the law) on the food product's packaging under "**INGREDIENTS:**" or "**CONTAINS:**" section, usually next to "Nutrition Information" but the code numbers or names of these additives can be printed on in a small font.

In my opinion placement of the text can be somewhat hidden or even misleading. Any dangerous additives added in the food, if the product contains any, really should be listed visibly and labeled on the pack for instance as "**Nasty Additives**".

Food additives give flavor. For any foods, flavoring is added so that these meals are pleasing to the palate when they come out of the microwave or the oven.

Preservatives are added for shelf life. Cakes can look great and so may canned and bagged foods when additives keep them fresh in their wrappings for weeks on end.

Here is a new list with identifying code numbers of the nasty food additives that we should avoid eating. Artificial food preservatives, food colors and flavor enhancers, these are dangerous chemicals added to our food and are known to be linked to Hyperactivity, Attention-Deficit Disorder (ADD), Asthma, Cancer and other medical conditions (these are just the ones tested for specific disorders, who knows what scientists will find after more rigorous testing!).

All the food colorings in the list below can end up under the label "artificial" or "natural" colors; there can be dozens of them at once or just a few, it's like playing the toxin lottery. If you see the words "artificial colors" or even "natural colors," it is better to avoid that product altogether. I have highlighted the additives you are most likely to encounter.

Dangerous Food Additives table

Additive Number	Name of Food Additive	Hyper-activity	Asthma	Cancer
102 & E102	Tartrazine (food color)	H	A	C
104 & E104	Quinoline Yellow (food color)	H	A	C
107 & E107	Yellow 2G (food color)	H	A	C
110 & E110	Sunset Yellow (Yellow food color #6)	H	A	C
120 & E120	Carmines, Cochineal (food color)	H	A	-
122 & E122	Azorubine, Carmoisine (food color)	H	A	C
123 & E123	Amaranth (Red food color #2)	H	A	C
124 & E124	Ponceau, Brilliant Scarlet (food color)	H	A	C
127 & E127	Erythrosine (Red food color #2)	H	A	C
E128	Red 2G (Red food color)	H	A	C
129 & E129	Allura Red AC (food color)	H	A	C
E131	Patent Blue (food color)	H	A	C
132 & E132	Indigotine, Indigo Carmine (food color)	H	A	C
133 & E133	Brilliant Blue (food color)	H	A	C
142 & E142	Acid Brilliant Green, Green S, Food Green (food color)	H	A	-
143	Fast Green (food color)	-	A	-
150 & E150	Caramel (food color)	H	-	-
151 & E151	Activated Vegetable Carbons, Brilliant Black (food color)	H	A	C
154	Food Brown, Kipper Brown, Brown FK (food color)	H	A	C

155 & E155	Chocolate Brown HT, Brown HT (food color)	H	A	C	
160b & E160b	Bixin, Norbixin, Annatto Extracts (yellow, red to brown natural colors)	H	A	-	
E173	Aluminium (preservatives)	-	-	C	
E180	Latol Rubine, Pigment Rubine (preservatives)	H	A	C	
200 & E200-203	Potassium & Calcium Sorbates ,Sorbic Acid (preservatives)	H	A	-	
210 & E210	**Benzoic Acid** (preservatives)	H	A	C	
211 & E211	**Sodium Benzoate** (preservatives)	H	A	-	
212 & E212	**Potassium Benzoate** (preservatives)	-	A	-	
213 & E213	Calcium Benzoate (preservatives)	-	A	-	
E214	Ethyl Para Hydroxybenzonate (preservatives)	-	A	-	
E215	Sodium Ethyl Para Hydroxybenzonate (preservatives)	-	A	-	
216 & E216	Propyl P Hydroxybenzonate, Propylparaben (preservatives)	-	A	-	
E217	Sodium Propyl P Hydroxybenzonate (preservatives)	-	A	-	
220 & E220	**Sulphur Dioxide also Sulfur dioxide** (preservatives)	H	A	-	
221 & E221	**Sodium Sulfite** or Sodium Sulphite (preservatives)	-	A	-	
222	**Sodium Bisulfite** or Sodium Bisulphite (preservatives)	-	A	-	
223 & E223	Sodium Metabisulfite or Sodium Metabisulphite (preservatives)	-	A	-	
224 & E224	Potassium Metabisulphite or	-	A	-	

	Potassium Metabisulfite (preservatives)				
225 & E225	Potassium Sulfite or **Potassium Sulphite** (preservatives)	-	A	-	
E226	Calcium Sulfite or **Calcium Sulphite** (preservatives)	-	A	-	
E227	Calcium Hydrogen Sulphite or Calcium Hydrogen Sulfite (preservatives)	-	A	-	
E228	Potassium Bisulfite, Potassium Hydrogen Sulfite or Potassium Bisulphite, Potassium Hydrogen Sulphite (preservatives)	H	A	-	
E230	Diphenyl, Biphenyl (preservatives)	-	-	C	
E231	Orthophenyl Phenol (preservatives)	-	-	C	
E236	Formic Acid (preservative)	-	-	C	
E239	Hexamine, Hexamethylene Tetramine (preservatives)	-	-	C	
249 & E249	**Potassium Nitrate** (preservative)	-	A	C	
250 & E250	**Sodium Nitrite** (preservative)	H	A	C	
251 & E251	Sodium Nitrate (preservative)	H	-	C	
252 & E252	Potassium Nitrate (preservative)	H	-	C	
260 & E260	**Acetic Acid**, Glacial (preservatives)	-	A	-	
280 to 283	Calcium or Potassium or **Sodium Propionates**, Propionic Acid (preservatives)	H	A	-	
310 & E310	Propyl Gallate (Synthetic Antioxidant)	-	A	C	
311 & E311	Octyl Gallate (Synthetic Antioxidant)	-	A	-	
312 & E312	Dodecyl Gallate (Synthetic	-	A	-	

	Antioxidant)				
319 & E319	TBHQ, Tert Butylhydroquinone (Synthetic Antioxidants)	H	A	-	
320 & E320	Butylated Hydroxyanisole (**BHA**) (Synthetic Antioxidants)	H	A	C	
321 & E321	Butylated Hydroxytoluene (**BHT**) or Butylhydroxytoluene (Synthetic Antioxidants)	H	A	C	
330 & E330	Citric Acid (**NOT DANGEROUS** naturally occurring e330 & 330 citric acid additive – can contain sulfites and mold.)	-	-	-	
407 & E407	**Carrageenan** (Thickening & Stabilizing Agent)	-	A	C	
413 & E413	Tragacanth (thickener & Emulsifier)	-	A	-	
414 & E414	Acacia Gum (Food Stabilizer)	-	A	-	
416	Karaya Gum (Laxative, Food Thickener & Emulsifier)	-	A	-	
421 & E421	**Mannitol** (Artificial Sweetener)	H	-	-	
430	Polyxyethylene Stearate (Emulsifier)	-	-	C	
431	**Polyxyl Stearate** (Emulsifier)	-	-	C	
E432 – E435	Polyoxyethylene Sorbitan Monostearate (Emulsifiers Gelling Stabilisers Thickeners Agents)	-	-	C	
433 – 436	**Polysorbate** (Emulsifiers)	-	-	C	
441 & E441	**Gelatine** (Food Gelling Agent)	-	A	-	
466	Sodium CarboxyMethyl Cellulose	-	-	C	
507 & E507	Hydrochloric Acid (Hydrolyzing Enhancer & Gelatin Production)	-	-	C	
518 & E518	**Magnesium Sulphate** (Tofu Coagulant)	-	-	C	

536 & E536	Potassium Ferrocyanide (Anti Caking Agent)	-	A	-	
553 & E553 & E553b	Talc (Anti Caking, Filling, Softener, Agent)	-	-	C	
620 – 625	<u>**MSG Monosodium Glutamate**</u>, Glutamic Acid, all Glutamates (Flavour Enhancers)	H	A	C	
627 & E627	**Disodium Guanylate** (Flavour Enhancers)	H	A	-	
631 & E631	Disodium Inosinate 5 (Flavour Enhancers)	-	A	-	
635 & E635	Disodium Ribonucleotides 5 (Flavour Enhancers)	-	A	-	
903 & E903	Camauba Wax (used in Chewing Gums, Coating and Glazing Agents)	-	-	C	
905 & 905 a,b,c	Paraffin and Vaseline, White Mineral Oil (Solvents, Coating and Glazing, Anti Foaming Agents, Lubricant in Chewing Gums)	-	-	C	
924 & E924	Potassium Bromate (Agent used in Bleaching Flour)	-	-	C	
925 & E925	Chlorine (Agent used in Bleaching Flour, Bread Enhancer and Stabiliser)	-	-	C	
926	Chlorine Dioxide (Bleaching Flour and Preservative Agent)	-	-	C	
928 & E928	Benzoyl Peroxide (Bleaching Flour and Bread enhancer Agent)	-	A	-	
950 & E950	Potassium Acesulphame (Sweetener)	-	-	C	
951	**Aspartame** (Sweetener)	H	A	-	
952 & E952	Cyclamate and Cyclamic Acid (Sweeteners)	-	-	C	
954 & E954	**Saccharine** (Sweetener)	-	-	C	

1202 & E1202	Insoluble Polyvinylpyrrolidone Insoluble (Stabiliser and Clarifying Agent added to Wine, Beer, Pharmaceuticals)	-	-	C	
1403	Bleached Starch (Thickenner and Stabiliser)	-	A	-	

These additives do a great job of making our food look good and taste good while it's sitting on a grocery store shelf for weeks, months, or even years. This is extremely unnatural, and you can just imagine what these additives do to your health. Even the idea that something has already been proven to cause cancer, or any disease for that matter, and is still considered "safe" and allowed to be put into our food is ridiculous. This is an industry folks, they have absolutely no regard for your health; to them it's all about their profits.

Let's vote with our wallets, stop polluting our bodies, and send a clear message to these greedy, selfish companies that we demand healthy, natural food!

Chapter One

Refined Flour, Pasta, Cookies, Crackers, Bread etc.

In 1911, the bread which made up 40 percent of the diet of the impoverished people of Britain was blamed for widespread poor health. Modern nutritional science confirms the accuracy of this assessment.

Refined white flour contains almost no natural minerals and vitamins. In particular, vitamin B deficiency from poor diet resulted in a range of illnesses that the Victorians called 'wasting diseases'. And white flour at the time was usually laced with alum, which made bad flour look whiter.

According to the Daily Mail:

"[In modern times], the Real Bread Campaign, a non-profit pressure group, claims that bread has actually gotten worse since 1911 in terms of secret adulterants -- enzymes that do not have to be declared on labels -- still being smuggled into it. Today, despite the modern fashion for healthy eating, 'nutritionally empty' white bread accounts for more than 50 percent of what we buy."

Today, there's a whole new breed of health-harming ingredients to contend with in your typical store-bought bread, including:

Processed salt	High fructose corn syrup	Trans fats (hydrogenated oils)
Soy	Treatment agents (oxidant chemicals)	Reducing agents
Emulsifiers	Preservatives	Enzymes (typically from fungi or bacteria)

Many of these ingredients are hidden, as they're not required to be listed on the label due to lobby groups from giant corporations which persuaded government to be very lenient on rules and regulations regarding ingredient labels and food in general.

Refined Foods are Devoid of Nutrients

It's important to realize that when food is refined, vital nutrients are destroyed. In some cases it's questionable whether what remains is even fit to be considered food... at least if the term "food" implies something of nutritional value.

In terms of bread, once you remove the most nutritious part of the grain, it essentially becomes a form of sugar. Processed white flour, or “enriched wheat flour” or just “wheat flour” is missing the most important and nutritious part of the seed; the outside bran layer and the germ (embryo).

Consider what gets lost in the refining process:

Half of the beneficial unsaturated fatty acids	50 percent of the calcium	80 percent of the iron	50-80 percent of the B vitamins
Virtually all of the vitamin E	70 percent of the phosphorus	98 percent of the magnesium	And many more nutrients are destroyed -- simply too many to list.

How Processed Grains Can Deteriorate Your Health

The end result of the excessive consumption of white bread and other processed forms of grain products can be seen all around you in the form of:

Obesity	Diabetes	Heart disease
Allergies and asthma	Gluten intolerance and Celiac disease	Vitamin deficiencies and related health problems

Vitamin B deficiencies in particular contribute to a wide range of illnesses, and vitamin B deficiencies are pervasive around the world. For example, an estimated 25 percent of American adults are deficient in B12 (more than half of the population of U.S. is deficient in the bare minimum RDA, or recommended dietary allowance, of vitamins and minerals)

We've also seen an extraordinary rise in digestive illnesses, such as gluten intolerance and Celiac disease, and modern industrial baking methods are likely a major contributor to these widespread problems. The rise in asthma and allergies may also be related to our modern food processing and manufacturing practices. For example, one of the enzymes commonly used in modern bread making is amylase, which is known to cause asthma.

Many also forget that most commercial wheat production is, unfortunately, a "study in pesticide application," beginning with the seeds being treated with fungicide. Once they become wheat, they are sprayed with hormones and pesticides. Even the bins in which the harvested wheat is stored have been coated with insecticides. These chemicals all contribute to increasing the average person's toxic load, which is a contributing factor to virtually every possible disease imaginable. I can't think of any illness that is not made worse by frequent toxic exposure, such as what we get through conventionally-grown foods and unfiltered water.

Whereas old time mills ground flour slowly, today's mills are designed for mass-production, using high-temperature, high-speed steel rollers. Next, the wheat hit with another chemical insult--a chlorine gas bath (chlorine oxide). This serves as a whitener, as well as an "aging" agent. Flour used to be aged with time, improving the gluten and thus improving the baking quality. Treating it with chlorine instantly produces similar qualities in the flour (with a disturbing lack of concern about adding another dose of chemicals to your food).

The resulting white flour is nearly all starch, and now contains a small fraction of the nutrients of the original grain. Additionally, the chemical treatments on the grain results in the formation of a by-product, alloxan—a poison used in the medical research industry to induce diabetes in healthy mice. Alloxan causes diabetes by spinning up enormous amounts of free radicals in pancreatic beta cells, thus destroying them. Beta cells are the primary cell type in areas of your pancreas called islets of Langerhans, and they produce insulin; so if those are destroyed, you develop diabetes.

Eating even moderate amounts of white flour and foods high in starch devoid of nutrition will make you feel fatigued, irritable, depressed, and lead to chronic illness. This white flour also digests into sugar raising insulin levels, making your body acidic, promoting fat storage, and making you even hungrier.

Why a High-Carb Diet Can be Disastrous to Your Health

Overconsumption of carbs is the primary driving factor for insulin resistance and type 2 diabetes. Unfortunately, the dietary establishment has unwisely been praising the virtues of carbohydrates while warning you to avoid fats. But anyone who bought into the high-carb, low-fat diets has likely struggled with their weight and health, wondering what they're doing wrong...

The truth of the matter is that a diet high in grain carbs (as opposed to vegetables) and low in fat may be **dangerous** to your health, and if you want to shed excess weight and improve your health, the opposite diet is what you're looking for!

Why are high-carb diets so bad?

To put it simply, overeating carbohydrate foods prevents fats from being used for energy, and lead to an increase in fat storage. It also raises your insulin levels, which in short order can cause insulin resistance, followed by diabetes. Insulin resistance is also at the heart of virtually every disease known to man.

Contrary to popular belief, eating fat does **NOT** make you fat—carbohydrates, such as sugar and white flour **do**. Your body has a limited capacity to **store** excess carbohydrates, but it can easily **convert** those excess carbohydrates into excess body fat. Any carbohydrates not immediately used by your body are stored in the form of glycogen (a long string of glucose molecules linked together). Your body has two storage sites for glycogen: your liver and your muscles. Once the glycogen levels are filled in both your liver and muscles, excess carbohydrates are converted into fat and stored in your adipose, or fatty tissue.

So, although carbohydrates are fat-free, excess carbohydrates end up as excess fat.

But that's not the worst of it. Any meal or snack high in carbohydrates will also generate a rapid rise in blood glucose. To adjust for this rapid rise, your pancreas secretes insulin into your bloodstream, which then lowers the levels of blood glucose. The problem is that insulin is essentially a storage hormone, evolved to put aside excess carbohydrate calories in the form of fat in case of future famine. So the insulin that's stimulated by excess carbohydrates *aggressively promotes the accumulation of body fat!*

To Summarise:

Too Much Wheat or Grain Gets Converted Into Fat
In other words, when you eat too much bread, pasta, and any other grain products, you're essentially sending a hormonal message, via insulin, to your body that says "store fat."

Additionally, increased insulin levels also:

- Make it virtually impossible for you to use your own stored body fat for energy
- Suppress two important hormones: glucagon and growth hormone. Glucagon promotes the burning of fat and sugar. Growth hormone is used for muscle development and building new muscle mass.

- Increases hunger: As blood sugar increases following a carbohydrate meal, insulin rises with the eventual result of lower blood sugar. This results in hunger, often only a couple of hours (or less) after the meal.

So, all in all, the excess carbohydrates in your diet not only make you fat, they make sure you **stay fat**. Cravings; usually for sweets, are frequently part of this cycle, leading you to resort to snacking, often on more carbohydrates. Not eating can make you feel ravenous shaky, moody and ready to "crash." If the problem is chronic, you never get rid of that extra stored fat, and your energy and overall health is adversely affected.

Below is a list of some of the most common complaints of people with insulin resistance (IR). Many of these symptoms may occur immediately following a meal of carbohydrates; others may be chronic:

Does this sound like you?

Fatigue. Some are tired just in the morning or afternoon; others are exhausted all day.	**Brain fogginess.** The inability to concentrate is the most evident symptom. Loss of creativity, poor memory, failing or poor grades in school often accompany insulin resistance, as do various forms of "learning disabilities."	**Hypoglycemia.** Feeling jittery, agitated and moody is common in IR, with an almost immediate relief once food is eaten. Dizziness is also common, as is the craving for sweets, chocolate or caffeine.

Yeast

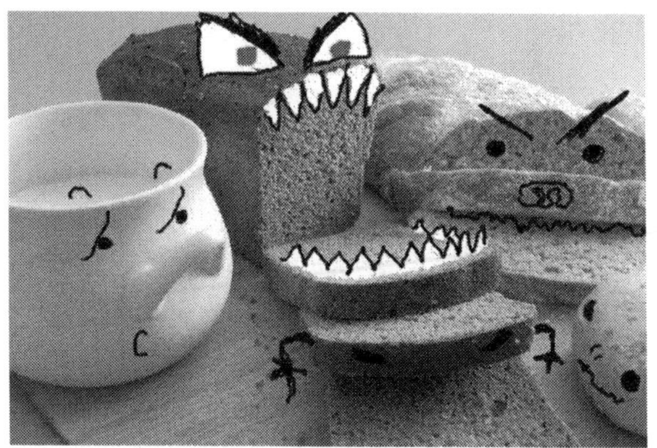

Yeast (living bacteria) currently used in breads is not the same healthy ferments or sourdough used much earlier in our history. The yeast currently used is a "science lab experiment gone wrong" type of product synthetically created in a lab through genetic modification. This yeast does break apart during cooking, and does not digest **at all** with our saliva or in our system, clogging our digestive tract, disturbing proper immune system function, leading to asthma, **cancer**, allergies, constipation, poor digestion, and provides food for fungus, candida, and other yeast infections in our body.

These killer yeast bacteria destroy other sensitive and less protected cells of our body by discharging a toxic substance which is made up of proteins which increase the permeability (ability to penetrate) of cellular membranes (cell walls) to viruses and pathogens. This killer bacteria divide exponentially at an astounding rate infecting the cells of the digestive tract, then moving on to the blood stream spreading pathogenic bacteria and allowing it to live and thrive while destroying beneficial bacteria (beneficial bacteria under proper nutrition and pH levels are able to produce B vitamins and even essential amino acids!). This leads to illnesses of the digestive tract, and all digestive organs like the stomach, gall bladder, pancreas, and liver.

The stomach is covered with a mucous membrane which provides protection against stomach acid. A diet high in yeast, sugar, and acidifying foods (coffee, sugar, white flour, alcohol, meat products, pasteurized milk products etc.) progressively destroy the mucous lining leading to ulcers, indigestion, and acid reflux. Such a diet also leads to formation of plaque deposits and stones in the gall bladder, liver, pancreas, and constipation. The mucous lining in the digestive tract also takes a giant hit by the pathogenic bacteria slowing down toxin removal, damaging the fine lining of the digestive tract, reducing its defence functions and reducing its ability to digest and use vitamins and minerals from the food as well as seriously hinder its ability to synthesize vitamins (again, our intestinal bacteria are able to synthesize soluble vitamins and even essential amino acids).

So instead of completely changing ones diet, many uninformed consumers just cover up this dangerous concoction brewing in their stomach with acid reflux medicine like pepto bismol. It's like putting a band-aid on a broken leg.

Bacterial, fungal, and parasitic infections easily penetrate the digestive walls migrating to the blood stream and from here to the entire body leading to severe decreases in cellular metabolism, biochemical changes of the blood, putrid slime deposits in the plasma of the blood, slower and more viscous blood flow, micro thrombi develop (blood clots), lymphatic system overstress, nervous tissue changes, irritable bowel syndrome, and many other serious health conditions.

The most serious of all is **acidosis** (high acid or pH level in the body). This leads to fatigue, fibromyalgia, lupus, irritability, mental fatigue, nausea, digestive problems, acid mouth, a white or grey film on the tongue, gastritis, black rings under the eyes, muscle pain from excess acid, and many other nasty ailments. The body uses colossal energy to try and restore the acid-base balance and increase pH levels to normal amounts (7.4 pH is normal; pathogenic bacteria/fungus/yeast thrive at anything lower. MOST ferments and enzymes can only function in a basic environment, in an acidic environment cholesterol coagulates and becomes plaque and debris, in an acidic environment amino acids deteriorate) by using its own alkaline minerals like calcium, magnesium, selenium, and iron from bones and teeth leading to poor tooth health and osteoporosis and bone/joint issues.

A French scientist named Étienne Wolff studied the effects of yeast on cancerous tumors. After a 37 month experiment he cultured a tumor growth with fermentative yeast and his results showed that the tumor growth increased two and three fold in just one week! As soon as yeast was removed from the solution, the tumor died. He concluded that **yeast contains something which stimulates the growth of cancerous tumors**. (You will learn more about cancer and how it forms in Part 2)

If you see "yeast" in the ingredient list **avoid that product like the plague**! (This sadly means that if you value your health, most mainstream breads are out of the question). Start looking for sour-dough or rye breads made by smaller bakeries.

Given the raging epidemic of cancer and other chronic diseases in this country, it may be unwise to include this white bread and yeast in your diet, even if it is present in small amounts. Replace the white bread or "enriched white flour" with whole wheat multigrain bread that has only a few ingredients, does not contain any yeast, sugar, acids, preservatives, and preferably locally made. Buy bread that is darker in color, and the more whole grains it contains the better (many breads these days have more than one grain like a "7 Grain" bread for example). If your finances allow it, it is also better to buy as much of your produce as possible to be Organic.

Foods To Avoid Containing Refined Flour/Sugar

- White bread/white flour
- Muffins
- Buns
- Cookies, crackers, cakes, cake mixes
- Sugary cereal
- Pre-packaged microwave meals, sauces, gravies
- Instant/ramen noodles (sugar bombs leading to nothing but extreme fat storage)
- Corn chips/tortillas

Anything that has refined white or non whole-grain flour, anything with yeast, sugar, and additives/preservatives is all toxic ingredients that poison your system and stop weight loss dead in its tracks – it's your choice.

Chapter Two

HFCS – High Fructose Corn Syrup

What is it?

HFCS is a derivative of corn, a highly processed and highly toxic sweetener that is one of the cheapest and most readily available sweeteners; hence its extremely wide usage and 4000% increase since 1973 now being one of America's most common sweeteners.

And average American consumes over 42 pounds of HFCS each year according to the USDA (the actual figures might be much higher today). Counting that in calories, that's over 75,200 extra calories per year coming at over 22 pounds a year per person! And that is JUST from soda, energy drinks, and juice drinks alone!

If the average American cut down just one soft drink or sugary drink a day they would instantly lose 10 pounds a year! Teenagers usually get around 15-20 teaspoons of added sugars in their soft drinks. Some studies show that sodas have replaced milk as a dietary staple and have become the third most common breakfast food. Drinking this sugar bomb at any time leads to a major crash in a few hours causing more hunger, insulin spikes, insulin resistance, and heavy weight gain. It is not surprising at all that so many teenagers are so overweight!

Contrary to popular belief, HFCS is not a natural substance, it is refined from corn and it does **not** occur in nature. There are a lot of natural substances that when refined become detrimental to our health. Just because it is made from corn does not mean it is good for you. It is an artificial ingredient just like sucrose (table sugar), it must be refined in a lab to take shape; it does not occur naturally by itself!

The stupidity of the argument "It occurs in nature, then it must be totally safe!" is beyond belief. Hydrocyanic acid, perhaps one of the most poisonous organic acids known, exists in minute traces in the fruit of peaches and plums, associated often with benzaldehyde, a flavoring agent. It exists in some varieties of cassava in such proportions that even fatal effects have resulted from eating the cassava starch. Salicylic acid is present in a flavoring product known and may exist, in traces, also in other food products. Another organic poison, arsenic is a widely distributed poisonous material which is often found in our foods, due to absorption from the soil. It is to our own benefit to REDUCE these substances not isolate them and add them to our foods!

The same can be said of preservatives, additives, colorants, taste enhancers etc. Yes they occur in nature, but that doesn't mean we need to isolate them and add them to our food in high amounts.

Research proves that our highest caloric intake comes from HFCS's, which are empty, unhealthy, even toxic calories which we absolutely do not need. If we take into account just how much of it we intake, then it becomes a serious issue. The reason why it is used? It is cheaper to make and almost twice sweeter than regular sugar.

There are a lot of studies out there showing that HFCS behaves much differently in our bodies than regular table sugar. HFCS is different than the fructose in corn, it is high fructose syrup. What they do is extract the glucose from the corn and add a chemical to it to turn it back into fructose. The fructose seen naturally in fruits and vegetables on the other hand is completely different, gets digested much easier, and is not harmful to our bodies.

However, a Princeton research team has again demonstrated that all sweeteners are NOT equal when it comes to weight gain -- rats with access to high-fructose corn syrup gained significantly more weight than those with access to table sugar, even when their overall caloric intake was the same.

Additionally, *Science Daily* quotes Professor Hoebel, a specialist in the neuroscience of appetite, weight and sugar addiction, as saying:

"Some people have claimed that high-fructose corn syrup is no different than other sweeteners when it comes to weight gain and obesity, but our results make it clear that this just isn't true, at least under the conditions of our tests.

When rats are drinking high-fructose corn syrup at levels well below those in soda pop, they're becoming obese -- every single one, across the board.

Even when rats are fed a high-fat diet, you don't see this; they don't all gain extra weight."

People who have struggled with their weight for years; examining their diets, avoiding fat and counting calories, yet not getting anywhere and wondering what they're doing wrong, you need to pay very close attention to this issue.

Long-term consumption of high-fructose corn syrup also led to abnormal increases in body fat, especially in the abdomen, and a rise in circulating blood fats called triglycerides. Making matters even worse, two other recent studies have also linked HFCS to liver disease.

Science Daily writes:
"We found that increased consumption of high fructose corn syrup was associated with scarring in the liver, or fibrosis, among patients with non-alcoholic fatty liver disease (NAFLD)," said Manal Abdelmalek, MD, MPH, associate professor of medicine in the Division of Gastroenterology/Hepatology at Duke University Medical Center.

The researchers found only 19 percent of adults with NAFLD reported no intake of fructose-containing beverages, while 52 percent consumed between one and six servings a week and 29 percent consumed fructose-containing beverages on a daily basis.

After following up on nearly 16, 000 people over the course of three to nine years, the risk of chronic kidney disease increased by over **150 percent** in those who consumed more than one soft drink per day.

Part of what makes HFCS such an unhealthy product is that it is metabolized to fat in your body far more rapidly than any other sugar, and, because most fructose is consumed in liquid form, its negative metabolic effects are significantly magnified. When you eat a fruit or vegetable the transition from sugar to fat is not so quick and your blood sugar level does not rise at such a monstrous rate. The fact is our bodies are not designed to ingest pure sugar in its raw form in such quantities!

"We have identified an environmental risk factor that may contribute to the metabolic syndrome of insulin resistance and the complications of the metabolic syndrome, including liver injury." - Abdelmalek.

This means something from our environment (sugar) is the cause of insulin resistance and liver damage amongst other diseases; this includes type 2 diabetes, or adult onset diabetes as it was before children began developing it.

The reason for the increased sugar and in turn HFCS is because of farm subsidies. In 2002 the Bush administration signed a 190 billion dollar farm subsidy act which paid farmers to grow more corn. The United States already had a surplus of corn; they had more corn than they knew what to do with. So why on earth did the government decide to subsidize them even more?

Well, the market price for a bushel of corn is 2$, but it costs the farmer about 3$ to grow that bushel. This means someone has to pay the farmer that extra dollar. So the American peoples' tax dollars, about 14 billion per year, pay for the remaining dollar. You would think that this subsidy is helping farmers right? Not so. This action of sending tax dollars to help pay for corn brings the price of corn down. But for whom? Not the sweet corn on your grocery shelves, but the corn (which is all genetically modified) that is used for HFCS that is found in virtually all foods on your grocery shelves, but mostly soft drinks and candy bars which are produced by the giant corporations like Coca-Cola, PepsiCo, Mars etc.

So the regular people, through their tax dollars, are helping the giant corporations save a few bucks when they use the genetically modified corn to make HFCS and poison you. Pause for a second to really understand this. Even if you don't eat junk food, your tax dollars are still subsidizing this poison so it can end up in more foods.

It's a never-ending circle. You pay to subsidize this poison that is causing an epidemic obesity, diabetes, heart disease, and cancer. You then pay again for all the medical procedures, drugs, pills, doctors and hospitals that treat these diseases. All the while, the only people making billions of dollars are the junk food producers and the pharmaceutical companies that sell you drugs, pills and medical procedures to treat your new diseases. Absolutely mind-boggling.

So while the companies are getting a better deal on their sweetener, the population is seeing an epidemic of obesity, diabetes, heart disease, and cancer, in part helped by your own tax dollars.

HFCS is the only caloric sweetener in U.S. soft drinks and it constitutes over 60 percent of the calories in apple juice. HFCS is used as a base for many fruit drinks. The primary source of HFCS in the American diet is soda and juice--about two-thirds of all HFCS consumed in the United States is in beverages.

So why is HFCS killing you?

Fructose is Metabolized to Fat

The digestive and absorptive processes for glucose and fructose are different. Unlike glucose, fructose converts to fat more than any other sugar. It is also known to raise triglycerides significantly.

A study published in the *Journal of Clinical Investigation*, comparing the effect of ingesting glucose vs. fructose found the following.

The investigators divided 32 overweight men and women into two groups, and instructed each group to drink a sweetened beverage three times per day. They were told not to eat any other sugar. The drinks were designed to provide 25% of the participants' caloric intake. That might sound like a lot, but the average American actually gets about 25% of her calories from sugar! That's the average, so there are people who get a third or more of their calories from sugar. In one group, the drinks were sweetened with glucose, while in the other group they were sweetened with fructose.

After ten weeks, both groups had gained about three pounds. But they didn't gain it in the same place. The fructose group gained a disproportionate amount of visceral fat, which increased by 14%! Visceral fat is the most dangerous type; it's associated with and contributes to chronic disease, particularly metabolic syndrome, the quintessential modern metabolic disorder. You can bet their livers were fattening up too.

The bad news doesn't end there. The fructose group also saw a worsening of blood glucose control and insulin sensitivity. They also saw an increase in small, dense LDL particles and oxidized LDL, both factors that associate strongly with the risk of heart attack and may in fact contribute to it. Liver synthesis of fat after meals increased by 75% meaning most of the sugar was converted to fat right away, an occurrence not seen in glucose digestion. It's clear that the fructose group experienced a **major metabolic shift**, and the glucose group didn't. Practically every parameter they measured in the fructose group changed significantly over the course of the 9 weeks. It's incredible.

Graph found here: http://www.jci.org/articles/view/37385/table/4

Fructose, and glucose for that part, is not meant to be consumed by itself as in HFCS or regular sugar. Fruits and vegetables have countless other substances that allow for proper digestion of the natural sugars in fruit. Yes, regular sugar, brown sugar, even HFCS is natural, but as discussed earlier, that doesn't mean it's good for the body and is healthy for you. Don't be fooled by the "natural" statement, just because its natural doesn't mean it is good for you.

Most Fructose is Consumed as a Liquid

The fact that most fructose is consumed in a liquid form significantly magnifies its negative metabolic effects because it is much easier to digest liquids than solids, meaning it absorbs quicker and in larger quantities. The devastation it has on our biology would be significantly lessened if it were consumed in solid food, but as I mentioned earlier, it is best to avoid all sugars in their free form.

Fructose Does Not Stimulate Insulin Secretion

In addition, unlike glucose, fructose does not stimulate insulin secretion or enhance leptin, a hormone thought to be involved in appetite regulation and production. Because insulin and leptin act as key signals in regulating how much food you eat and body weight, this suggests that dietary fructose may contribute to increased food intake and weight gain. This means the mechanism that tells your body that you've had enough food doesn't work, so you end up eating more.

Fructose Has no Enzymes, Vitamins or Minerals

Fructose, like all other free sugars, has no enzymes, vitamins or minerals so it must take micronutrients from the body to absorb itself for use. However, eating a small piece of whole fruit on the other hand, which contains natural fructose, is not likely to be a problem for most people because fresh fruits contain the enzymes, vitamins and minerals that are needed for the fructose to get properly digested and absorbed in the body.

In an excellent book, *The Saccharine Disease*, Dr. T. L. Cleave demonstrates that many of the diseases that presently afflict us are relatively modem plagues. In his view, and what many other scientists around the globe believe, is that these diseases of civilization are due largely to the incredible increase in sugar consumption during the past century.

Cleave shows that many diseases that are common today were virtually unknown until the introduction of refined sugar. These conditions include constipation, diverticular disease, varicose veins, thrombosis, hemorrhoids, dental caries (cavities), the twin plagues of obesity and diabetes, E.coli infections, and peptic ulcers. He also touches on the subject of colon cancer.

Cleave rules out the possibility that these diseases were caused by the refining of wheat, since the wide-scale use of white bread dated from 1800, while the onslaught of these common modem diseases only happened in the early 20th century.

It is hard to comprehend the massive increase in sugar use in our society. In 1815, the average resident of Great Britain consumed about 15 pounds of sugar per year. When Cleave's book was published in England in 1974, this had risen to about 120 pounds per year. In the United States in 1999, each person consumed about 158 pounds of sugar every year! That's a pound of sugar every two to three days!

Since high-fructose corn syrup was developed more than 30 years ago, consumption of the sweetener, which flavors everything from soda pop to ranch dressing, has skyrocketed. Now Americans down more than **160 pounds** a year each. Since 1950, soft-drink consumption per capita has quadrupled, from about 11 gallons per year to about **46 gallons** in 2003--nearly a gallon a week per person. With all that sugar-eating, it's no wonder people don't have much room for their vegetables. In 2003, during the entire year, the average American consumed a dismal **8.3 pounds** of broccoli and just over **25 pounds** of dark lettuce (the kinds that are really good for you). How is your body supposed to be healthy when all you eat is nutrient and vitamin deficient foods full of sugar year after year?

The average American consumes about 20 teaspoons (almost one-half cup) of sugar per day, which accounts for 16 percent of our daily intake of calories. For teenagers, sugar consumption accounts for a full 20 percent of calories per day. In 1977 sugar accounted for "only" 11 percent of our caloric intake.

This is the catch folks. A lot of the calories today come from sugar, and not the good sugar from fruits and vegetables (which is filled with enzymes, vitamins, and minerals). These empty sugar calories get converted straight to fat, rob your body from its dwindling supply of nutrients, promote an acidic environment, and become food for the bacteria in your body. It's like eating poison in a fancy wrapper.

The total amount of food available for each person to eat increased 16 percent from 1,675 pounds in 1970 to 1,950 pounds in 2003. The increase in food available for consumption resulted in a corresponding jump in calories, from

2,234 calories per person per day in 1970 to 2,757 calories in 2003 (after adjusting for plate waste, spoilage, and other food losses).

Believe it or not, even toddlers are being primed for a lifetime of sugar addiction. According to the Center for Science in the Public Interest (CSPI), major manufacturers "encourage feeding soft drinks to toddlers by licensing their logos to a maker of baby bottles, Munchkin Bottling, Inc. Infants and toddlers are four times likelier to be fed soda pop out of those bottles than out of regular baby bottles." We have not yet spoken about the link between sugar and cancer. However, "the affinity of cancerous tissue for sugar (glucose) is well known."

I'm going to repeat that quote one more time; "The affinity for cancerous tissue for sugar is well known." The fact is that cancer cells feed on sugar. If you create an acidic, oxygen-less environment, fill that environment with sugar and you are pretty much creating a breeding ground for cancer, bacteria, yeast infections (candida) and a body full of disease. This isn't some wacky conspiracy theory; these are cold hard scientific facts and simple biology. It is much simpler to prevent cancer than look for the cure in the form of drugs or surgical procedures. If you don't eliminate the CAUSE of cancer then it can never be cured. It is like trying to use chemicals to destroy bacteria that live in a dirty pond, the bacteria live there because the pond is dirty, clean the pond and there will be no bacteria. Instead we use chemicals to destroy everything in that pond and hope that the bacteria will be destroyed as well.

Sugar and Your Health

The "glycemic index" is a measure of how a given food affects blood-glucose levels, with each food being assigned a numbered rating. The lower the rating, the slower the absorption and digestion process, which provides a more gradual, healthier infusion of sugars into the bloodstream. On the other hand, a high rating means that blood-glucose levels are increased quickly, which stimulates the pancreas to secrete insulin to drop blood-sugar levels. These rapid fluctuations of blood-sugar levels are not healthy because of the stress they place on the body.

One of sugar's major drawbacks is that it raises the insulin level, which inhibits the release of growth hormones, which in turn depresses the immune system. This is not something you want to take place if you want to avoid disease.

An influx of sugar into the bloodstream upsets the body's blood-sugar balance, triggering the release of insulin, which the body uses to keep blood-sugar at a constant and safe level. Insulin also promotes the storage of fat, so that when you eat sweets high in sugar, you're making way for rapid weight gain and elevated triglyceride levels, both of which have been linked to cardiovascular disease. Complex carbohydrates tend to be absorbed more slowly, lessening the impact on blood-sugar levels. The reason free sugar has such an effect is because it is in its free form and not bound to anything which explains the sudden rise in insulin after a sugary snack or drink. Fruits and vegetables do have sugar, but it is bound to a variety of vitamins, minerals, enzymes, and fiber which ensures a **natural** digestion and absorption process.

Our bodies were never meant to ingest sugar in its free form!

Sugar depresses the immune system.

It was only in the 1970's that researchers found out that vitamin C was needed by white blood cells so that they could phagocytise (destroy) viruses and bacteria. White blood cells require a 50 times higher concentration of vitamin C inside the cell as outside so they have to accumulate vitamin C.

Glucose and vitamin C have similar chemical structures, so guess what happens when the sugar levels go up? They compete with one another to get absorbed into the cells of the body. And the thing that allows the entry of glucose into the cells is the same thing that allows the entry of vitamin C into the cells. If there is more glucose around, there is going to be less vitamin C allowed into the cell. It doesn't take much: a blood sugar value of 120 reduces the phagocytic index by 75%. So when you eat sugar, think of your immune system slowing down to a crawl. Dr Cochrain revealed that **just one *tea*spoon of sugar will lower your immune resistance by 50% for up to 24 hours.** (Coke or any soda beverage has 8 ***table*spoons** of sugar in one can).

Another problem with soft drinks is the tremendous amount of PHOSPHORUS that's contained in them. Large amounts of phosphorous are bad news for the body because they combine with other minerals (like Calcium) and tie them up for eventual excretion. Calcium is a mineral that your body needs in large amounts in your bloodstream for daily use. If your soft drink is yanking the calcium out of your blood stream, where does the body get the calcium it needs? It gets it from your teeth, bones, hair, and nails! This is partly the reason for the tremendous increase in osteoporosis in our society.

"There are many research studies which allude to the fact that high **phosphorus** and/or phosphoric acid (found in meat and soft drinks) pulls calcium out of the bony structures (bones, teeth and nails) in the process of digestion and assimilation. This has a disastrous effect on bone density, leaving them porous and spongy. When calcium is pulled from the bones, it is released through the kidneys, resulting in stone formation (kidney stones) before it is excreted," The Greenleaves of Barley, Dr. Mary Ruth Swope, 1987

There is something called a "phagocytic index" which tells you how rapidly a particular macrophage or lymphocyte (different types of immune system fighter cells) can gobble up a virus, bacteria, or cancer cell. It was in the 1970's that Linus Pauling realized that white blood cells need a high dose of vitamin C and that is when he came up with his theory that you need high doses of vitamin C to combat the common cold.

Here we are getting a little bit closer to the roots of disease. It doesn't matter what disease we are talking about, whether we are talking about a common cold or about cardiovascular disease, or cancer or osteoporosis, the root is always going to be at the cellular and molecular level, and more often than not insulin is going to have its hand in it, if not totally controlling it.

The health dangers created by ingesting sugar on a daily basis are certain. Simple sugars have been observed to aggravate asthma, move mood swings, provoke personality changes, muster mental illness, nourish nervous disorders, deliver diabetes, hurry heart disease, grow gallstones, hasten hypertension, and add arthritis.

Because refined dietary sugars lack minerals and vitamins, they must draw upon the body's micro-nutrient stores in order to be metabolized into the system. When these storehouses are depleted, metabolization of cholesterol and fatty acid is obstructed, contributing to higher blood serum triglycerides, cholesterol, promoting obesity due to higher fatty acid storage around organs and in sub-cutaneous tissue folds.

Because sugar is devoid of minerals, vitamins, fiber, and has such a deteriorating effect on the endocrine system, major researchers and major health organizations (American Dietetic Association and American Diabetic Association) agree that sugar consumption in America is one of the 3 major causes of degenerative disease.

Honey is a simple sugar

There are 4 classes of simple sugars which are regarded by most nutritionists as "harmful" to optimal health when prolonged consumption in amounts above 15% of the carbohydrate calories are ingested: Sucrose, fructose, honey, and malts.

Some of you may be surprised to find honey here. Although honey is a natural sweetener, it is considered a refined sugar because 96% is a simple sugar: fructose, glucose and sucrose. It is little wonder that the honey bear is the only animal found in nature that has a problem with tooth-decay (honey decays teeth faster than table sugar). Honey has the highest calorie content of all sugars with 65 calories/tablespoon, compared to the 48 calories/tablespoon found in table sugar. The increased calories are bound to cause increased blood serum fatty acids, as well as weight gain, on top of the risk of more cavities.

Pesticides used on farm crops and residential flowers have been found in commercial honey. Honey can be fatal to an infant whose immature digestive tracts are unable to deal effectively with Botulinum Spore growth. What nutrients or enzymes raw honey does contain are destroyed by manufacturers who heat it in order to give it a clear appearance to enhance sales. If you are going to consume honey, make sure it is raw, unheated, that the farmer does not use any pesticides, and make sure the honey has a high concentration of natural enzymes.

The reason honey is regarded as being just as bad as sugar is because honey today is much, much different from the honey even 50 years ago. With mass production, lower standards, lack of knowledge on proper honey farming, pesticides, herbicides, polluted air etc. the honey today has lost most of its healing properties. 100 years ago in Russia, honey was given out only by prescription in a pharmacy because of its tremendous healing properties on many disease and ailments. Honey that is on your grocery store shelf is nothing more than a sugary syrup devoid of all the beneficial enzymes, minerals, and vitamins. If you can find a good beekeeper who produces high quality honey, then this honey will be better than any sweetener, and you may eat it as much as you like.

How sugar can affect you:

- Sugar can suppress the immune system.
- Sugar can upset the body's mineral balance.
- Sugar can contribute to hyperactivity, anxiety, depression, concentration difficulties, and crankiness in children.
- Sugar can produce a significant rise in triglycerides.
- Sugar can cause drowsiness and decreased activity in children.
- Sugar can reduce helpful high density cholesterol (HDLs).
- Sugar can promote an elevation of harmful cholesterol (LDLs).
- Sugar can cause hypoglycemia.
- Sugar contributes to a weakened defense against bacterial infection.
- Sugar can cause kidney damage.
- Sugar can increase the risk of coronary heart disease.
- Sugar may lead to chromium deficiency.
- Sugar can cause copper deficiency.
- Sugar interferes with absorption of calcium and magnesium.
- Sugar can increase fasting levels of blood glucose.
- Sugar can promote tooth decay.
- Sugar can produce an acidic stomach.
- Sugar can raise adrenaline levels in children.
- Sugar can lead to periodontal disease.
- Sugar can speed the aging process, causing wrinkles and grey hair.
- Sugar can increase total cholesterol.
- Sugar can contribute to weight gain and obesity.
- High intake of sugar increases the risk of Crohn's disease and ulcerative colitis.
- Sugar can contribute to diabetes.
- Sugar can contribute to osteoporosis.
- Sugar can cause a decrease in insulin sensitivity.
- Sugar leads to decreased glucose tolerance.
- Sugar can cause cardiovascular disease.
- Sugar can increase systolic blood pressure.
- Sugar causes food allergies.
- Sugar can cause free radical formation in the bloodstream.
- Sugar can cause toxemia during pregnancy.
- Sugar can contribute to eczema in children.
- Sugar can overstress the pancreas, causing damage.
- Sugar can cause atherosclerosis.
- Sugar can compromise the lining of the capillaries.
- Sugar can cause liver cells to divide, increasing the size of the liver.
- Sugar can increase the amount of fat in the liver.
- Sugar can increase kidney size and produce pathological changes in the kidney.

- Sugar can cause depression.
- Sugar can increase the body's fluid retention.
- Sugar can cause hormonal imbalance.
- Sugar can cause hypertension.
- Sugar can cause headaches, including migraines.
- Sugar can cause an increase in delta, alpha and theta brain waves, which can alter the mind's ability to think clearly.
- Sugar can increase blood platelet adhesiveness which increases risk of blood clots and strokes.
- Sugar can increase insulin responses in those consuming high-sugar diets compared to low sugar diets.
- Sugar increases bacterial fermentation in the colon.

Is Sugar More Addictive than Cocaine?

According to a new research study, **refined sugar is far more addictive than cocaine** -- one of the most addictive and harmful substances currently known.

An astonishing 94 percent of rats who were allowed to choose mutually-exclusively between sugar water and cocaine, chose sugar. Even rats who were addicted to cocaine quickly switched their preference to sugar, once it was offered as a choice. The rats were also more willing to work for sugar than for cocaine.

The researchers speculate that the sweet receptors (two protein receptors located on the tongue), which evolved in ancestral times when the diet was very low in sugar, have not adapted to modern times' high-sugar consumption.

Therefore, the abnormally high stimulation of these receptors by our sugar-rich diets generates excessive reward signals in the brain, which have the potential to override normal self-control mechanisms, and thus lead to addiction.

Additionally, their research found that there's also a cross-tolerance and a cross-dependence between sugars and addictive drugs. As an example, animals with a long history of sugar consumption actually became tolerant (desensitized) to the analgesic effects of morphine.

Sugar and cancer

Of the over 4 million cancer patients being treated in the U.S. today, almost none are offered any scientifically guided nutrition therapy other than being told to "just eat good foods." Many cancer patients would have a major improvement in their conditions if they controlled the supply of cancer's preferred fuel: GLUCOSE. By slowing the cancer's growth, patients make it possible for their immune systems to catch up to the disease. Controlling one's blood-glucose levels through diet, exercise, supplements, and prescription drugs - when necessary - can be one of the most crucial components to a cancer treatment program. There is even a saying that "Sugar feeds cancer".

German Otto Warburg, Ph.D., the 1931 Nobel Prize winner for his work on cancer, was the first to discover that cancer cells have a fundamentally different energy metabolism compared to healthy cells.

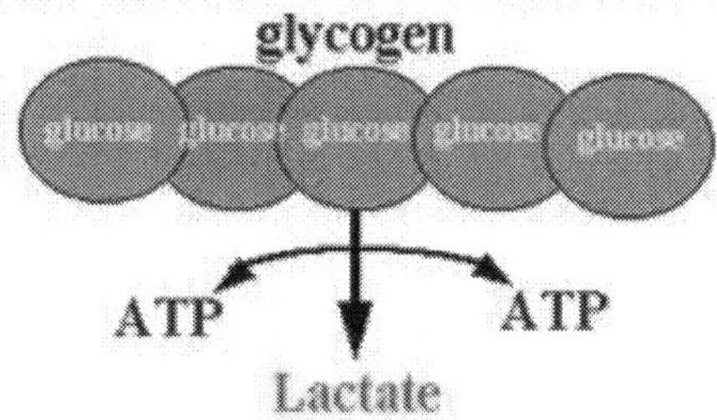

The essence of his Nobel thesis was this: malignant tumors frequently exhibit an increase in "anaerobic glycolysis" - a process whereby glucose is used by cancer cells as a fuel with lactic acid as an anaerobic by-product - compared to normal tissues.

Normal cells on the other hand function through "aerobic glycolysis" and use oxygen instead of sugar for energy production.

The large amount of lactic acid produced by this fermentation of glucose from the cancer cells is then transported to the liver. This conversion of glucose to lactate creates a lower, more acidic PH in cancerous tissues as well as overall physical fatigue from lactic acid build-up. Therefore, larger tumors tend to exhibit a more acidic PH.

Hence, cancer therapies should attempt to regulate blood-glucose levels through diet, supplements, exercise, and stress reduction. Since cancer cells derive most of their energy from anaerobic glycolysis, the goal is not to eliminate sugars or carbohydrates entirely from the diet but rather to control what you eat to help starve the cancer cells and boost immune function.

Otto Warburg showed that cancer cells use sugar for energy and do not respire the normal way like healthy cells. This fact is the basis of the high-tech diagnostic tool known as positron emission tomography (PET). PET scans are x-rays that reveal areas of heightened glucose metabolism in the body, which indicate the presence of cancer. PET scans are used today to detect cancer, its spread in the body, the effectiveness of treatment etc. Can you make the connection? The scanning tool checks for heightened sugar metabolism which should raise a few eyebrows, if heightened sugar metabolism which indicates cancer in a body part, maybe sugar is the problem? But again, the medical mafia is not looking for a cure, they are busy making billions treating the symptoms of an acidic, sugar filled, and oxygen depleted body.

It certainly is suspicious that, like the other diseases I have mentioned, the incidence of cancer increased tremendously at the same time as sugar consumption went sky-high.

Again and again you can see the connection. Cancer, as well as most other diseases, thrive in a toxic, acidic, oxygen-less environment. Fast food, meat, GMO, additives, preservatives, sugar, and sodas all create such an environment. The only question is which disease will you get first?

If you want to avoid obesity, diabetes, liver dysfunction, increased cholesterol levels, autoimmune disease, cancer, and countless other diseases then stop drinking sodas and anything with high fructose corn syrup or high sugar content. This is the easiest and simplest way to begin weight loss and avoid disease. Thousands of people took the change, have you?

Is brown sugar healthier? Nope. Brown sugar, cane sugar, sugar crystals are the same bad sugar you should avoid at all costs.

I also get questions regarding the sugar in fruits and vegetables. The difference between isolated sugar (regular sugar) and sugar found in all other foods is the sugar that's in foods is bound to a myriad of enzymes, vitamins, minerals, nutrients, and fiber, which ensure absolute perfect absorption and metabolism. Free sugar is nutrition less and gets converted to fat and leads to diabetes, not to mention that table sugar is not found in nature and is toxic to our bodies.

What to do?

HFCS and regular sugar is being added to more products than you thought; like ketchup, dressings, soups, sauces, cereals, cookies and many more. Read the label of your favorite grocery item, you are bound to find HFCS, glucose-fructose or sugar on the label.

There are many sugar alternatives out on the market, the best one in my opinion is Stevia which comes from a sweet leaf. Now you can find a derivative of Stevia called Rib-A which should not be used, only whole leaf stevia powder is acceptable. Another alternative is raw agave syrup, coconut crystals, raw natural honey that has NOT been pasteurized or filtered. Once honey is fine-filtered and pasteurized, it loses ALL of its beneficial properties and turns into regular sugar. So make sure to always read the label!

Chapter 3

Artificial Sweeteners – Splenda, NutraSweet, Aspartame

Are artificial sweeteners the answer to sugar? Do they really help you lose weight?

The belief that eating artificially sweetened foods and drinking artificially sweetened beverages will help you to lose weight is a carefully orchestrated deception. So if you are still opting for sugar-free choices for this reason, you are being greatly misled.

For years now studies have shown that consuming artificial sweeteners breaks the connection between a sweet sensation and a high-calorie food, thereby changing your body's ability to regulate intake naturally.

In one study by psychologists at Purdue University's Ingestive Behavior Research Center, rats that ate yogurt sweetened with an artificial sweetener consumed more calories (and didn't make up for it by cutting back later), gained more weight, and put on more body fat than rats that ate yogurt sweetened with sugar.

Other studies, too, have shown that eating artificial sweeteners might hinder your body's ability to estimate calorie intake, thus boosting your inclination to overindulge. Your body and your brain simply do not have the same biological response to artificial sweeteners that they do to regular sugar, and this can pose some serious problems.

The truth is artificial sweeteners are toxic substances which not only trick your brain and make you gain weight, but have been linked to numerous neurological disorders, swelling and redness of the skin, heart palpitations and other very serious conditions.

In reality there is absolutely no evidence to show that zero calorie artificial sweeteners actually help you lose weight, on the contrary, evidence shows they may actually be stimulating your appetite and insulin response.

First of all, lab made artificial sweeteners trick your brain into thinking you have just eaten a sugary, carbohydrate rich meal. What normally happens when we eat sugars or complex carbohydrates like starches is they are broken down into glucose which enters the blood stream (glucose is small chain sugars, while carbohydrates and starches are long chain sugars). Our pancreas then releases insulin which "unlocks" our cells and allows glucose to be transported into the cell for energy and to normalize blood sugar levels.

Since there are no actual sugars to be broken down, your body feverishly activates the hunger response to try and get some actual sugars into your system to get rid of all that insulin floating around in your system. Appetite is activated, you get hungry and want to eat even more than before, and if you don't, this leads to insulin resistance, and diabetes! Artificial sweeteners make you gain much more weight.

The other negative effects of artificial sweeteners are even worse.

There are 6 artificial sweeteners approved by the FDA. Saccharin (Sweet-n-Low), sucralose (Splenda), aspartame (NutraSweet), acesulfame potassium (Ace-K, Sunett, Sweet One, Neotame), and a natural non artificial sweetener Stevia (Truvia) or Rib-A derived from the herb Stevia rebaudiana.

Saccharin, aka benzoic sulfinide or E954, was the first artificial sweetener on the market, and just like the others it has no calories. It is a synthetic white powder, has absolutely no nutritional value and is not easily digestible by our bodies. Interestingly enough it was discovered in 1879 when a researcher was looking for a coal tar derivative! This guy was not looking for anything related to food, but somehow came upon this substance (maybe accidentally tasted it?) then he commercialized it, and ever since then controversy rages on over its safety.

In 1977, a study accused saccharin of being a carcinogen after it was linked to bladder tumors in mice. The US National Toxicology Program put saccharin on their cancer causing list, officially labeling it as a carcinogen. Cyclamate, an earlier version of saccharin, was banned in 1970 for similar reasons. The FDA later ruled that saccharin should carry a warning label regarding its cancer connection. These labels were soon removed due to inconclusive evidence, but it was most likely due to heavy corporate lobbying due to financial interest, as it is usually done.

What is Aspartame?

Aspartame is 100 times sweeter than sugar, but has been linked to over 90 different side effects!

Brain tumors, seizures, joint problems, and even death! These and 92 other dangerous side effects come from this commonly used artificial sweetener with a terrible history of poor research, cover-ups and other nonsense. But that hasn't stopped this toxic poison from invading thousands of different foods and beverages we eat every day.

Back in 1965, while people were protesting the Vietnam War and rocking out to the Rolling Stones, Bob Dylan, and Jimi Hendrix, scientist James Schlatter tripped over one of today's most commonly used and accepted chemical concoctions: aspartame.

While recrystallizing a chemical compound (aspartylphenylalanine-methyl-ester), some of the powder spilled and got onto Schlatter's fingers. Not realizing his, he licked his fingers inadvertently and noticed the sweet taste.

Four years later, in 1969, the *Journal of the American Chemical Society* reported on aspartame, discussing the "accidental discovery of an organic compound with a profound sucrose (table sugar) like taste."

Sugar-like taste is an understatement. Aspartame is 100 to 200 times sweeter than sugar, depending on concentration. But what, exactly, is this chemical sweetener?

A Sweet Mess

Whether you are talking about the little yellow packets of Equal or NutraSweet, aspartame remains a laboratory creation. It is composed of three elements: aspartic acid (40 percent), phenylalanine (50 percent), and methanol (10 percent).

Both aspartic acid and phenylalamine are amino acids, which sounds good, right? Not really. See, aspartic acid is a known excitotoxin, meaning it over stimulates your nervous system.

Phenylalanine is the precursor to tyrosine, which is used to make excitatory neurotransmitters. (Notice a pattern here?) Excitatory transmitters energize you and speed up process in your body.

Now add in the methanol. Methanol is used to make formaldehyde, which is a colorless, poisonous gas. It is commonly used to make resin adhesives, paint, disinfectants, and embalming fluid. Ah, yeah. And if you drink it straight, you can go blind.

Mix them all together and this combination has been found to have potent excitatory effects on brain chemistry, often leading to a whole host of health problems, including headaches, dizziness, anxiety, and depression.

Clearly, the answer to "is aspartame safe" question is a resounding NO. So how is it that aspartame is even legal? Tricky maneuvering seems to be the answer.

Fast forward to 1996, when the FDA gave aspartame blanket approval as a "general purpose sweetener," despite ongoing concerns regarding its habitual, long-term use, and long list of side effects.

This is particularly odd when you consider that **75 percent of all adverse reactions to food additives reported to the FDA are due to aspartame!**

Thanks to the Freedom of Information Act, the FDA has been required to keep of list of reactions and related aspartame side effects, all 92 of them. They include:

- Death,
- Headaches and seizures,
- Vision loss,
- Seizures,
- Hearing loss,
- Joint pain, and
- Breathing difficulties.

And these issues are mild compared to the other dangers of aspartame consumption. Turns out, many conditions are worsened or even brought on by aspartame, including cancer, brain tumors, Parkinson's disease, and Alzheimer's disease.

What about Splenda? It is marketed as "natural" and "made from sugar." Dirt is also natural, and arsenic, and lead, etc. but that doesn't mean we should ingest it! Deceiving marketing tactics have made people believe this toxic substance is safe to eat. Splenda is made from sucralose which is a natural sugar, but after heavy processing there is nothing resembling sugar at all. It is a chemically created synthetic compound, modified by adding chlorine atoms to sugar.

According to Shane Ellison (www.thepeopleschemist.com), a well-known Organic Chemist:

"Splenda's manufacturer claims that the chlorine added to sucralose is similar to the chlorine atom in the salt (NaCl) molecule. When combined with sodium, chlorine forms a harmless "ionic bond" to yield table salt. Sucralose makers often point this out to defend its safety. Apparently, they missed day 2 of Chemistry 101 - the day they taught about "covalent" bonds. Unlike ionic bonds, covalently bound chlorines are not meant for the human body. Sucralose is covalently bonded with chlorine and much more like ingesting tiny amounts of chlorinated pesticides, but we will never know the real harm, without long-term, independent human research. Sucralose, incidentally, was discovered in the 1970s by researchers looking to create a new pesticide. It wasn't until the young scientist who developed it accidentally tasted his new "insecticide" that he learned it was sweet."

Pesticides are not that marketable as food products, but a no calorie sweetener with such an innocent name as "Splenda" sure is. This synthetic product was once something resembling a bug-killer, and if it kills bugs, seems that it would be quite dangerous to humans as well.

Sound like something you want to be drinking or eating?

Even the studies funded by Splenda's manufacturers send chills down my spine (usually these studies are extremely carefully done, meticulously prepared and executed to show the product in the most favorable light with only positive benefits, and even so, studies **still showed scary side effects**). Their studies showed that animals fed Splenda suffered horrific side effects like enlarged livers, kidneys, and shrunken thymus glands. The crazy part is that these were **short term** studies; can you imagine what would happen in the long run?

There are no long term studies on Splenda ever conducted except one: you! Seems like we are the guinea pigs trying out all these different chemicals, and what are the results? Obesity, cancer, diabetes, heart disease, and every single disease on the rise **year after year**.

According to Dr. Joseph Mercola (www.mercola.com), the following symptoms have been
observed within 24-hours of eating Splenda products:

• Redness, itching, swelling, blistering, weeping, crusting, rash, eruptions, or hives. This is
the most common allergic symptom that people have.
• Wheezing, tightness, cough, or shortness of breath.
• Swelling of the face, eyelids, lips, tongue, or throat; headaches and migraines.
• Stuffy nose, runny nose, sneezing.
• Red, itchy, swollen, or watery eyes.
• Bloating, gas, pain, nausea, vomiting, diarrhea, or bloody diarrhea.
• Heart palpitations or fluttering.
• Join pains or aches.
• Anxiety, dizziness, spaced-out sensation, depression.

Although Splenda is not as toxic as aspartame, it is not something that is fit for your consumption unless you want to be sick and overweight. There are plenty of other sugar substitutes that have no side effects other than positive ones, the best ones being Stevia and raw unpasteurized honey.

Sugar Free Foods to Avoid

- Diet sodas
- Sugar free sport drinks
- Sugar free snacks and desserts
- Sugar free ice cream
- Sugar free jams, spreads
- Sugar free gum
- Sugar free candy
- Anything that says “sugar free” is guaranteed to contain one or more of these artificial sweeteners

Chapter 4

Trans Fats, Vegetable Oils, Margarines etc.

Most of us believe, as told by the media, that fat is the biggest thing we should be avoiding. It has the most calories per gram (fat has 9 calories per gram, carbs/proteins has 4) so it should be the most fattening, right? Wrong. Eating the **right kind** of fats will not only make you healthier but will actually make you **lose weight**. Saturated fats and cholesterol are not unhealthy as we have been led to believe, but the culprits are actually vegetable oils and trans/hydrogenated fats.

Simply speaking, a fat is a combination of carbon molecules combined together to form a chain. Various combinations of the carbon molecules make different types of fats. There are saturated and unsaturated fats. Saturated fats can only have a straight structure, unsaturated fats on the other hand can be have a bent shape (cis mono or polyunsaturated fats like omega 3, 6) or a straight shape (trans unsaturated fat). The reason trans fats and saturated fats are considered bad is because their molecular structure is straight, and can clump together and clog arteries. Hydrogenated and trans fats are artificial fats that have added hydrogen to make them straight in shape, increasing their melting point, and thus making them much more stable for increased shelf life.

Naturally occurring fatty acids generally have the *Cis* configuration which means the molecular structure of the fat is bent.

When the fat is *Trans*, then it is straight in shape.

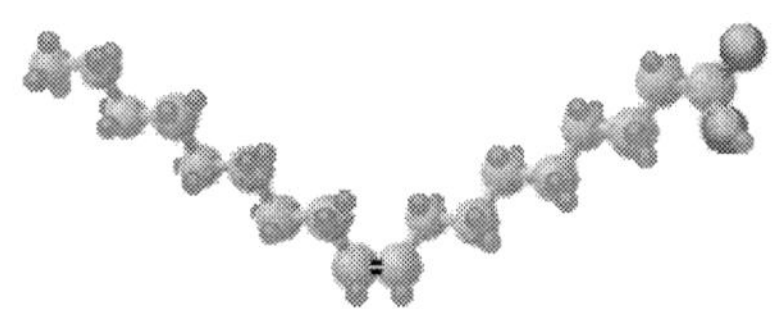

Cis-9-octadecenoic acid
(Oleic acid)

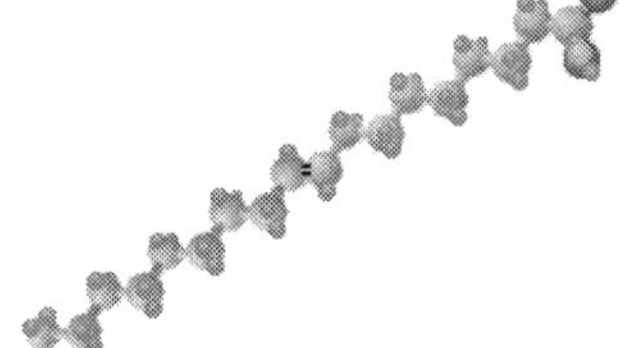

Trans-9-octadecenoic acid
(Elaidic acid)

The walls of the cells in our bodies are made up of fats, mostly from the good essential fats (essential fats are those that cannot be manufactured by the body) like omega 3 (hemp, walnut, coconut, flaxseed), omega 6 (soybean oil, corn oil, safflower oil, sunflower oil , peanut oil, cottonseed oil, rice bran oil) which combine together to form the cellular membrane.

When the essential fatty acids are missing from the diet (essential fatty acids are very volatile and are removed from our foods to get a longer shelf life), cells have no choice but to substitute inappropriate fats (margarine, shortenings, fried fats, animal fats) into their structure, resulting in type II diabetes and perhaps cancer. This makes cells brittle and hard like an eggshell instead of a healthy, soft, porous membrane.

These fats when used in the cell wall interfere with the absorption of nutrients and damage the mitochondria (an organelle inside our cells that produces energy needed for the cell to live), thereby interfering with production of ATP (the energy source or "food" for our cells), then this can cause significant damage to the cell because ATP is needed for important cellular processes such as membrane transport, lipogenesis and protein synthesis. This causes cells to become dysfunctional blocking proper metabolism, nutrient absorption, oxygenation, and a poor ability to respond to glucose.

Despite these dangers, trans and hydrogenated fats are widely used in all sorts of processed foods; cookies, crackers, pastries, cakes, chips, fast food, margarine, popcorn, pretty much most of what is found on your grocery store shelves.

What about vegetable oils? Yes, they are better than trans fats but they also have some very negative effects on the body. These oils like canola, soybean, sunflower, safflower, and others contribute to major inflammation (the main cause of disease and aging) due to the upset in the ratio of omega 3 and omega 6 fatty acids.

Before the age of food processing people had a good balance of fats, especially omega 3 and 6, with a ratio of about 2:1 or 3:1 (2 parts omega 6, to 1 part omega 3). The ratio now is about 20:1! This high imbalance leads to inflammatory related diseases such as autoimmune, cardiovascular, and oncologic. Consuming large amounts of vegetable oils wrecks havoc on the natural balance damaging our whole body, leading to irritability, learning disabilities, liver toxicity, decreased immune function, mental and physical growth problems, increased acidity, and they have been linked to mental disorders like Alzheimer's, dementia as well as accelerated aging - all signs of inflammation and acidity in the body. A 1994 study appearing in a leading medical journal showed that almost three quarters of the fat clogged in arteries was unsaturated. This means it was not the "artery clogging" saturated fats, but vegetable oils!

On the same note, high heat applied to oils during frying turns them into hydrocarbons that can cause cancer. Typical frying temperature is about 400 degrees F (200 c) and can reach up to 600-700 degrees F. When fats / oils are heated to such temperatures the good healthy fats (CIS fatty acid) are converted to the bad TRANS fats. The unsaturated good fats then begin to behave like saturated bad fats. Trans fats also interfere with the body's usage of omega 3 fats.

When heated, they raise rather than lower serum cholesterol levels (about 50% of the cholesterol increasing effect of saturated fat) and can raise LDL cholesterol by nearly as much as saturated fat. Besides the extra fat consumed, this is another reason why fried foods contribute to hardening of the arteries.

The inflammation and acidity caused by the vegetable oils damages blood vessels and so the body starts manufacturing "cement" to repair the damaged vessels. This cement is **cholesterol** which has been wrongly accused as the culprit behind heart disease when it is actually omega 6 fats, trans/hydrogenated oils, sugars, chemical additives and other inflammatory and acidifying foods in our diet.

When oil is reheated to frying temperatures (as in deep fryers), the fat is more likely to develop the cancer producing agents acrolein and benzopyrene. Very hot temperatures also destroy vitamins and alter major proteins. Temperatures up to 1000 degrees F especially when one re-uses cooking oil (as in fast-food restaurants), breaks down the polyunsaturated molecule and free radicals then form.

Simply speaking; a free radical is a free floating molecule that is unstable, and to become stable it steals electrons from other healthy cells turning those healthy cells unstable. When a healthy cell becomes unstable, it begins to age very quickly and can die. The free radicals are toxic due to their strong oxidizing (rusting) capacity, as they damage and destroy cells. Antioxidants are molecules that donate their electrons to the free radicals so they don't have to steal them from your cells; thereby preventing damage and destruction to your body.

These fats that have been changed by heat are incorporated into the cell wall where they interfere with the respiration and oxygen transport of the cell. This means they invade your cell and prevent it from working properly.

Acrolein, nitrosamines, hydrocarbons and benzopyrene are generated when fats are heated. They are all carcinogenic, cancer causing substances.

Deep-fried foods are the worst; such as fried chicken, French fries, onion rings, potato chips, corn chips, cooked beef, chicken and just about all cooked meats due to their high fat content. Cancer is the number one killer of children in the United States and this is one significant reason why.

Paul Addis, professor of food science and nutrition at the University of Minnesota, says "Rancid oils are one of the factors that are important in heart disease. Oils turn rancid when the fats are broken down in cooking, and it's unarguable, these fats are toxic" Addis says.

Avoid Margarine, Shortening, and Spreads at All Costs!

There are a myriad of unhealthy components to margarine and other butter imposters, including:

- **Trans fats**: These unnatural fats in margarine, shortenings and spreads are formed during the process of hydrogenation, which turns liquid vegetable oils into a solid fat

- **Trans fats** contribute to heart disease, cancer, bone problems, hormonal imbalance and skin disease; infertility, difficulties in pregnancy and problems with lactation; and low birth weight, growth problems and learning disabilities in children.

- A U.S. government panel of scientists determined that man-made trans fats are unsafe at any level. (Small amounts of natural trans fats occur in butter and other animal fats, but these are not harmful.)

- **Free radicals**: Free radicals and other toxic breakdown products are the result of high temperature industrial processing of vegetable oils. They contribute to numerous health problems, including cancer and heart disease.

- **Synthetic vitamins**: Synthetic vitamin A and other vitamins are added to margarine and spreads. These often have an opposite (and detrimental) effect compared to the natural vitamins in butter.

- **Emulsifiers and preservatives**: Numerous additives of questionable safety are added to margarines and spreads. Most vegetable shortening is stabilized with preservatives like BHT.

- **Hexane and other solvents**: Used in the extraction process, these industrial chemicals can have toxic effects.

- **Bleach**: The natural color of partially hydrogenated vegetable oil is grey so manufacturers bleach it to make it white. Yellow coloring is then added to margarine and spreads.

- **Artificial flavors**: These help mask the terrible taste and odor of partially hydrogenated oils, and provide a fake butter taste.

- **Mono- and di-glycerides**: These contain trans fats that manufacturers do not have to list on the label. They are used in high amounts in so-called "low-trans" spreads.

- **Soy protein isolate**: This highly processed powder is added to "low-trans" spreads to give them body. It can contribute to thyroid dysfunction, digestive disorders and many other health problems.

- **Sterols**: Often added to spreads to give them cholesterol-lowering qualities, these estrogen compounds can cause endocrine problems; in animals these sterols contribute to sexual inversion.

Foods To Avoid

- Margarine/Crisco/Butter substitutes
- Pastries, Cookies
- Cookie dough
- Doughnuts
- Frozen dinners (toxic mixture of everything mentioned above)
- Fried foods/fast foods
- Cheese spreads
- Whipped Cream

Substitute with REAL vegetables, coconut oil, and butter (more on that later).

Chapter 5

Commercial Pasteurized Dairy Products

Milk is touted everywhere as a health food, but not many people know the difference between real raw milk products and commercial pasteurized milk products. The issue here is pasteurization which if we are to be compelled to drink pasteurized milk, we should at least understand what pasteurization means. It set out to accomplish two things: Destruction of certain disease-carrying germs and the prevention of souring milk. These results are obtained by keeping the milk at a temperature of 145 degrees to 150 degrees F. (~64 c) for half an hour, at least, and then reducing the temperature to not more than 55 degrees F.

The human race existed way before anyone even heard of Pasteur (the man who invented pasteurization) and even as a child I drank raw milk from grass fed cows without antibiotics, vaccines, hormones, or pus which is all what is found in regular commercial milk, and millions of people across the world have been consuming raw milk for thousands of years. In reality, raw milk from **free grass fed cows** is one of the **most beneficial foods on the planet**. It is so nutritious that you can survive solely on milk products even if there was nothing else to eat.

The dairy industry is passing off pasteurized milk from sick cows fed hormones and antibiotics as a wholesome and healthy drink - but this is far from the truth. Countless studies have shown that commercial milk plays a key role in many health problems including: diabetes, prostate cancers, arthritis, atherosclerosis, anemia, MS, leukemia, ovarian cancer, excess mucous, and many others.

There are dozens of reports and studies available that show the dangers of commercial pasteurized milk which can cause intestinal colic, intestinal irritation, intestinal bleeding, anemia, allergies, and sinus problems from excess mucous. A big concern is the contamination of milk by pus, hormones, chemicals, and pesticides which are all found in the milk on your grocery store shelves.

Fifty years ago a cow produced 2000 pounds of milk per year. Today a cow can produce up to 50,000 pounds! They achieve this through a toxic mix of drugs, antibiotics, growth hormones, force feeding, and specialized breeding. These chemicals go through the cow's system and end up in your milk.

Another issue is bovine growth hormone which stimulates milk production but has been linked to cancer and tumor growth. Large corporations lobbied the government so organic companies who don't use bovine growth hormone (BGH) **CAN NOT** even state this fact on the label, because if people actually **knew** what was in their milk, no sane person would drink it.

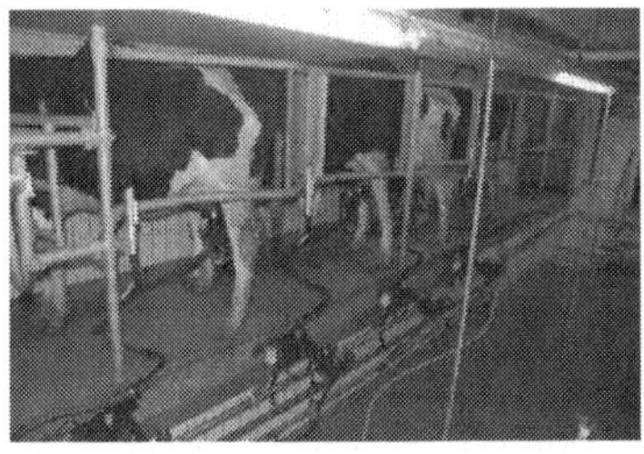

BGH dramatically increased a cow's milk production, and with that, it also increases mastitis (udder infection) of the dairy cow's udders by 50-70%. They then have to fill the cow with huge amounts of antibiotics and drugs for the various infections the cows get while spending their entire lives in a tiny cage being fed genetically modified corn meal while their calves are being sent to slaughterhouses. That is not healthy milk if you ask me, and I don't want to be part of this chemical experiment.

Did you know that over FIFTY percent of all antibiotics produced in the United States go directly to animal feed! Antibiotics which ideally should only be used very rarely in case of serious infections are being used CONSTANTLY because of poor, dirty, filthy conditions the cows live in. By drinking this milk we are also drinking all these antibiotics. If you tested the milk you are drinking you would find traces of up to **80 different antibiotics**! Not only that but you are also drinking pesticides and chemicals found in their feed, and hormones used on the cows.

Commercial milking is a horrible ordeal. In order to keep a steady supply of milk, the cows are repeatedly impregnated. Several times a day, dairy cows are hooked by their udders to electronic milking machines that can cause the cows to suffer electrical shocks, painful lesions, and mastitis. Some spend their entire lives standing on concrete floors; others are crammed into massive mud lots.

Cows have a natural lifespan of about 25 years and can produce milk for eight or nine years, but the stress caused by factory farm conditions leads to disease, lameness, and reproductive problems that render cows worthless to the dairy industry by the time they are four or five years old, at which time they are sent to the slaughterhouse.

Due to the constant infections and mastitis of commercials cows, white blood cells (in other words; pus) make it into your milk. Due to this fact, the USDA allows milk to contain from one to one and a half million white blood cells per milliliter (0.03 oz) of milk. The milk you drink contains cow pus, sounds delicious doesn't it.

The 9 million cows in America, for the most part, are not healthy. Half the herds in America have cows affected with bovine leukemia virus, half the herds have cows infected with a disease called Crohn's disease, which is caused by a bacterium called mycobacterium paratuberculosis, which has infected 40 million Americans and caused irritable bowel syndrome. Every person with Crohn's disease tests positive for mycobacterium paratuberculosis. Every one! One hundred percent! And this was published in 1965 for the Proceedings for the National Academy of Science.

What was once a wholesome, delicious, and nutritious beverage has transformed into a disgusting cocktail of antibiotics, chemicals, hormones, and pus. Commercial pasteurized milk products should be avoided at all costs. Let's stop supporting these cruel and unhealthy methods, and stop giving our money to these corporations who have not a care in the world about the animals or **about you**!

But wait there's more! Sounds like a horrible infomercial... Not only do you get the antibiotics, chemicals, hormones and pus, but you also get milk that is totally changed in composition from the raw milk in grass fed cows. Since dairy cows these days are raised for profit, meaning with total disregard for health and nutrition and as cheaply as possible, that means they are raised on an unnatural diet of grains and corn, not grass like Mother Nature intended. Because of this very unnatural diet, the composition of milk fat changes reducing the healthy omega 3 and Conjugated Linoleic Acid to almost nothing.

Pasteurization began in the early 1900's to kill pathogens in the milk that caused various illnesses caused by poor animal nutrition and dirty production methods. If a cow is given the freedom to graze freely, has her natural diet of grass, is raised in a clean environment, and the milk handled properly then there is absolutely no reason to doubt the cleanliness of milk.

Raw milk sours, pasteurized milk rots.

According to Sally Fallon of the Weston Price Foundation:

"Heat alters milk's amino acids, lysine and tyrosine, making the whole complex of proteins less available; it promotes rancidity of unsaturated fatty acids and destruction of vitamins. Vitamin C loss in pasteurization usually exceeds 50 percent; loss of other water-soluble vitamins can run as high as 80 percent. Pasteurization alters milk's mineral components such as calcium, chlorine, magnesium, phosphorus, potassium, sodium and sulphur as well as many trace minerals, making them less available. There is some evidence that pasteurization alters lactose, making it more readily absorbable."

When any food, including milk, is heated up above 42 degrees Celsius/106 degrees Fahrenheit, protein/carbohydrate molecules as well as vitamins and nutrients actually change their shape and composition, making it much harder for our bodies to digest and use them. The more any food item is heated, the more destruction occurs on the molecular level making it less and less usable. This is the reason why the human body cannot live if our temperature goes above 42 degrees Celsius/108 f (as in a high fever) because our protein molecules that make up our whole body begin to break apart and change their shape, slowly destroying the body. The usability of any food heated above the maximum temperature is about 5%, meaning 95% of it clogs your system and goes out the opposite end. As opposed to raw, unheated, and unprocessed food where the usability is around 90-100%. This is partly the reason we eat so much, our body can't use most of it so it is always hungry for nutrients.

In the case of milk, during pasteurization all the enzymes and proteins are completely destroyed leading to partial or incomplete indigestion, lactose intolerance, gastric colitis, gas, bloating, allergic reactions, chronic fatigue, allergies, mucous formation, and other degenerative diseases. Also, since the enzymes are destroyed (enzymes help digest food), calcium is not fully digested and absorbed, fats like CLA and omega 3 are not digested and absorbed leading to a useless disease causing liquid that is best to be avoided altogether if you value your health.

Homogenization also plays a destructive role in milk production. Due to pus and other impurities milk manufacturers send milk at high speeds through micro membranes which break apart fat globules into micro globules and make milk seem cleaner and better looking. These tiny fat molecules are now more susceptible to be oxidized by air increasing spoilage and turning the good fat into bad fat.

Homogenization today is usually a two step process. The first stage, similar to Gaulin's early device, pushes milk through small, tapered tubes or pores. As the diameter shrinks and the flow of milk remains constant, pressure builds up and fat globules break apart in the turbulence.

The higher the pressure, the smaller the particles. How much pressure? Typically 2,000-3,000 pounds per square inch (psi), although some super homogenizers work at over 1000 times atmospheric pressure- 14,500psi and higher!

You can jam milk through pretty small holes with force like that. Before homogenization, fat globules range in size from 1-10 microns (a micron = ~0.00004 inch). After, the size range is reduced to 0.2-2 microns.

As the much smaller fat globules begin to reassemble, they include fragments of whey and casein in their walls. Some are completely surrounded by a layer of protein. The tendency is for these new, chemically altered globules to clump together. Stage two of the homogenization process breaks up this unwanted assembly and makes sure everything stays in solution.

Some researchers believe that these protein-heavy fat globules can potentially increase homogenized milk's ability to cause allergic reactions. Numerous studies confirm this, at least with rodents as test subjects. Other known effects on milk quality include increased viscosity (the milk is thickened in consistency) whiter appearance, lowered heat stability, increased sensitivity to light-triggered oxidation and less pronounced milk flavor.
It is no wonder that so many people are allergic to milk, this toxic substance causes diarrhea, vomiting, stomach pains, depression, cramps, nausea, headaches, sinus and chest congestion, acne, sore throats and other symptoms of an allergic reaction.

What about the calcium? Many sources recommend ingesting dairy for calcium, but the Physicians Committee cites a longitudinal study by Harvard University found that women who drank more milk had **more bone fractures** than those who drank less, as well as other studies with similar findings. Many studies show that drinking pasteurized milk actually leeches calcium **OUT** of the bones!

What about the whey or casein protein found in protein bars or protein powder? If you see the word “whey” it’s better to stay away. "Casein," "sodium caseinate," "calcium caseinate" that's the milk powder protein that you don't want in your body. When you take milk and you get rid of the fat and you get rid of the water and you're just left with protein, and basically they're blood proteins, milk protein, 90% of it is casein. Casein, when it's extracted from milk, is actually used as a glue to attach labels to bottles. It's the glue used to hold together the wood in your furniture. When you eat this casein, your body sees it as a foreign particle and begins to produce histamines creating an allergic reaction and mucous. And that's why it is mucus-forming. Proteins that were not heated as in **raw** milk are totally digestible and usable.

An excerpt from an interview done by The Health Ranger Mike Adams with a prominent activist and author against milk:

"**Mike Adams**: Can you give a brief summary of -- you've mentioned a few here, diabetes and acne, heart disease is mentioned in your book quite prominently -- but what other chronic diseases are, say, aggravated or even caused by chronic milk consumption?
Robert Cohen: Well, you know, that's an interesting question. Let's look at the Big Five -- in America, the number one killer is heart disease, and then we've got osteoporosis and cancer, and diabetes and asthma. We look at nations where they drink milk, we find these diseases are common. We look at nations where cheese consumption has tripled in the last 30 years, like England and France and Canada and the United States, we find also a tripling of asthma and breast cancers. Guess what country has the highest rate of breast cancer? Number one in breast cancer rate, Denmark, followed by Norway, followed by Holland, followed by Sweden -- are you detecting a trend?
Mike: Milk consumption.
Robert Cohen: Let's play some more trivia with you, Mike. We know breast cancer -- what country has the highest rate of heart disease?
Mike Adams: Well, I'm still thinking the United States.
Robert Cohen: Nope! Denmark, Norway, Holland and Sweden -- you're going to get it sooner or later! Bone disease, heart disease, breast cancer -- see where are we going with this? --highest rates of dairy consumption. We're seeing absolute correlations between these diseases and dairy consumption, and I can give you the reason. We have much more than just national epidemiological studies -- we have mechanisms by which these diseases occur, in breast cancer and every cancer, thousands of things cause cancer. Every time we pick up a newspaper there's a new thing identified as causing cancer."
Learn more: http://www.naturalnews.com/002695.html#ixzz1nMJ5djKF

The consensus is clear, if you want to be much healthier and lose weight quicker, avoid this toxic substance! More on the miraculous benefits of **Raw** milk a little later.

Commercial Milk Products To Avoid

- Pasteurized milk, even organic milk
- Pasteurized yogurt
- Pasteurized sour cream
- Pasteurized cottage cheese
- Pasteurized processed cheese
- Pasteurized chocolate milk
- Pasteurized cream
- Ice cream (make from pasteurized dairy)
- Any commercially available milk product will lead to terrible health and is best avoided

Chapter 6

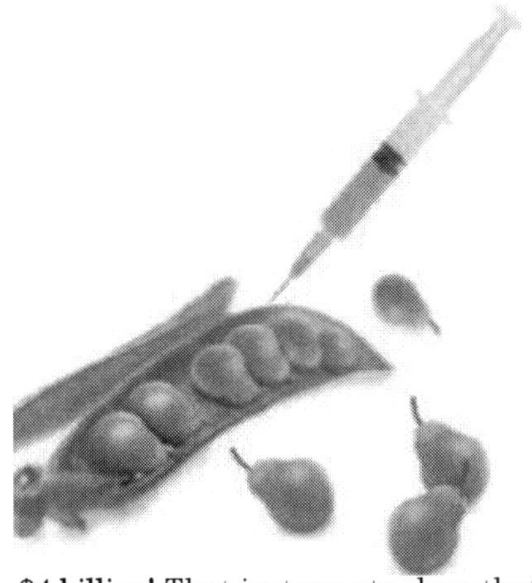

Genetically Modified Soy

A new health craze has taken over, who hasn't heard of the marvels of soy? The marketing bandwagon has touted soy as the next perfect health food for decades. In fact, its health benefits have been aggressively pushed in advertisements on national TV.

And from **1992 to 2006**, soy food sales increased from **$300 million to nearly $4 billion**! That just goes to show that soy has fast become synonymous with healthy eating.
But could something that sounds so healthy be actually dangerous?

Nowadays you don't have to stomach the "beany" flavored, drab soy products of the past to gain these supposed benefits because today you can find chocolate-flavored soymilk, soy burgers, soy ice cream, soy cheese, and just about any other soy food you could imagine. But those aren't the only sources of soy. Soy is now in just about every processed food out there -- even those that you'd think have nothing to do with soy, like condiments, yogurt, bread, sausages, and pasta sauce -- often in the form of soybean oil or the emulsifying agent soy lecithin (which is made from the **sludge** left over after crude soy oil is processed).

In fact, you may be surprised to learn that soybeans provided a whopping 75 percent of the edible consumption of fats and oils in the United States in 2006.

Why such a massive increase in consumption? Well the media did a great job advertising it as a "cure all health miracle." This couldn't be farther from the truth.

Back in 1999, the U.S. Food and Drug Administration approved a health claim for soy, and suddenly -- after a heavy marketing campaign from the soy industry -- an onslaught of "healthy" soy products bore the logo: "Diets low in saturated fat and cholesterol that include 25 grams of soy protein a day may reduce the risk of heart disease."

The resulting fanfare over the soybean has been every marketing director's dream: Eat soy, they say, and you can lose weight, protect your heart, lower your cholesterol, have more energy, and reduce the symptoms of menopause, among many other reported benefits.

Consider these facts from the Soyfoods Association of North America:

As of 2007, 85 percent of consumers perceive soy as healthy (up from 82 percent in 2006)
33 percent of Americans eat soy foods or beverages once a month or more
70 percent of consumers believe soybean oil is a healthy oil
Over half of consumers have tried soy foods or beverages in a restaurant
Over three in five consumers believe that eating soy-based foods can help to reduce obesity, and 84 percent agree with (or would like more information about) the FDA's claim that consuming 25 grams of soy protein per day reduces your risk of heart disease

Marketing has done a great job convincing the people that soy is a health food, but the truth is SOY IS NOT THE HEALTH FOOD YOU BELIEVE IT IS (the exception here is fermented soy which will be explained below).

Far from being the health cure-all it's purported to be, "thousands of studies link soy to malnutrition, digestive distress, immune-system breakdown, thyroid dysfunction, cognitive decline, reproductive disorders, and infertility -- even cancer and heart disease," says Dr. Kaayla Daniel, author of the book The Whole Soy Story: The Dark Side of America's Favorite Health Food.

The following is a breakdown of unfermented soy's major problems.

Unfermented soy contains natural toxins known as "antinutrients."
These antinutrients are large quantities of inhibitors that prevent your enzymes needed for protein digestion

Soy contains hemagglutinin.
Hemagglutinin is a clot-promoting substance that causes your red blood cells to clump together inhibiting oxygen uptake, growth, and cellular metabolism.

Soy contains growth depressing substances.

Soy contains goitrogens
Goitrogens lead to a depressed or less functioning thyroid.

Soy contains phytates
Phytates prevent the absorption of minerals including calcium, magnesium, iron, and zinc which play key roles in the biochemistry of your body. It doesn't matter how many vitamins you may be taking, if you eat soy products those vitamins don't get absorbed! If you are a vegetarian and regularly eat soy products like tofu/soy milk as a substitute for meat you are causing yourself serious mineral deficiencies which present themselves as suppressed normal body functions, suppressed immune function, and cravings of not-so-healthy foods.

Soy is full of phytoestrogens (isoflavones), genistein, and daidzein.
These compounds mimic and sometimes block our natural hormone estrogen, and have been found to have serious adverse effects on various human tissue.

Did you know that drinking even as little as two glasses of soymilk daily for one month has enough of these chemicals to alter a woman's menstrual cycle!? Phytoestrogens have also been linked to a disruption of endocrine function, infertility, and may even promote breast cancer in women.

Soy has high levels of aluminum
Soy beans are made into a slurry, combined with a solution to remove the fiber, then separated using an acid wash, neutralized in an alkali solution, and all of this is washed in large aluminum tanks which leach aluminum into the soy. During drying, nitrites are also created (a potent cancer-causing agent), and a toxin called lysionalanine is formed during the alkalizing process. Doesn't sound like something you would want to eat.

Soy puts your baby at serious risk.
Almost 20% of U.S. infants are fed soy formula. This chemical slurry full of antinutrients and hormones harm your baby's future sexual development, reproductive function, mineral balance, hormonal balance, and promote negative health conditions.

Pesticides and GMO.
Soy foods are heavily sprayed with pesticides, and more than 80% of soy grown in the U.S. is genetically modified.

Experiments using soy isolate created vitamin and mineral deficiencies. Deficiencies in vitamin E, D, B12, calcium, magnesium, manganese, molybdenum, copper, iron, and zinc were found after ingestion of soy protein isolate by animals who also developed enlarged organs such as the pancreas, thyroid gland, and fatty livers.

Questionable benefits on cholesterol
Scientists are questioning soy's positive effects on the levels of cholesterol after some doubtful studies.

Soy has been linked to the following health effects, and this is not a complete list:

Breast cancer

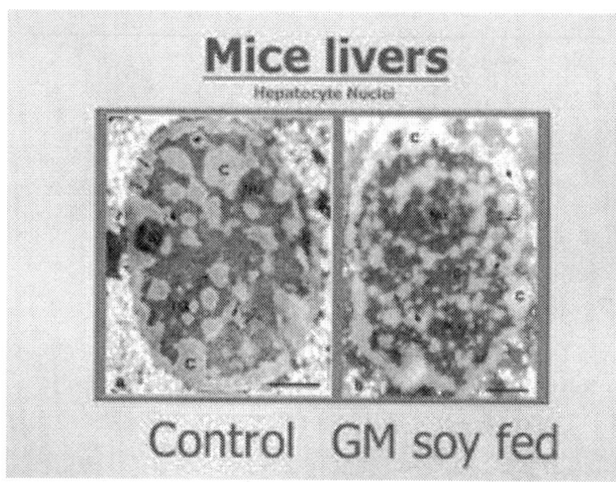

Brain damage
Infant abnormalities
Thyroid disorder
Fatty liver
Kidney stones
Immune system impairment
Severe, potentially fatal, food allergies
Infertility
Dangers during pregnancy and nursing

It is quite evident that soy is not a miracle food, nor is it anything even remotely resembling a "health food." The only exception here is **fermented** soy products. Soy was not even considered a food until fermentation techniques were discovered about a thousand years ago. ONLY fermented soy has any benefits as a food product. During fermentation the phytate and "antinutrients" are reduced, and their beneficial properties become available for our digestive system.

The only soy products that are fine to eat are **tempeh** (a fermented soybean cake with firm texture and a nutty-mushroom like flavour, **miso** (fermented soybean paste commonly used in miso soup), **natto** (fermented soybeans with a sticky texture and cheese-like flavour), and **soy sauce** (traditional soy sauce is made by fermenting soybeans, salt, and enzymes, but be very cautious because most brands on the market today use a chemical process instead of old fashioned fermentation). Tofu is NOT fermented and is NOT recommended for eating. To be honest I would not recommend any soy products due to them being GMO and still having residue of phytates, "antinutrients," and the negative qualities mentioned above. Eat it only if you have to, substitute it whenever possible.

Soy Foods To Avoid

- Soy milk
- Soy baby formula
- Soy protein
- Soy protein/energy bars
- Tofu
- Soy ice cream
- Textured vegetable protein (used as a filler and texturizer in meatless products)
- Soy snacks like chips, rice cakes etc.
- Anything "meatless" has high amount of soy and better be avoided

Chapter 7

Energy and Protein Bars

Energy and protein bars are advertised as something healthy, and the trend has caught on. They are sweet, filling, seem to be nutritious, and have plenty of protein, but are they as healthy as they claim to be?

When cheap soy protein became available on the market, protein bar sales exploded. Balance Bars, Zone Perfects Bars, and Atkins bars were first on the scene to be taken over by dozens of different companies promoting their new "meal replacement." Most bars these days are made with soy protein, and as the previous chapter discussed, soy protein is a potent mixture of phytic acid, enzyme inhibitors, isoflavones, growth suppressors, and blood clotting factors. Not to mention all the soy, if not organic, is genetically modified and highly processed and heated, meaning the protein is degraded to a point that it cannot be digested and used in our bodies becoming totally useless.

Soy protein? Bodybuilders beware: because many weight gainer powders, bars and shakes contain this dangerous ingredient and it can cause troubling side effects such as diminished libido and erectile dysfunction. It is important to become a label and ingredient list reader. There are so many different names for soy additives, you could be bringing home a genetically modified soy-based product without even realizing it. Dr. Daniel offers a report, "Where the Soys Are," on her Web site. It lists the many "aliases" that soy might be hiding under in ingredient lists -- words like "boullion," "natural flavor" and "textured plant protein."

Here are a few other names soy tends to hide under:
Mono-diglyceride
Soya, Soja or Yuba
TSF (textured soy flour) or TSP (textured soy protein)
TVP (textured vegetable protein)
Lecithin
MSG (monosodium glutamate)

Not all textured vegetable protein is made from soy, but a great deal of it is. Lecithin can be made from soy, eggs, sunflower or corn. Be sure to contact the manufacturer to find out which is in your product if the label doesn't reveal this information.

The whey protein in bars is also heavily processed and heated, which destroys the protein making it totally unusable by the body (any protein heated above 42 Celsius/106 Fahrenheit is denatured, or fused together, making it totally unusable by our body – more on this in part 2 of the book). During the old days, when raw milk products were processed, the whey and skim milk were given to pigs and chickens. Nowadays with large scale industrial production the dairy industry has an overabundance of whey, it is their waste product, so they decided to use it in protein powders and protein bars as a cheap alternative to good quality proteins.

High fructose corn syrup is commonly used in energy bars and has been shown to be much worse than sugar. Whether HFCS, sugar, or artificial sweeteners they all cause terrible health consequences like insulin spikes, more hunger, and increased fat storage.

In reality, protein bars are just candy bars in disguise full of waste by products intended to provide a cheap alternative to actual food. To list the dangers of these ingredients would be too many, it is much better for your health to avoid these at all costs. You may substitute them with raw nuts, raw dried fruits, or a green shake which has fully digestible protein, vitamins and minerals that have not been altered or processed and are in their original form without any side effects. The more things you eat raw, the more energy you will have, the less cravings you will get, and the more weight you will lose!

The best quality proteins are leafy green vegetables (spinach, kale etc.) and hemp protein. And the best protein/energy bars are organic or RAW energy bars which are very delicious and provide organic, wholesome ingredients to fuel your body.

Energy Bars To Avoid
Luna, Kashi, Powerbar, Quaker, Kudos, MetRX, Balance Bars, Cliff Bars, Genisoy, Soy Sensations and anything with soy, HFCS, sugar, refined flours, colors, and preservatives.

Chapter 8

Soft Drinks and Juices

Huge increases in soft drink consumption have not happened by chance-they are due to intense marketing efforts by soft drink corporations. Coca Cola, for example, has set the goal of raising consumption of its products in the US by at least 25 percent per year. The adult market is stagnant so kids are the target.

Soft drink companies spend billions on advertising. Much of these marketing efforts are aimed at children through playgrounds, toys, cartoons, movies, videos, charities and amusement parks; and through contests, sweepstakes, games and clubs via television, radio, magazines and the internet. Their efforts have paid off. Last year soft drink companies grossed over $57 billion in sales in the us alone, a colossal amount.

In 1998 the Center for Science in the Public Interest (CSPI) warned the public that soft drink companies were beginning to infiltrate our schools and kid clubs. For example, they reported that Coca-Cola paid the Boys & Girls Clubs of America $60 million to market its brand exclusively in over 2000 facilities. Fast food companies selling soft drinks now run ads on Channel One, the commercial television network with programming shown in classrooms almost every day to eight million middle, junior and high school students. In 1993, District 11 in Colorado Springs became the first public school district in the us to place ads for Burger King in its hallways and on the sides of its school buses. Later, the school district signed a 10-year deal with Coca-Cola, bringing in $11 million during the life of the contract. This arrangement was later imitated all over Colorado. The contracts specify annual sales quotas with the result that school administrators encourage students to drink sodas, even in the classrooms. One high school in Beltsville, Maryland, made nearly $100,000 last year on a deal with a soft drink company.

The ingredients in soft drinks is a witches brew concoction that has absolutely no nutritional value and seriously degrades health.

High Fructose Corn Syrup, now used in preference to sugar, is associated with poor development of collagen in growing animals, especially in the context of copper deficiency. All fructose must be metabolized by the liver. Animals on high-fructose diets develop liver problems similar to those of alcoholics.

Aspartame, used in diet sodas, is a potent neurotoxin and endocrine disrupter. **Caffeine** stimulates the adrenal gland without providing nourishment. In large amounts, caffeine can lead to adrenal exhaustion, especially in children.

Phosphoric acid, added to give soft drinks "bite," is added to mask the extreme amounts of sugar which would otherwise be almost undrinkable. Phosphoric acid is just that, an acid, and leeches minerals from our bones and teeth like calcium and magnesium. Over the last 30 years a virtual tome of information has been published linking soft drink consumption to a rise in osteoporosis and bone fractures.

Citric acid often contains traces of MSG, a neurotoxin.

Artificial Flavors may also contain traces of MSG.

All carbonated drinks are highly acidic. Carbon must be in balance with oxygen in our body since carbon is acidic and oxygen is alkaline. With all the acids, and sugar, our body fights really hard to keep alkalizing our system by taking minerals from our bones and teeth.

Sport drinks are no exception. Usually they are full of sugar or artificial sweeteners which we have already learned are toxic to our system. According to body physiology, if you are not working out heavily for 45 minutes or more, there are no benefits of drinking sport drinks. The best sport drink you can have is water with a little bit of honey and sea salt added which will give you the exact same effect as a sport drink, and for much cheaper and without any extra chemicals.

Juices

Most people think that commercially available juice is "healthy." This could not be farther from the truth. Just like milk, juices are pasteurized, meaning heated to boiling temperatures for prolonged periods of time. As we already know, this procedure destroys everything beneficial from the original ingredient. Raw juices are full of amazing nutrients, enzymes, vitamins, and minerals. Pasteurization destroys all that, and turns real juice into a sugar bomb that will make you gain weight and develop diabetes.

The juices you see on your grocery store shelves are nothing more than colored sugar water. Commercially produced fruit juice is probably more calorific than you are aware. Most 200 – 250 ml glasses or bottles contain at least a couple hundred calories mainly due to the added sugars. The sugars that acidify your body, wreak havoc on your insulin balance and metabolism, and create the perfect grounds for ill health.

Pasteurization is considered to be a 'safe' method to treat juice and milk, even though the process alters the products in a negative way.

Despite this, if you continue drinking pasteurized juice or milk products, then commercial companies will continue using the process of juice pasteurization. But one thing is definite – when you juice your own fresh, thoroughly washed (and you know that because you're the one washing it) fruit and vegetables, you can be certain that you can make a healthier juice than any juice available in your supermarket or local grocery store. In addition to that of course, it'll undoubtedly be delicious!

Maybe once you've tried your very own juice, you will see the difference between store bought orange juice, preserved in a treated carton, for untold months, compared to a freshly prepared orange juice with all of its flavor and nutrients fully intact - **you most definitely won't go back once you've discovered the benefits of juicing for yourself!**

Chapter 9

Animal Products and Farm Raised Fish

Ever since giant multinational corporations got a hold of the food market, things changed for the worse. Profits became the ultimate goal, with the quality of the product taking a backseat. For example light bulbs are made specifically to last a certain amount of hours and then break down so you buy new ones; while some 50 years ago light bulbs were built to last for decades. Computer hard drives are programmed for a specific number of hours or rounds so you are **forced** to buy new things over and over again. The food industry is no different than any other industry; it keep pumping out cheap products as fast as possible for as much profit as possible.

Ever since the 1980s when giant multinational companies took hold of the food market, more than 80% of the 35 million beef cattle slaughtered annually in the U.S. ended up being concentrated into the greedy hands of only four corporations. Small time country farming has turned into an industrial machine pumping out toxic products and calling it "food."

Many of today's farms are actually large industrial facilities, not the green pastures and red barns that most Americans imagine. These consolidated operations are able to produce food in high volume but have little to no regard for the environment, animal welfare, or food safety. In order to maximize profits, factory farms often put the health of consumers and rural communities at risk.

Cattle raised for beef are subjected to numerous painful procedures during their lives. These include the repeated infliction of third degree burns (branding), having their testicles ripped out (castration), and the removal of their horns. To minimize costs, all of these practices are routinely conducted without any painkillers.

The majority of cattle spend their lives on overcrowded feedlots, "standing ankle deep in their own waste eating a diet that makes them sick", as Michael Pollen writes in the *New York Times*.

The grains that they are fed (often contaminated with fungus and fungicides), which is a totally unnatural food for the cow, are used to fatten up livestock as quickly as possible and as cheaply as possible. Usually they are fed genetically modified, lowest quality grain, corn, which the animals cannot properly digest, and "fillers" such as **municipal garbage, stale pastry, chicken feathers, gum, candy**, **sawdust**, **chicken manure**.

This unnatural diet can lead to an array of health problems, such as bloat, acidosis (bovine heart burn), diarrhea, ulcers, liver disease, and general weakening of the immune system. The normal pH of 7 in cows that are supposed to graze on grass is lowered to a highly acidic pH of 4 from a grain diet which is perfect breeding ground for deadly bacterial strains like E.coli which sickens and even kills many people who then eat this cow meat. High acidity also stops the production of omega 3 fatty acids and CLA and increases omega 6 fatty acids which Americans already consume way too much of.

During transport to feedlots, auctions, and slaughterhouses, cattle also endure extreme cruelty. Food is not given to the animals during transport or the day before since it will not be converted into profitable flesh. Some cattle succumb to pneumonia, dehydration, or heat exhaustion, and many have their flesh get frozen to the sides of transport vehicles during long trips.

Dr. Lester Friedlander, a former USDA veterinarian, put it this way: "In the summertime, when it's 90, 95 degrees, they're transporting cattle from 12 to 15 hundred miles away on a trailer, 40 to 45 head crammed in there, and some collapse from heat exhaustion. This past winter, we had minus-50-degree weather with the wind chill. Can you imagine if you were in the back of a trailer that's open and the wind-chill factor is minus 50 degrees, and that trailer is going 50 to 60 miles an hour?"

These industrial facilities share many characteristics, including:

Excessive Size

- Unnaturally large numbers of animals are confined closely together. Cattle feedlots generally contain thousands of animals in one place, while many egg-laying businesses house one million or more chickens. The main animals for such operations are cows, pigs, chickens and turkeys, but this practice is also applied to sheep, goats, rabbits, and various types of poultry.

Disregard for Animal Welfare

- Metal buildings confine animals indoors, with minimal room for normal behaviors and little or no access to sunlight and fresh air.
- Animals are mutilated to adapt them to factory farm conditions. This includes cutting off the beaks of chickens and turkeys (de-beaking), and amputating the tails of cows and pigs (docking).
- Pens and cages restrict the natural behavior and movement of animals. In some cases, such as veal calves and mothering pigs, the animals can't even turn around.
- Due to the extreme volume of cattle being slaughtered (about 250 cattle per hour) it is almost impossible for any humane treatment and slaughtering procedures.

Misuse of Pharmaceuticals

- High doses of antibiotics for bacterial control and as a positive effect also used for the purpose of fattening up the cattle
- Fed all sorts of hormones to promote unnatural fast growth

Mismanagement of Waste

- Excessive waste created by large concentrations of animals is handled in ways that can pollute air and water.
- Man-made lagoons on industrial farms hold millions of gallons of liquid waste, from which contaminants can leach into groundwater. The manure is normally sprayed on crops, but often excessively, leading it to run off into surface waters.
- Nutrients and bacteria from waste can contaminate waterways, killing fish and shellfish and disturbing aquatic ecosystems.

Socially Irresponsible Corporate Ownership

- One corporation often owns or controls all aspects of the production process, including animal rearing, feed production, slaughter, packaging and distribution. Known as vertical integration, this approach leads to tremendous consolidation of power that is leveraged against small farmers and diminishes corporations' accountability for irresponsible practices.

- Contract growing indentures independent farmers to grow livestock for a corporation. In the contract system, the corporation dictates all aspects of raising the animals, while the farmer is left with the risk, overhead, waste, and the disposal of any animals that don't survive until slaughter.

Information gathered from
http://www.sustainabletable.org/issues/factoryfarming/

The cows are born in a stressful environment, fed an unnatural diet; genetically modified grains with toxic garbage "fillers," stuffed with hormones, pesticides, antibiotics, forced to extreme confinement and dirty conditions, and to top it off slaughtered in the most inhumane horrible way possible. Then the meat is processed with toxic preservatives and colors like nitrites (which preserve the meat and turn it a more appealing red in color) that have been widely studies and shown to promote cancer, respiratory diseases, immune diseases, skin problems, and a host of other terrible illnesses.

Is that something you want inside of you?

Farmed Vs. Wild Caught Fish

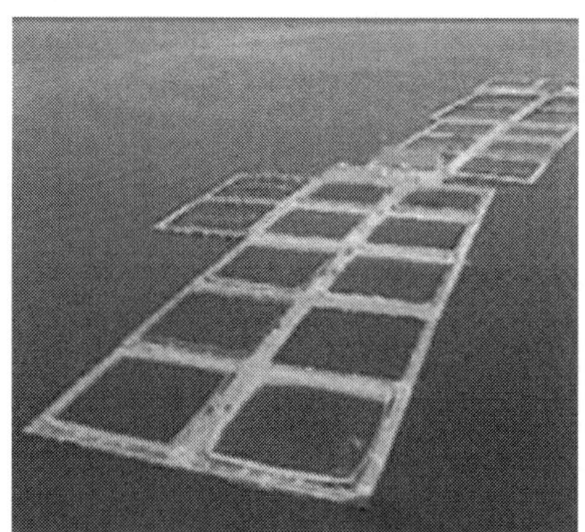

There are a few very important differences between wild caught fish and the fish found in your supermarket and restaurants.

Farmed fish are held in small pens, or cages, not being allowed the freedom of movement or feeding on their natural diet.

Farmed fish are much higher in fat content since they are not spending any time vigorously swimming through ocean waters or leaping up rocky streams like their wild brothers. Lazily swimming through crowded pens eating unnatural grain-based fish meal makes them far less nutritious, and even toxic.

Farmed fish have much more inflammatory omega 6 content which creates a heavy imbalance of omega 3 to omega 6 levels. Farmed fish have more than double the omega 6 content than wild species. The healthy omega 3 levels are also much smaller in farmed fish.

Farmed fish are also given high levels of antibiotics and pesticides to get rid of infections and sea lice which run rampant in densely packed fish lots. In the end you are the one eating all these toxins!

Studies have shown that farmed salmon accumulates far more cancer causing PCBs and poisonous dioxins than wild salmon. Tests on grocery store farmed salmon showed that they contain up to twice the fat and 16 times the PCB levels as compared to wild salmon. These toxins are stored in the fat and end up on your plate.

Farmed salmon are also given dyes in the food to make them pink in color; otherwise they would be grey in color. These dyes contain toxic ingredients that are not fit for human consumption.

Uneaten pellets and excrement from fish farms leeches onto the ocean floor stimulating pathogenic bacteria which pollute the ocean floor destroying marine life and many sea dwelling creatures. A good sized salmon farm produces the amount of excrement equivalent to the sewage of a city of 10,000 people.

We get most of our fish from China. They do 61% of the world aqua farming.. As we eat more fish, their ponds become increasingly packed with more fish to accommodate the demand. A more tightly packed pond means more disease and pollution from fish waste. Antibiotics and other drugs are liberally used to combat this problem including malachite green, an antifungal and potential carcinogen. Safety standards and practices are much less stringent in other countries, and the fish being sold to us from overseas is full of toxins, pesticides, mercury, and other cancer causing agents, all in the name of profit. They pollute lakes, oceans, promote the use of toxic substances, and sell us food full of chemicals that only harm our body. Vote with your wallets folks, only your purchase habits can put a stop to terrible practices.

What You Can Do

We can all help put an end to the factory farming system by buying our food from smaller, sustainable farms, or fish that is "wild caught". These businesses still aim to profit from their labor, but that's not their only objective. They have essentially a triple bottom line - of social, environmental and financial gain - which means they won't sacrifice the health of the land or the quality of food simply to make a few dollars more.

- When you buy local fruits, vegetables, and meat products, you support your local economy. More of the money you spend goes directly to the farmers themselves because less goes to transportation and middlemen. Buying locally also means burning less fossil fuel to get food from the farm to the table, which benefits the environment.

Health Concerns of Meat Products

There is no longer any doubt about the fact that eating meat is bad for your health.

The list of diseases which are more common among meat eaters looks like the index of a medical textbook.

Anaemia, appendicitis, arthritis, breast cancer, cancer of the colon, cancer of the prostate, constipation, diabetes, gall stones, gout, high blood pressure, indigestion, obesity, piles, strokes and varicose veins are just some of the well known disorders which are more likely to affect meat eaters than vegetarians.

The meat industry is a multi-billion dollar powerhouse that has its profits at stake. It does everything in its power to make people believe that meat is healthy, nutritious, and a good source of protein. These are all lies. Meat products have been linked to cancer, heart disease, diabetes, immune disorders, high blood pressure and to so many other horrible diseases that it is a shame people still don't know about its dangers.

We have been falsely led to believe that people can't survive without meat and that it has something no other food product has. These are all unfounded lies brought to you by huge corporations that ONLY HAVE PROFITS in their mind. They don't care about your health and they do everything possible that you don't get true information regarding their products.

Have you ever heard of "The China Study"? Not many people have, yet it is only the ***largest most comprehensive study of human nutrition ever conducted.***

The China Study was a HUGE study that went on for 30 years; it resulted in over 8,000 statistically significant correlations between diet and disease. It surveyed a vast range of diseases and diet and lifestyle factors in rural China, and more recently, in Taiwan.

A monumental nationwide survey was conducted in China in the 1970s on cancer death rates from twelve different types of cancer. More than 2,400 Chinese counties and 880 million citizens were involved. This resulted in a color-coded atlas showing where certain types of cancer were high, and where they were non-existent. This provided information on over four dozen different kinds of disease, including cancers, heart diseases, and infectious diseases.

The China Study was a grand design; it gathered data on 367 variables, and compared each variable to the others. They went into 65 counties across China and administered blood tests and questionnaires to 6,500 adults. They took urine samples, and directly measured everything families ate over a three day period. And they analyzed food samples from markets across the country.

When they were done, they had an unmatched comprehensive study.

Early in his career as a researcher with MIT and Virginia Tech, Dr. Campbell, the author of *The China Study* worked to promote better health by eating more meat, milk and eggs -- "high-quality animal protein ... It was an obvious sequel to my own life on the farm and I was happy to believe that the American diet was the best in the world."

He later was a researcher on a project in the Philippines working with malnourished children. The project became an investigation for Dr. Campbell, as to why so many Filipino children were being diagnosed with liver cancer, predominately an adult disease. The primary goal of the project was to ensure that the children were getting as much protein as possible.

"In this project, however, I uncovered a dark secret. Children who ate the highest protein diets were the ones most likely to get liver cancer..." He began to review other reports from around the world that reflected the findings of his research in the Philippines.

Although it was "heretical to say that protein wasn't healthy," he started an in-depth study into the role of nutrition, especially protein, in the cause of cancer.

The research project culminated in a 20-year partnership of Cornell University, Oxford University, and the Chinese Academy of Preventive Medicine, a survey of diseases and lifestyle factors in rural China and Taiwan. More commonly known as the China Study, "this project eventually produced more than **8000 statistically significant associations** between various dietary factors and disease."

The findings? "People who ate the most animal-based foods got the most chronic disease ... People who ate the most plant-based foods were the healthiest and tended to avoid chronic disease. These results could not be ignored," said Dr. Campbell.

In *The China Study*, Dr. Campbell detailed the connection between nutrition and heart disease, diabetes, and cancer, and also its ability to reduce or reverse the risk or effects of these deadly illnesses.

I go into a great more detail about this issue in Part 2 of my book, but here are the main issues:

Animal protein promotes the growth of cancer. The book author T. Colin Campbell, PhD., grew up on a dairy farm, so he regularly enjoyed a wholesome glass of milk. Not anymore. In multiple, peer-reviewed animal studies, researchers discovered that they could actually turn the growth of cancer cells on and off by raising and lowering doses of animal protein. The huge population studies showed almost perfect correlations between the amount of animal products eaten and the amount of cancers, heart disease and other serious health conditions present.

Poor nutrition switches on disease. The food you eat affects the way your cells interact with carcinogens, making them more or less dangerous. "The results of these, and many other studies, showed nutrition to be far more important in controlling cancer promotion than the dose of the initiating carcinogen." He showed that nutrition was a **far greater controlling factor** in disease than the actual carcinogen!

The study findings are bulletproof. After years of controversial lab results on animals, the researchers had to see how they played out in humans. The study they created included 367 variables, 65 counties in China, and 6,500 adults (who completed questionnaires, blood tests, etc.). "When we were done, we had more than 8,000 statistically significant associations between lifestyle, diet, and disease variables." In other words, there's no arguing with the findings.

The results are simple: Eat plants for health. "People who ate the most animal-based foods got the most chronic disease. People who ate the most plant-based foods were the healthiest."

Heart disease can be reversed through nutrition. Caldwell B. Esselstyn, Jr., M.D., a physician and researcher at the best cardiac center in the country, The Cleveland Clinic, treated 18 patients with established coronary disease with a whole foods, plant-based diet. Not only did the intervention stop the progression of the disease, but 70 percent of the patients saw an opening of their clogged arteries. Dr. Dean Ornish, a graduate of Harvard Medical School, completed a similar study with consistent results.

Plants are powerful. It's not just cancer and heart disease that respond to a whole foods, plant-based diet. It may also help protect you from diabetes, obesity, autoimmune diseases, bone, kidney, eye, and brain diseases.

Plants do it better. "There are virtually no nutrients in animal-based foods that are not better provided by plants." Protein, fiber, vitamins, minerals—you name it, they've got it, plus all the health benefits.

Lessons from The China Study

1) Breast cancer is associated with consumption of animal fat (but not plant fat).
2) Heart disease is associated with animal protein consumption. Stop eating animal protein, and most heart disease will reverse.
3) Type 1 diabetes is associated with consumption of pasteurized cow's milk (raw milk was not studied).
4) Type 2 diabetes is associated with increased fat intake.
5) Colon cancer is associated with meat consumption.
6) Multiple Sclerosis is associated with pasteurized cow's milk consumption (raw milk was not studied).
7) Increased hip fractures from osteoporosis are associated with increased pasteurized milk consumption (raw milk was not studied).
8) Kidney stones are associated with animal protein intake.
9) Macular degeneration and cataracts, forms of eye disease, occur when we fail to eat enough highly colored fruits and vegetables. Both diseases are likely to be increased by animal based foods.

10) Cognitive impairment, memory loss, and Alzheimer's disease are associated with an animal-based diet.

His findings across 65 countries and thousands of people clearly showed that animal products can turn cancer on and off. It is a very comprehensive study and I greatly recommend you read the book called *The China Study*. I go into a great more detail in Part 2 of my book on this topic, so keep reading☺

The biggest myth concerning meat is that a vegetarian diet is somehow deficient in protein and nutrients. Athletes, pregnant women and parents often justify the desire to eat meat by saying that they need animal protein in order to be healthy human beings. This is probably the biggest myth in all of nutrition, and is completely false and untrue.

Dr. T. Colin Campbell, professor emeritus at Cornell University and author of The China Study, explains that in fact, we only recently (historically speaking) began eating meat, and that the inclusion of meat in our diet came well after we became who we are today. He explains that "the birth of agriculture only started about 10,000 years ago at a time when it became considerably more convenient to herd animals. This is not nearly as long as the time [that] fashioned our basic biochemical functionality (at least tens of millions of years) and which functionality depends on the nutrient composition of plant-based foods."

That is similar with what Physicians Committee for Responsible Medicine President Dr. Neal Barnard says in his book, *The Power of Your Plate*, in which he explains that "early humans had diets very much like other great apes, which is to say a largely plant-based diet, drawing on foods we can pick with our hands. Research suggests that meat-eating probably began by scavenging--eating the leftovers that carnivores had left behind. However, our bodies have never adapted to it.

To this day, meat-eaters have a higher incidence of heart disease, cancer, diabetes, and other problems."

There is no more authoritative source on anthropological issues than paleontologist Dr. Richard Leakey, who explains what anyone who has taken an introductory physiology course might have discerned intuitively--that humans are herbivores. Leakey notes that "you can't tear flesh by hand, you can't tear hide by hand.... We wouldn't have been able to deal with food source that required those large canines" (although we have teeth that are called "canines," they bear little resemblance to the canines of carnivores).

In fact, our hands are perfect for grabbing and picking fruits and vegetables. Similarly, like the intestines of other herbivores, ours are very long (carnivores have short intestines so they can quickly get rid of all that rotting flesh they eat). We don't have sharp claws to seize and hold down prey. And most of us (hopefully) lack the instinct that would drive us to chase and then kill animals and devour their raw carcasses." Dr. Milton Mills builds on these points and offers dozens more in his essay, A Comparative Anatomy of Eating.

The point is this: Thousands of years ago when we were hunter-gatherers, we may have needed a bit of meat in our diets in times of scarcity, but we don't need it now. Says Dr. William C. Roberts, editor of the *American Journal of Cardiology*, "Although we think we are, and we act as if we are, human beings are not natural carnivores. When we kill animals to eat them, they end up killing us, because their flesh, which contains cholesterol and saturated fat, was never intended for human beings, who are natural herbivores."

Non-meat eaters have always been known to have **more endurance and stamina** in the sport world. And there are, and have been, many vegetarian athletes and bodybuilders.

Many people will still say that our "ancestors" ate meat, but this is simply not true. Let's look at the actual data from anthropologists. Hunter-gatherers typically ate a diet that is **80% or more plant matter**. Early anthropologists studying hunter-gatherer tribes (Amazonian, African etc) assumed that meat is more important than it is because they spent most of their time interacting with the men of the tribes, and the men liked to talk about hunting. But in fact, meat is a **small** percentage of overall diet in most hunter-gatherer societies (excluding cultures like the Inuit where meat is the only food available) and women provide most of the food through gathering wild plants. A real Paleo diet would consist largely of roots, nuts, vegetables, fruit, leaves, and seeds, and would include a smaller percentage of mammal meat, bird meat, seafood, insects, and eggs. It would include no dairy at all (except for breastfeeding infants), and would be very high in fiber and nutrients and come from a much wider variety of plants than what we eat in our society. As any competent nutritionist will tell you, this is an ***extremely healthy diet***.

What about vitamin B12 which many nutritionists will tell you only comes from meat? Even the Encyclopedia of Dietary Supplements, put together by a blue ribbon committee of scholars from the National Institutes of Health says "Because vitamin B12 is found only in animal source foods, strict vegetarianism has long been associated with a greater risk of deficiency of this vitamin." These "scholars" obviously have never heard of spirulina which contains ***750%*** of the daily recommended intake of vitamin B12 in only ***5 grams***! Let's see any animal product even come close.

Old habits die hard, and it's convenient for people who like to eat meat to think that there is evidence to support their belief that eating meat is "natural" or the cause of our evolution. For many years, I too, clung to the idea that meat was good for me; I realize now that I was probably comforted to have justification for my continued attachment to the traditions I grew up with.

But in fact **top nutritional and anthropological scientists** from the most reputable institutions unanimously agree that humans are natural herbivores, and that we will be healthier today if we stick with our herbivorous roots. It may be inconvenient, but it is the truth.

Vegetarian bodybuilders: http://www.treehugger.com/slideshows/culture/10-superstar-athletes-who-dont-eat-meat/page/2/

What do Alicia Silverstone, Alanis Morissette, Barry White, Bif Naked, Casey Affleck, Ellen Degeneres, Jason Mraz, Jenny McCarthy, Liv Tyler, Mike Tyson, Tobey Maguire, Vanessa Williams, Woody Harrelson, Anne Hathaway, B.B King, Bill Clinton, Brad Pitt, Bryan Adams, Carrie Ann Moss, Chris Martin (Coldplay), Christina Applegate, Claudia Schiffer, Demi Lovato, Deepak Chopra, Diane Keaton, Dustin Hoffman, George Harrison (Beatles), Ian McKellan (Lord of the Rings), Jane Goodall, Kelly Clarkson, Kim Basinger and hundreds of other stars have in common? Yep, they are all either vegans or vegetarians. For a full list you may visit this web site: http://www.happycow.net/famous_vegans2.html

There is a whole site dedicated to vegan bodybuilding; you can check it out and see some amazing examples for yourself: http://veganbodybuilding.com/

The verdict? "*Eat a whole foods, plant-based diet, while minimizing the consumption of refined foods, animal products, and pasteurized milk products.*" **The less meat, pasteurized milk products, and refined foods you eat, the more healthier you will be, the more amazing you will feel and the more weight you will lose; period.**

Chapter 10

Raw Organic Grass Fed Dairy

Raw, unpasteurized, unhomogenized, free range, grass-fed milk has been used for millennia as a nutritious drink and even as medicine up until just after World War II. Due to the potent nutritional content of raw milk, you could totally live on milk products if you had no other source of food! Raw cow's milk has all 8 essential amino acids in varying amounts, depending on stage of lactation with about 80% of them caseins; slow but easily digestible proteins, ; but only if **not pasteurized**. The other 20% are whey proteins which are easily digested in their raw form but very heat sensitive meaning they are destroyed very easily with heat. Also the enzyme content is very high, high immunoglobulin count (immune factors), and vitamin/mineral binding proteins allowing for perfect digestion.

Milk in its raw state has specific anti microbial agents that provide protection from outside invaders. Lactoferrin, an iron-binding protein, has numerous beneficial properties including improved absorption and assimilation of iron, anti-cancer properties and anti-microbial action against several species of bacteria responsible for dental cavities. Recent studies also reveal that it has powerful antiviral properties as well.

Two other players in raw milk's antibiotic protein/enzyme arsenal are **lysozyme** and **lactoperoxidase**. Lysosome can actually break apart cell walls of certain undesirable bacteria, while lactoperoxidase teams up with other substances to help knock out unwanted microbes too.
The immunoglobulins, an extremely complex class of milk proteins also known as **antibodies**, provide resistance to many viruses, bacteria and bacterial toxins and may help reduce the severity of asthma symptoms. Studies have shown significant loss of these important disease fighters when milk is heated to high processing temperatures during pasteurization.

As you can see, milk is a natural bacterial and virus fighting machine that can adapt to specific invaders creating a perfect immune drink, but only in its **RAW** state.

Let's look at the carbohydrates found in milk. Lactose, or milk sugar, is the primary carbohydrate in cow's milk. Made from one molecule each of the simple sugars glucose and galactose, it's known as a disaccharide. People with lactose intolerance for one reason or another (age, genetics, etc.), no longer make the enzyme lactase and so can't digest milk sugar. This leads to some unpleasant symptoms, which, needless to say, the victims find rather unpleasant at best. Raw milk, with its lactose-digesting **Lactobacilli** bacteria intact, make digestions of lactose an easy process allowing people with lactose intolerance to find that they can drink raw milk just fine!

The end-result of lactose digestion is a substance called lactic acid (responsible for the sour taste in fermented dairy products and the **same** acid produced in our muscles during exercise which leads to muscle fatigue). Besides having known inhibitory effects on harmful species of bacteria, lactic acid **boosts the absorption** of calcium, phosphorus and iron, and has been shown to make milk proteins more digestible.

What about milk fat? Approximately two thirds of the fat in milk is saturated. Saturated fats play a number of key roles in our bodies: from construction of cell membranes and key hormones to providing energy storage and padding for delicate organs, to serving as a vehicle for important fat-soluble vitamins (see below).

All fats cause our stomach lining to secrete a hormone (cholecystokinin or CCK) which, aside from boosting production and secretion of digestive enzymes, lets us know we've eaten enough. With that trigger removed, non-fat dairy products and other fat-free foods can potentially help contribute to overeating.

Now consider that prior to 1900, very few people died from heart disease. The introduction of hydrogenated cottonseed oil in 1911 (as trans-fat laden Crisco) helped begin the move away from healthy animal fats found in raw milk products, and toward the slow, downward trend in cardiovascular health from which millions continue to suffer today.

CLA, short for *conjugated linoleic acid* and abundant in milk from grass-fed cows, is a heavily studied, polyunsaturated Omega-6 fatty acid with promising health benefits. Among CLA's many potential benefits: it raises metabolic rate, helps remove abdominal fat, boosts muscle growth, reduces resistance to insulin, strengthens the immune system and lowers food allergy reactions. As luck would have it, grass-fed raw milk has from 3-5 times the amount found in the milk from feed lot cows

Volumes have been written about the two groups of vitamins; water and fat soluble, and their contribution to health. Whole raw milk has **all 37 of them**, and they're completely available for your body to use. Whether regulating your metabolism or helping the biochemical reactions that free energy from the food you eat, they're all present and ready to go to work for you. Unlike the milk we drink today which has absolutely nothing beneficial left in it after processing; in order to make it somewhat healthy, the milk producers add synthetic indigestible vitamins back into it.

Just to repeat, nothing needs to be added to raw milk, especially milk from free range grass-fed cows. No vitamins. No minerals. No enriching. It's a **complete food**.

Minerals

Our bodies, each with a biochemistry as unique as our fingerprints, are incredibly complex, so discussions of minerals, or any nutrients for that matter, must deal with ranges rather than specific amounts. Raw milk contains a broad selection of completely available minerals ranging from the familiar calcium and phosphorus down to trace elements, the function of some, as of yet, is still rather unclear.

A sampling of the health benefits of calcium, an important element abundant in raw milk includes: reduction in cancers, particularly of the colon: higher bone mineral density in people of every age, lower risk of osteoporosis and fractures in older adults; lowered risk of kidney stones; formation of strong teeth and reduction of dental cavities, to name a few.

An interesting feature of minerals as nutrients is the delicate balance they require with other minerals to function properly. For instance, calcium needs a proper ratio of two other macronutrients, phosphorus and magnesium, to be properly utilized by our bodies. Guess what? Nature codes for the entire array of minerals in raw milk (from cows raised on properly maintained pastures) to be in proper balance with one another thus optimizing their benefit to us.

Probably pasteurization's worst offence is that it makes the calcium insoluble (indigestible, unusable). This frequently leads to rickets, bad teeth and nervous troubles, for sufficient calcium content is vital to children; and with the loss of phosphorus also associated with calcium, bone and brain formation suffer serious setbacks. So much for the “calcium and milk” marketing campaign.

Enzymes

The 60 plus (known) fully intact and functional enzymes in raw milk have an amazing array of tasks to perform, each one of them essential in facilitating one key reaction or another. Some of them are native to milk, and others come from beneficial bacteria growing in the milk. Just keeping track of them would require a post-doctoral degree!

To me, the most significant health benefit derived from food enzymes is the burden they take off our body. When we eat a food that contains enzymes devoted to its own digestion, it's that much less work for our pancreas. Given the choice, I'll bet that busy organ would rather occupy itself with making metabolic enzymes and insulin, letting food digest itself.

The amylase, bacterially produced lactase, lipases and phosphatases in raw milk, break down starch, lactose (milk sugar), fat (triglycerides) and phosphate compounds respectively, making milk more digestible and freeing up key minerals. Other enzymes, like catalase, lysozyme and lactoperoxidase help to protect milk from unwanted bacterial infection, making it safer for us to drink. Pasteurized milk has none of these enzymes, which are destroyed by heat, making it virtually indigestible.

Cholesterol

Milk contains about 3mg of cholesterol per gram - a decent amount. Our bodies make most of what we need, that amount fluctuating by what we get from our food. Eat more, make less. Either way, we need it. Why not let raw milk be one source?

Cholesterol is a protective/repair substance. A waxy plant steroid (often lumped in with the fats), our body uses it as a form of water-proofing, and as a building block for a number of key hormones.

It's natural, normal and essential to find it in our brain, liver, nerves, blood, bile, indeed, every cell membrane. The best analogy I've heard regarding cholesterol's supposed causative effects on the clogging of our arteries, is that blaming it is like blaming crime on police because they're always at the scene. Cholesterol is the "concrete" which repairs our vessels that get damaged by acidic blood. Our body makes cholesterol in regards to its needs and is NOT the culprit! The culprit is a poor, acidic, sugar filled, preservative/artificial color and flavor laced diet.

Raw milk also has a plethora of beneficial bacteria that help digest all the sugars, carbs, fats, and even make enzymes that help break proteins apart- a real benefit for people with weakened digestion whether it be from age, pharmaceutical side-effects or illness

Raw milk is a living food with remarkable self-protective properties, but here's the kick: most foods tend to go south as they age, raw milk just keeps getting **better**. Raw milk sours, pasteurized milk **rots**. As milk sours (turning into kefir, cottage cheese) it becomes even more "miraculous" with an increase in enzymes, vitamins, mineral availability, and overall digestibility.

The stories of people becoming sick from raw milk are unfounded and not directly linked to the milk but to some other condition. Poorly raised sick dairy cows, dirty conditions, and unsanitary procedures are the likely causes of pathogenic bacteria in milk. One thing is quite clear, pasteurized milk has thousands of reports from sick individuals. The huge dairy business has fought for years to invent some non-existent dangers from drinking raw milk to preserve their business making raw milk illegal to sell in most states and in Canada, but there **are** ways to get raw milk!

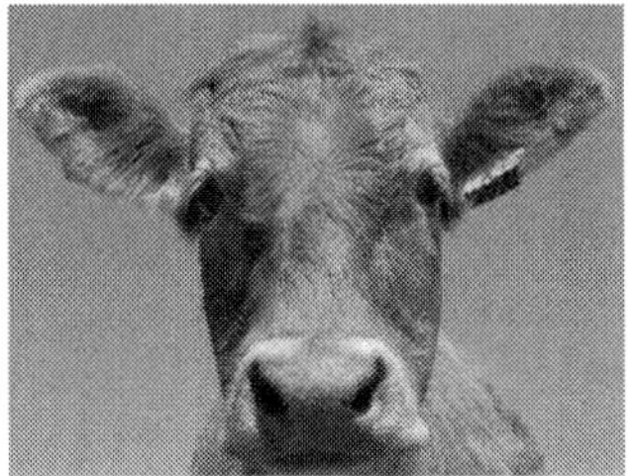

Raw milk is a complete food, and as mentioned above you can survive solely on milk and raw milk products if you had to. Raw milk also tastes absolutely amazing, much different than the bland liquid sold under the name of pasteurized milk these days.

To find a raw milk provider near you, visit this website:

http://www.realmilk.com/

Chapter 11

Beneficial Fats, Hemp Oil, Butter, and Coconut Oil

There is a lot of misconception regarding fat and oils these days and to answer the question of what is good and what is bad you need to know what fat is in the first place.

The subject of fats is downright confusing, no doubt about it. To understand fats, you need to be willing to endure a little bit of chemistry. Don't worry! I'll keep it simple and use lots of pictures. This is very simple and just the very basics.

Let's start with the raw materials for all fats: carbon, hydrogen and oxygen. Certain atoms can hold on to, or 'bond' with other elements. Carbon, for instance, has 4 bonds available. Oxygen has two, hydrogen, only one. In other words, carbon can have 4 friends, oxygen 2, and poor old hydrogen only 1 friend.

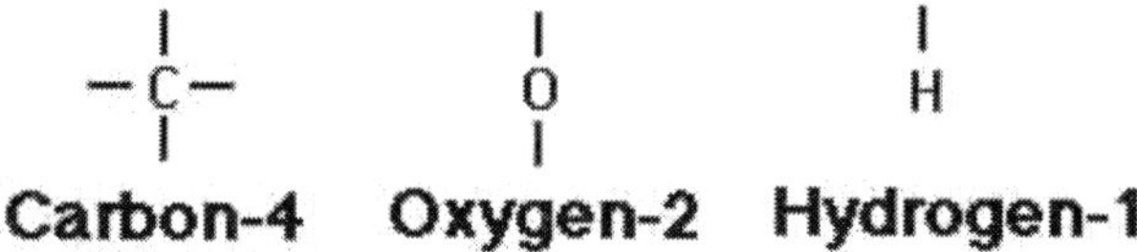

Seems simple enough, but what a dizzying array of things you can make with just these three simple elements! We'll stick with the fats for now, though, and consider one last thing about carbon. Two carbon atoms next to each other can share either one or two bonds in the fats you're likely to find in raw milk:

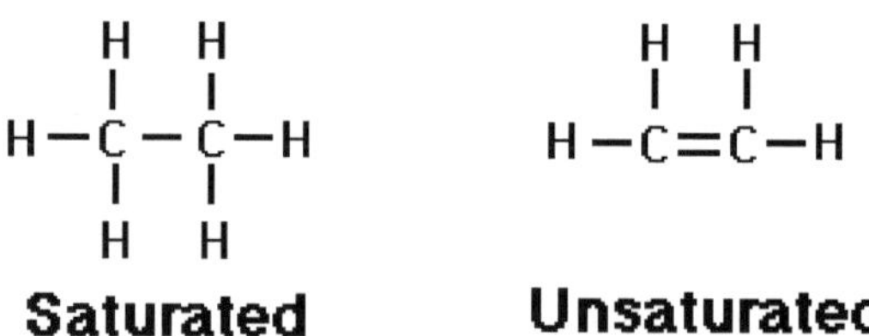

The type of bond determines the number of hydrogens each carbon can hold. The two carbons to the left, above, held together by a single bond, are said to be ***'saturated'*** because they're holding all the hydrogens they can. That's all saturated means.

The two carbons above on the right, connected by a double bond, are ***'unsaturated'*** because each could possibly hold on to one more hydrogen if they weren't busy being so friendly with one another. In other words, saturated carbons can have no more friends, they are full, unsaturated carbons have some extra spaces for a few extra friends.

The building blocks of all fats are called ***fatty acids***. Simply put, they're chains of carbon atoms connected like beads on a string.

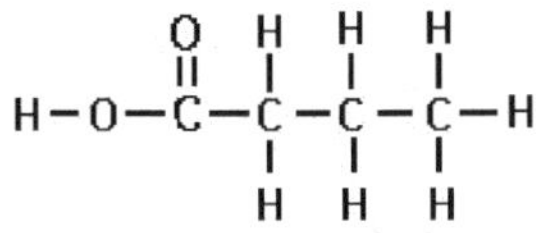

```
        O  H  H  H
        ‖  |  |  |
  H-O-C-C-C-C-H
           |  |  |
           H  H  H
```

Butyric Acid-Saturated Fatty Acid

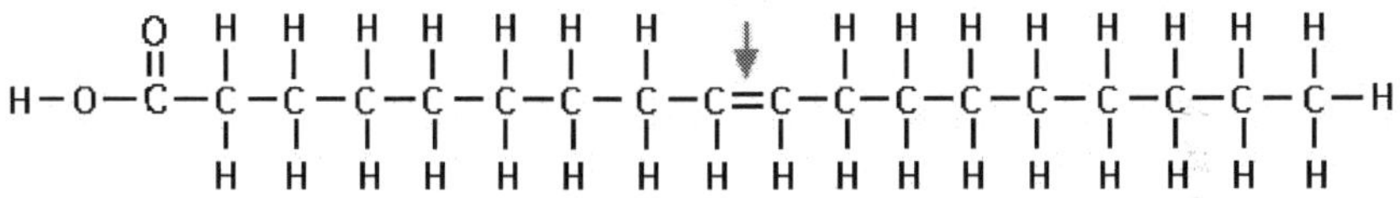

```
      O  H  H  H  H  H  H  H   ↓   H  H  H  H  H  H  H  H
      ‖  |  |  |  |  |  |  |       |  |  |  |  |  |  |  |
H-O-C-C-C-C-C-C-C-C-C=C-C-C-C-C-C-C-C-C-H
         |  |  |  |  |  |  |  |  |  |  |  |  |  |  |  |  |
         H  H  H  H  H  H  H  H  H  H  H  H  H  H  H  H  H
```

Oleic Acid- Monounsaturated Fatty Acid

```
      O  H  H  H  H   ↓   H   ↓   H  H  H  H  H  H  H  H
      ‖  |  |  |  |       |       |  |  |  |  |  |  |  |
H-O-C-C-C-C-C-C=C-C-C=C-C-C-C-C-C-C-C-C-H
         |  |  |  |  |  |  |  |  |  |  |  |  |  |  |  |  |
         H  H  H  H  H  H  H  H  H  H  H  H  H  H  H  H  H
```

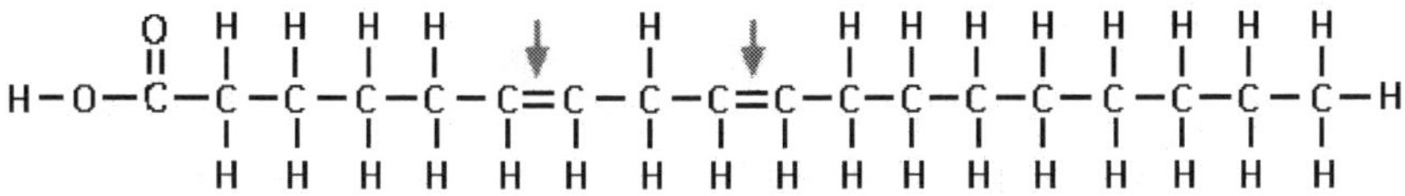

Linoleic Acid- Polyunsaturated Fatty Acid

There are two types of fats; saturated and unsaturated.

- **Saturated** have no double bonds. Only straight in shape.

- **Unsaturated** can have either one double bond (monounsaturated) or many double bonds (polyunsaturated). Can be bent (natural fats like olive oil, hemp oil, etc.) or straight (commercially made, hydrogenated, or after heat or cooking)

What are triglycerides? Most fats in our bodies and foods come in bunches of three:

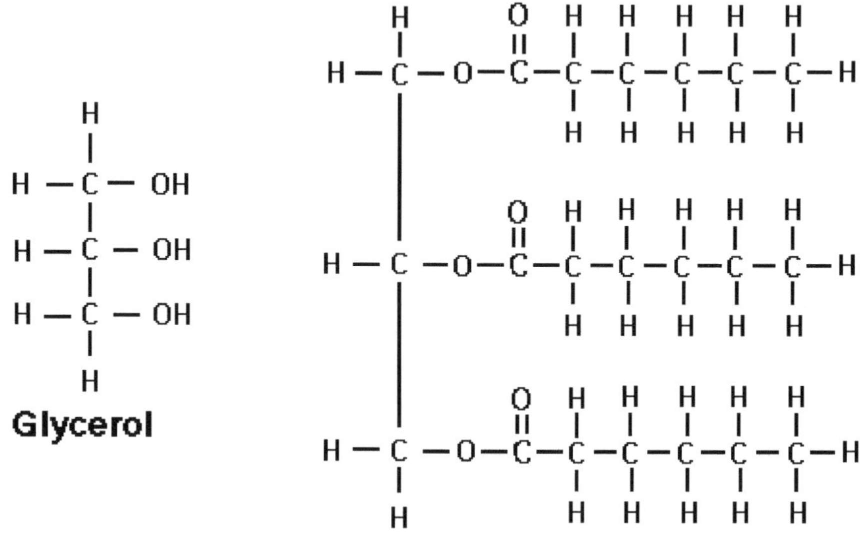

Meaning three fatty acids on a backbone of sugar, simply speaking. This is how fat tends to be stored, in packages of three. High levels of triglycerides in the blood have definitely been linked to the potential for heart disease. Their source is **not** from fats in the diet though, but rather from **excess carbohydrates not burned for energy**.

Overeating sugar or white flour products causes a spike in insulin, the hormone which, besides controlling blood sugar, also triggers the formation of fats destined for storage.

Why hydrogenate oils? When vegetable oil processors thought it would be cool to make their products stay solid at room temperature, like butter and lard, they came up with a process called ***hydrogenation*** which yielded margarine and shortening. This makes fat more stable meaning it can last longer without spoiling and allows it to have a more "pretty" texture and taste.

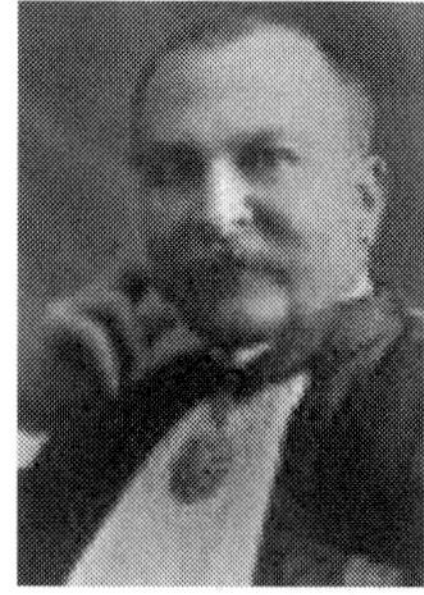

Nobel Prize winner Paul Sabatier (1854-1941, **at right**) is considered the father of the hydrogenation process. He discovered in 1897 that the metal, nickel, catalyzes, or facilitates, the attachment of hydrogen to carbon compounds.

In the actual process, workers heat the oil to very high temperatures and bubble hydrogen gas through it in the presence of nickel or some other catalytic metal. Since the vegetable oils are unsaturated, they can take on a few more hydrogens.

When they do, the molecule stiffens, and the fat is now closer to a solid. They can control just how firm it gets by how long they pump the gas through. That's why you'll sometimes see the term 'partially hydrogenated' on ingredient labels.

What also happens during hydrogenation, or later, during high heat cooking with the processed oils, is the formation of molecules so strangely configured that they're completely unsuitable for use in our bodies.

As an added "bonus", the double bonds in these foreign fatty acids are easily broken, allowing the formation of free radicals- highly reactive molecules with an unpaired electron, just looking for something to destroy.

Promotion of breast cancer, heart disease, diabetes, weakened immune systems and hormonal dysfunction are just some of the maladies for which studies have implicated these unnatural trans fats.

New medical studies are surfacing showing it is **not** the cholesterol and saturated fats that we eat that contributes to heart attacks, but the **trans fats** like Crisco, margarine, shortening, and highly processed omega 6 fats (soybean oil, sunflower oil, corn oil, safflower oil and other vegetable oils) that increase the inflammation that causes our bodies to send out cholesterol to mend the inflamed blood vessel walls.

Our bodies badly **need** saturated fats; they make up half or more of our cell walls, they bolster our immune systems, nourish our heart muscle, carry important fat soluble vitamins and antioxidants, and, in the case of butter, contain anti-fungal, anti-microbial and anti-cancer agents. We NEED both **saturated** and **unsaturated** fats, as long as they are UNPROCESSED, NATURAL, and in their RAW form.

To butter or not to butter?

Butter made from unpasteurized cream is a wonder food, just like raw milk. Margarine on the other hand is a man made refined oil full of inflammatory trans fat that is not fit for human consumption and leads to a host of terrible health issues. High temperature, high pressure and the use of solvents make margarine more into a petroleum oil rather than something resembling food.

Butter on the other hand has been used for millennia with usage recorded back over 5000 years ago! Butter made from unpasteurized milk from grass fed cows is a natural super food stock full of nutrients:

- Butter contains conjugated linoleic acid (CLA), a powerful fat burner, muscle builder, anti-cancer agent, and immunity booster.
- Butterfat is a source of good clean energy.
- Unpasteurized butter contains more omega 3 than regular butter.
- Butter is a great source of easily absorbable vitamin A which benefits the thyroid and adrenals both of which aid in fat loss and extra energy.
- Butter contains short and medium chain fatty acids that have strong anti-tumour effects.
- Grass fed butter contains a very important vitamin K2 which is required in absorbing calcium, maintaining arterial health, protecting the joints, prevents cataracts, and calcification of the pineal gland
- Butter contains a substance called the "Wulzen Factor," or "anti-stiffness factor," discovered by researcher Rosalind Wulzen. This compound protects against degenerative arthritis, hardening of the arteries, cataracts, and calcification of the pineal gland. The Wulzen Factor is not present in dairy that is commercially available in grocery stores as it is totally destroyed during pasteurization.
- Butter contains a very important element selenium, which is a strong anti-cancer nutrient.
- Butter contains iodine in its highly absorbable form which is essential for a properly functioning thyroid and for proper fat metabolism.
- Butter is a source of lauric acid, important for your immune system and for treating fungal infections.
- Butter protects against tooth decay.
- Butter contains natural lecithin which is very important for brain function and cholesterol metabolism.
- Butter contains natural anti-oxidants which protect you against free radical damage.

- Butter contains glycospingolipids which protect agains gastrointestinal infection, especially in the very young and elderly
- Many factors in butter ensure optimal growth of children, especially iodine and vitamins A, D, and K2. Low fat diets have been linked to failure to thrive in children, and for some reason low fat diets are recommended for youngsters!
- Saturated fats in butter are critical to lung function and protection against asthma.
- CLA and short and medium chain fatty acids in butter help control weight gain.
- Butter contains many nutrients needed for fertility and normal reproduction.

Commercial butter made from pasteurized cream has almost none of the benefits listed above. If you can find a local farmer, cow share program, or anywhere you can get raw milk and butter from, these two miracle foods will boost your health and actually **increase** fat loss!

It is not just about "fats," it's what is ***around*** these fats that is important. Butter is not just a blob of fat, it is filled with nutrients, vitamins, minerals and health promoting factors while being an all natural, easy to digest fat that is beneficial for your health.

Coconut Oil – The Healthy Saturated Fat

You have probably heard for the last 60 years or so from health care officials and media that saturated fats are bad for you and lead to a plethora of negative health consequences like high cholesterol, obesity, heart disease, and Alzheimer's disease.

At the same time during the last 60 years the American population has witnessed the levels of heart disease, obesity, high cholesterol, and Alzheimer's disease skyrocket compared to our ancestors and even primitive societies that use saturated fats as their dietary staple.

Studies on the Pacific Island population who get around 30-60% of their total caloric intake from fully saturated coconut oil have shown almost non-existent rates of cardiovascular disease. Something does not add up here.

The fact is, **not all saturated fats are created equal**. The key word here being "created" because some fats are naturally saturated and full of nutrients, while other fats are artificially saturated and have a host of negative health consequences, as already mentioned.

Hydrogenation adds a hydrogen atom to vegetable oils, manipulating them through a heating process and producing a rancid, thickened oil who's only benefits is longer shelf life and increased profits for the greedy corporations.

The medical and scientific community are pretty much united in the opinion that hydrogenated oils (called trans fats) fats should be avoided. And the concerning thing here is that these same damaging oils were proclaimed to be "healthy" and "heart friendly" for the past 60 years by giant multinational corporations protecting their greedy profits.

The science behind these damaging saturated fats came out, which is a good thing, but at the same time created a lot of confusion. If this artificial saturated fat is a bad thing, then ALL saturated fats are bad! Right? This is the confusion amongst the population. The GOOD saturated fats were thrown in with the nasty, lab made, artificial saturated fats.

Just like butter, coconut oil is a miracle food, and those who live in traditional tropic cultures will definitely agree on the health benefits of this oil which has been used for thousands of years.

Dr. Weston Price traveled throughout the South Pacific islands in the 1930's and examined the local population examining their diets and the effects on their dental and overall health. He found that coconut oil comprised a majority of their overall calories, but they were slim, healthy, and had virtually no heart disease. A similar study on two Polynesian atolls in 1981 revealed that even though coconut oil accounted for the majority of their calories but they had almost perfect vascular health.

There was absolutely <u>no</u> evidence to support the claim that <u>natural saturated fats</u> had any negative effect on health whatsoever.

This is definitely not what you have been hearing all these years; these people should be full of sickness, clogged arteries, obesity, and heart disesease.

Coconut oil has many positive benefits including:

- Promoting your heart health
- Promoting weight loss
- Supporting your immune system health

- Supporting a healthy metabolism
- Providing you with an immediate energy source
- Keeping your skin healthy and youthful looking
- Supporting the proper functioning of your thyroid gland

How does this happen? Well, coconut oil has a "magic" ingredient that is not found in other natural saturated fats. This secret ingredient is lauric acid.

50 percent of the fat content in coconut oil is made up of lauric acid, which is a "miracle" ingredient due to its potent health promoting properties. In your body, the lauric acid is converted into monolaurin, which has anti-viral, anti-bacterial, and anti-protozoa properties.

Monolaurin is a monoglyceride which can actually destroy lipid coated viruses such as:

- HIV, herpes
- Measles
- Influenza virus
- Various pathogenic bacteria
- Protozoa such as giardia lamblia.

Lauric acid is a powerful virus and gram-negative bacteria destroyer, and coconut oil contains the most lauric acid of any substance on earth!

Capric acid, another coconut fatty acid present in smaller amounts, has also been added to the list of coconut's antimicrobial components.

This is one of the key reasons you should consider consuming coconut oil, because there aren't many sources of monolaurin in our diet. But the health benefits of coconut oil don't stop there.

Coconut oil is composed of about 2/3 **medium** chain fatty acids (MCFAs), also called **medium** chain triglycerides (MCTs), which have a whole list of health benefits, and coconut oil is the richest source of these MCFA's. The reason vegetable oils are not as healthy is because vegetable oils are comprised of **long** chain fatty acids (LCFAs).

- LCFAs are difficult for your body to break down -- they require special enzymes for digestion.
- LCFAs put more strain on your pancreas, liver and your entire digestive system.
- LCFAs are predominantly stored in your body as fat.
- LCFAs can be deposited within your arteries in lipid forms such as cholesterol.
- In contrast to LFCAs, the MCFAs found in coconut oil have many health benefits, including the following beneficial qualities:
- MCFAs are smaller. They permeate cell membranes easily, and do not require special enzymes to be utilized effectively by your body.
- MCFAs are easily digested, thus putting less strain on your digestive system.
- MCFAs are sent directly to your liver, where they are immediately converted into energy rather than being stored as fat.
- MCFAs actually help stimulate your body's metabolism, leading to weight loss.

Another amazing benefit of coconut oil is its miraculous ability for weight loss and metabolism stimulation.

In the 1940s farmers used this relatively cheap oil to try and fatten up their livestock, and failed miserably. Instead, the oil made the animals lean, hungry, and more active than before!

Research demonstrates that replacing LCFAs (long chain fatty acids) with MCFAs (medium chain fatty acids) results in decreased body weight and reduced fat storage.

Coconut oil is now used by athletes because MCFAs are much more easily digested, and help stimulate the metabolism to be turned to energy much quicker. Coconut oil has now entered the athletic arena and is used to increase performance of the athlete.

Not only does coconut oil improve thyroid function which helps the body drop the extra pounds but the increased metabolism also stimulates the healing process, cell regeneration, and an immune system boost.

Do you want to look younger and reduce wrinkles and fine lines? When coconut oil is used on the skin, it absorbs into the connective tissue, and reduces the appearance of wrinkles and fine lines by helping the connective tissue be more strong and supple while acting as an exfoliant removing dead skin cells making your skin smoother.

Coconut oil is so beneficial and nutritious it is used in baby formulas, hospitals to feed the critically ill, those on tube feeding, and those with digestive problems. It is extra helpful for pregnant women, nursing moms, the elderly, those with digestive problems, athletes, and for anyone who is interested in absolute maximal health and wellbeing.

Hemp Oil

Surely no member of the vegetable kingdom has ever been more misunderstood than hemp. For thousands of years, humans have *used* parts of the *hemp* plant for food, textiles, paper, fabric, and fuel oil. In recent years, emotion, not reason, has guided our policy toward this crop. And nowhere have emotions run hotter than in the debate over the distinction between industrial hemp and marijuana. Hemp and marijuana are NOT the same thing!

If you would like to know more about the differences between hemp and marijuana you may read this article: http://naihc.org/hemp_information/content/hemp.mj.html

Hemp seed and oil has been called "Nature's Perfect Food for Humanity" - a wealth of health for everyone.

The oil can be used as part of a nutritional programme to maintain and improve good health. With a pleasant nutty flavour, Hemp Seed Oil is ideal for use in salad dressings, mayonnaise, dips etc. It is not suitable for frying as this reduces its benefits.

Hemp has had a long-standing relationship with humanity; modern science reveals that it contains all the essential amino acids and essential fatty acids necessary for human life, as well as a rare protein known as globule edestins that is very similar to the globulin found in human blood plasma.

Hemp seeds contain the most balanced and richest natural single source of essential oils for human consumption. The E.F.A.'s not only help to restore wasting bodies, but also improve damaged immune systems, so it is not so surprising that modern researchers have studied them in relationship to the modern immune attacking AIDS virus. (Eidlman, M.D., Hamilton, ED.D, Ph.D 1992).

Hemp oil is **nature's most balanced oil for human nutrition** (3:1 LA to LNA ratio) and is easily digestible; in fact this oil could provide all of our Essential Fatty Acid (EFA) requirements for **life**, due to the balanced 80% EFA content of the oil. Hemp oil is also **25% protein** giving your body most of the amino acids you need.

Research has shown that this nutritional oil was once a part of **worldwide** dietary intake, as it was **one of the first cultivated crops**. All natural foods contain some substances, which are essential to life. Oils for example, found in nuts and seeds, contain significantly higher amounts of essential fatty acids than other foods.

Much information about Hemp has been systematically removed from written texts since the 1930's and is now difficult to find. Many of the myths about hemp, perpetuated by governments to this day relating to hemp being a drug crop are incorrect and simply **propaganda created to make way for synthetic man made products**.

The seven-time Nobel Prize nominee, Dr. Johana Budwig, a pioneer of E.F.A research, reported success in treating heart infraction, arthritis, cancer and other common diseases with massive doses of E.F.A.'s. Budwig's research indicates that many of these killer and crippling diseases may be caused in part by our diet of saturated fat and trans-fat, which are present in much of the food we eat. According to this healing Doctor, saturated fat and trans-fat befuddle the electronic charge of the unsaturated oils, which are present in cell membranes.

'This decreases the cells ability to receive and store electrons from the sun, which according to Budwig is a key factor in human health.'

Alternatively, a balanced diet of E.F.A's keeps the charge of the unsaturated fats in the cells membranes working properly and electron rich. As Budwig herself explains:

"The sun's rays are very much in harmony with humans. It is no coincidence that we love the sun. The resonance in our biological tissue is so strongly tuned to the absorption of solar energy that physicists who occupy themselves with this scientific phenomenon, the quantum biologists say that there is nothing on earth that has a higher concentration of solar energy photons than humans. This enrichment with solar energy depends strongly on the like energy aspects, a wavelength that is compatible with humans, and this is

supported when we eat foods that have electromagnetic waves of solar rays--the photon. An abundance of these electrons, which are tuned to the solar energy frequency, exist, for example, in many seed oils. Scientifically these oils have even been designated as electron-rich, essential, highly unsaturated fats. (Budwig 1992)

Budwig states that when we began to homogenize vegetable oils so that they would last longer on store shelves, we unknowingly changed their E.F.A. content into saturated fats in the ensuing heating process. These E.F.A. robbed, thus electron poor "promote the emergence of cancer.... *They behave like tar, as insulators relative to the transport of electrons in living tissue."* Alternatively, *"electron-rich highly unsaturated oils... increase the absorption, storage and utilization of the sun's energy".*

Budwig relates that after her ailing patients have been treated with an E.F.A. rich diet and then "lie in the sun, they notice they feel much better-rejuvenated"; (Budwig 1992) "On the other hand, nowadays we frequently observe that the heart fails on sunny beaches, and not infrequently heart attacks occur. We can observe some individuals in our time experiencing stress from exposure to the sun's energy, whereas others respond with dynamic improvement in all vital functions. The stimulating effect that sunshine has on the secretions of the liver, gall bladder, pancreas, bladder, and salivary glands is easy to observe. These organs only dry out upon exposure to sunshine when the substance that stimulates secretions is missing. The decisive factor in all these observations is whether the surface-active, electron-rich, highly unsaturated fats are present as a resonating system for solar energy, or, if they are missing. The doctor tells cancer patients to avoid the sun; that they can't tolerate the sun. As soon as these patients--also cancer patients--were placed on my oil-Protein diet for just 2-3 days, i.e. a diet that contains an abundant supply of essential fats, they were able to tolerate the sun very well. Yes, they emphasize how well they suddenly feel in the sun, how the life forces are stimulated and that they feel dynamically energized."(Budwig 1992)

Benefits of Cold Pressing

Oils should be pressed with a minimum of heat because the higher the temperature of the oil the faster it is destroyed by light, oxygen and other chemical reactions. The shape and properties of Fatty-acid molecules can change lowering their nutritional and biological value.

In the UK there are no restrictions on pressing oil from live seed unlike America where the seed has to be killed by high temperatures to allow it to be imported. With this burned seed, it is not possible to press fresh living oil that remains stable with a long shelf life.

Because Hemp Seed Oil is such a rich source of both LA (Omega 6) and LNA (Omega 3) in balanced proportions, conditions caused by deficiencies in both can be treated with one oil.

The functions of LNA include: Production of smooth skin, increased stamina, faster healing, increased vitality, brings a feeling of calmness, reduces inflammation, water retention, platelet stickiness and blood pressure, enhances immune functions, reduces the pain and swelling of arthritis, can reverse pre-menstrual syndrome, can treat bacterial infections, brain development in children.

People who use hemp seed oil products have reported that after they begin to use hemp seed oil, they have seen smoother, thicker hair, stronger nails and softer skin. In addition, the balance of essential fatty acids in hemp seed oil have benefits for nearly every cell and helps your body to fight and ward off degenerative diseases including cancer and cardiovascular diseases.

Hemp seed oil is also a good source of gamma-linolenic acid (GLA) which makes the oil a rival to flax seed oil and Evening Primrose Oil. It is also an excellent alternative to fish oil supplements -- fish have been reported to be contaminated by mercury as well as other toxins. Nursing mothers and pregnant women may wish to use hemp seed oil instead of fish oil, as they reduce their intake of fish but maintain the level of essential fatty acids. Hemp seed oil has been found to be helpful in relieving pre-menstrual tension as well.

Hemp seed oil contains ingredients that give it unique anti-inflammatory properties that are not often found in other oils. This, added to its antioxidant properties, allows hemp oil to detoxify and clean your skin, as well as to even out your skin tone.

Hemp seed oil is used in cosmetics which takes care of skin lesions and blotches that may occur as a result of excessively dry skin. Since it won't clog your pores like many other oils, you can safely use hemp seed oil to moisturize your skin, and do so without any greasy build-up. Hemp seed oil is also a natural sun block, which helps people who use it to avoid diseases related to over-exposure to the sun's more harmful rays.

Hemp oil is truly a miracle oil that has benefits inside the body and on the skin. Hemp has been used for thousands of years as a food, for building materials, and as clothing from its beneficial fibre.

Here are some interesting facts about the uses of industrial hemp:

- **Hemp as a rotation crop & soil rejuvenation**

  Hemp is used as a rotation crop worldwide due to the quick growth and ability to grow in many environments. Hemp returns nutrients to the soil unlike many rotation crops because the nutrient levels are high in the roots and they are returned to the soil after each harvest.

- **The environmental advantages of Hemp**

  Fast growing
  Higher yields
  Simplest plant to grow
  Adapted to cultivation in all climates
  Hemp as Food.

- **Most nutritious and easily digestible food on the planet**
  Only complete source of protein, all 20 essential amino acids, and essential fatty acids. The only food that supplies virtually all man's dietary needs in one source.

- **Hemp as Clothing**
  Hemp fiber is longer, stronger, more absorbent and warmer than cotton. It is a very strong and soft fabric.

- **Hemp as Fuel**
  Making Fuel from hemp is very easy and can be turned into anything from fuel pellets to liquid fuel and gas.

- **Hemp as Paper**
  Hemp can produce more paper than trees can per acre and can be used for every quality of paper. Because paper can be made from hemp easier than from trees, more chemicals are used to make paper from trees, making hemp the eco-friendliest option.

- **Hemp as Paints and Plastics**
  Paint, varnish, and even plastic can be made from hemp oil.

- **Concrete from Hemp**
  When hemp hurds are mixed with limestone and water it forms a substance that is harder than concrete with only 1/6 the weight.

"The most cultivatable, optimum dry biomass plant species on earth, uniquely and immediately capable of the economical replacement of all mankind's use of high-pollutant costly fuels and uranium for energy, petrochemical products, gasoline and plastics." - FCDA Europe

Oils In Your Kitchen

If you have a choice between even pasteurized butter and margarine/spread, **always** choose butter because it will **always** be a better choice. However, it is best to avoid butter made from pasteurized cream, and just skip the spreads altogether before you can find yourself real raw butter, or even make some yourself! www.realmilk.com has places you can get raw milk and http://www.positron.org/food/butter/ has instructions on how you can make your own butter, enjoy!

There should only be a few oils in your kitchen; extra virgin cold pressed **olive oil** which is a much better monounsaturated fat that works great as a salad dressing and other cold dishes, raw unpasteurized organic **butter**, **coconut oil**, **flax oil**, and **hemp oil**.

For cooking do not use any unsaturated oils like vegetable oils which are highly reactive to heat and oxidative damage. Polyunsaturated oils like corn, soy, safflower, sunflower, and canola oils **are absolutely the worst oils to use for cooking**. Never ever use any vegetable oils for cooking! Not only are trans fats created from these relatively gentle oils, but they produce a plethora of toxic, cancer causing chemicals after they have been heated. Most vegetable oils are also GMO which by itself should be reason enough to completely exclude them from your diet, and they are high in omega 6 which creates inflammation and accelerates many chronic degenerative diseases.

I don't recommend cooking your food at all, because the more you cook and the higher the heat, the more proteins become denatured and destroyed, the more carbohydrates become fused together and unusable, the more fats become carcinogenic, practically all vitamins/minerals are destroyed or rendered useless and the seemingly healthy food has turned into something barely usable by the body.

These changes take time so if you will cook or worse yet, fry, there is only one oil that can stand up to the heat, and that is coconut oil. Butter or ghee/clarified butter is the next best thing.

For eating: raw unpasteurized butter, hemp oil, flax oil, and extra virgin olive oil.
For cooking: coconut oil or butter/ghee.

Chapter 12

Raw Unprocessed Nuts

Remember, it's not about the calories. It's about the nutrient density of foods that will make you lose weight and feel amazing. What I have not yet mentioned is another difference between raw and processed/cooked foods.

Nature has provided our body with a very simple, yet very effective, safety mechanism against overeating, and against absorbing things from our digestive tract that we don't need. Nobel Prize laureate Pavlov discovered that the relationship between the amount of hydrochloric acid in our digestive juices and our body's need for nutrients is directly correlated. In other words, if our body needs nutrients, we will have more hydrochloric acid in our stomachs for digestion, and if our bodies do not need any nutrients, there will be no hydrochloric acid for digestion. Simple. If our body does not need any nutrients, but we ingest some food, it will simply not digest and come out the same way it came in.

So how come people are still overweight and obese? Did the mechanism stop working? The mechanism is fine; it all has to do with the type of food we eat. Nutritionists, doctors, and chemists tell us that cooked food is much better absorbed because during the heating process, it breaks down, meaning complex structures are broken down into simple structures. This actually bypasses what your saliva and your stomach acid are supposed to do. So when we eat cooked food it comes as somewhat pre-digested, but here lies the ultimate evil. If raw food enters our digestive system and it is not needed, it is simply not broken down and exits in the same shape that it came in. But cooked food, since it is already broken down, **bypasses** this safety mechanism and is absorbed no matter what, whether it is needed or not!

Our body is completely defenseless against cooked food!

As an example let's look at raw protein and simplify what happens during digestion. As a raw form of protein enters your body, it is usually in a very tight roll that is quite large. If your body has no need for protein, no hydrochloric acid is produced, it is not digested, and it leaves your body the same way it came in. And since it is still raw, it does not rot or fester becoming food for the bad bacteria in your digestive tract and does not become a toxin.

On the other hand, if a denatured or broken down and dead protein enters your body, it will bypass the lack of hydrochloric acid safety mechanism, and some of it will bypass the mucous membrane (another safety mechanism will be discussed later) and get absorbed straight into the blood. These denatured, dead particles are treated as an invader by your body and will be attacked by the white blood cells. Some other particles will stick together forming plaques that will attach themselves to various capillaries, and day by day this garbage will pile up inside your body and clog up your arteries, kidneys, liver etc. Add to this the denatured, dead particles of carbohydrates, fats, inactive vitamins, inorganic minerals, all the additives like pesticides, preservatives, flavor enhancers, and other toxic substances, and you will have a poisonous concoction floating around your body (this will be discussed in great detail in Part 2).

What this means is you can never gain weight from raw foods, ever. If you eat bucket loads of fruits/veggies/nuts/sprouted live grains, you can never gain weight. This is something that is never talked about and completely missed, yet is one of the most important aspects of weight loss and health. The more Raw foods you eat the more weight you will lose and the better you will feel!

Raw nuts are nutrient powerhouses that are perfect as a snack pretty much at any time of the day (nuts/seeds/grains are more difficult to digest so eating them in the morning/night might lead to fatigue, sluggishness, sleepiness and loss of energy, it is best to eat them during the day).

Several studies over the past several years have shown the health benefits of nuts -- which contain monounsaturated fat, vitamin E, folic acid, magnesium, copper, protein, and fiber, and are rich in antioxidant phytochemicals.

They are a powerhouse of good nutrition that can dramatically reduce the risk of heart disease. They've also been shown to play an important role in helping to lower "bad" cholesterol levels and raise "good" cholesterol levels. In addition, they can help dilate blood vessels and prevent hardening of the arteries.

In the Nurses Health Study, which followed 86,016 nurses for 14 years, found those who ate 5 ounces or more of nuts per week reduced their risk of dying from heart disease by 35%. The researchers also noted that the nut-eaters tended to weigh less than the nurses who did not eat nuts.

Eating nuts is hailed for decreasing blood cholesterol levels. The lower the blood cholesterol levels, the less likely you are to suffer from heart disease.

Nuts are the preeminent source for manganese. Manganese is an essential nutrient and trace mineral that aids the enzyme systems in your body. The manganese compound is renowned for diminishing cholesterol absorption from food.

While all nuts are healthy, there a few superstars:

Brazil nuts contain a very high amount of selenium: about 70 to 90 micrograms per nut. So only 3-4 Brazil nuts will provide you with ample amounts of this essential nutrient. And, nuts do their part to keep bones strong by providing magnesium, manganese, and boron, essential for bone health.

In addition to healthy fats and vitamin E, a quarter-cup of **almonds** contains almost 99 mg of magnesium (that's 25% of the daily value for this important mineral), plus 257 mg of potassium. To know more about almonds, one of the healthiest nuts you can eat, you may read this article:
http://www.whfoods.com/genpage.php?tname=foodspice&dbid=20

Walnuts, pecans, and chestnuts have the highest antioxidant content of the tree nuts, with walnuts winning out over the others in antioxidant content. And, peanuts (although technically, a legume) also contribute significantly to our dietary intake of antioxidants.

Pistachios help to reduce the risk of macular degeneration, a common cause of visual loss in older individuals. Pistachios contain two important carotenoids, lutein and zeaxanthin, compounds which help prevent this common eye condition. Carotenoids are also strong antioxidants that help to offset cell injury and damage. A daily snack of pistachios could be a tasty and effective way to protect one of your most important senses - your vision.

Dieter's Dream Come True

To find a food that is delicious, nutritious, and filling, is a dieter's dream come true. Dieters who eat nuts tend to stick to their diets because the fat and fiber content of nuts makes them very filling. As a result, you are not as hungry and ultimately eat less.

Several studies have found that eating small amounts of nuts ***helps dieters lose weight***. One psychological benefit noted in a study done by Pennsylvania State researchers was that dieters did not feel like they were dieting when nuts were allowed in their eating plans - which helped them stay on their diets longer.

Your goal is to eat nuts *instead of* other sources of fat like cakes, cookies, or chips. You won't feel deprived when you top your apple or celery slices with raw nut butter! Try it out, next time you get food cravings, take a handful of nuts and munch away while watching the cravings disappear.

A study published in the journal "Obesity" that found persons who consume nuts twice a week are far less likely to amass unwanted pounds than those who don't include nuts in their diet. In fact, the study that involved 8,865 men and women in Spain discovered individuals that ate nuts twice a week were 31 percent less likely to add weight than their counterparts. The authors of the study were quoted as saying, "Frequent nut consumption was associated with a reduced risk of weight gain···11 pounds or more. These results support the recommendation of nut consumption as an important component of a cardio protective diet and also allay fears of possible weight gain."

"Nuts are very high in dietary fiber, and are one of the best plant sources of protein"
Here are some ways to add healthy "nut" fat to your diet:

Top hot or cold cereal with nuts for a nourishing breakfast.
Mix some dried fruit with your nuts for added flavor.
Use fat-free salad dressing and add nuts to your salads.
Use nuts to replace croutons in salads or soups.
Bring pasta to life by sprinkling it with chopped nuts.
Add great flavor to steamed veggies with a handful of nuts.

As long as the nuts are **raw** and are not mixed with too much other fats or sugars, which may create gas, bloating, indigestion, and reduce the benefits of this wonderful food, you can eat nuts as much as you like. Eat them by themselves or with some dried fruit, or a bit sprinkled here and there, they create a wonderful addition to your diet.

Chapter 13

Avocadoes

Avocadoes are in a nutrition league of their own with astounding levels of healthy monounsaturated fats, over 20 vitamins, minerals, and phytonutrients to keep your body in tip-top shape.

- Avocadoes are pretty much the only fruit that contains monounsaturated fat, the "good fat" which helps to reduce the risk of heart disease.
- Avocadoes contain 76 milligrams of beta sitosterol in a 3 oz serving. This nutrient helps to maintain healthy levels of cholesterol
- Avocadoes contain high levels of vitamin K which helps protect the blood, prevent bone fractures, and protects against liver and prostate cancer.
- High in potassium, a mineral that regulates blood pressure, and help guard against heart disease and stroke.
- High in fibre promoting healthy bowel movements, regulating cholesterol, and keeping blood sugar levels normal.
- Contain vitamin B6, folate, dietary copper, alpha and beta carotene, and antioxidants making this fruit one of the most nutritious.
-

Avocadoes go great with salad, by themselves, mixed with salsa, on a sandwich, or in a fresh delicious guacamole mix. Personally I love avocadoes so much I eat them with a spoon straight out of their shell sprinkled with some Himalayan or sea salt.

Chapter 14

Organic Dark Leafy Greens

Pound for pound, dark leafy vegetables are the most concentrated source of nutrition of any food.

They have every vitamin, mineral, and nutrient you can think of like iron, calcium, potassium, magnesium, selenium, vitamins K, C, E, B, A, D, phytonutrients like beta carotene, lutein, zeaxanthin, even healthy fats like omega 3.

Te definite heavyweight of superfoods are kale and spinach, no wonder Popeye loved his favorite vegetable so much! For example, kale has 1300 percent the daily requirement of vitamin K which is much more important than we actually thought. Because of their high magnesium content and low glycemic index, green leafy vegetables are also valuable for persons with type 2 diabetes.

- **Phytochemicals**

The bioactive non nutrient plant compounds in fruit, vegetables, grains, and other plant foods—have been linked to reductions in the risk of major chronic diseases. It is estimated that more than 5000 phytochemicals have been identified, but a large percentage still remain unknown and need to be identified before their health benefits are fully understood.

- **Chlorophyll**

Everyone is aware of the importance of eating green vegetables because of the **chlorophyll** content. It is well known that chlorophyll is recognized for its anti-inflammatory, anti-mutagenic, and antioxidant properties. Chlorophyll has been cited as strengthening the immune response; therapeutic for inflammation of the ear and the mucous membrane of the nose and sinuses; supportive of normal kidney function; accelerating wound and ulcer healing; and reducing fecal, urinary and body odor in geriatric patients. This makes chlorophyll very beneficial to diabetics. In addition, the chlorophyll in green vegetables detoxifies carcinogens found in cooked meats or barbecued foods.

Lutein and *zeaxanthin*, carotenoids found in dark-green leafy vegetables, are concentrated in the eye lens and macular region of the retina, and play a protective role in the eye. They protect against both cataract and age-related macular degeneration, the major cause of blindness in the elderly. Some studies suggest that lutein and zeaxanthin may help reduce the risk of certain types of cancer, such as breast and lung cancer, and may contribute to the prevention of heart disease and stroke.

Green veggies contain a variety of *carotenoids*, *flavonoids* and other powerful antioxidants that have cancer-protective properties. In a Swedish study, it was reported that eating 3 or more servings a week of green leafy vegetables significantly reduced the risk of stomach cancer, the fourth most frequent cancer in the world. Cabbage, cauliflower, Brussels sprouts, and broccoli are rich in indoles and *isothiocyanates*, which protect us against colon and other cancers. Broccoli sprouts have been reported to contain 10 or more times as much *sulforaphane*, a cancer protective substance, than does mature broccoli. A higher consumption of green leafy vegetables has been shown to **significantly decrease** the risk of breast cancer and skin cancer.

If you had a choice to pick only 2 food groups to eat for the rest of your life, organic raw leafy green vegetables (spinach, kale) and raw milk would sufficiently and perfectly give your body absolutely everything it needs, and more, to live a healthy life. Our ancestors ate up to 6 pounds of leafy greens daily and saw none of the "Western" diseases like cancer, heart disease or diabetes. You can eat pounds upon pounds of veggies, and gallons of milk, and you will never gain any weight. On the contrary you will be leaner, stronger, and healthier. Take note from Popeye☺

Note: Green powders have become very popular, but they are not the same as Green vegetables! Don't completely rely on green powders and avoid eating any greens!

Instead, look for creative ways to eat more greens, and use green powder to complement your nutritional program, i.e. mixed (steamed) veggies, salads, casseroles, stir-frys, smoothies, juicing, drinks.

Concerning green powder, make sure you're using a high quality green superfood powder supplement that is grown organically and does not contain chemicals. Also, ensure the supplement company selling the green powder is a reputable firm.

A powder of vegetables or algae can never compare in nutritional value to fresh green vegetables! Those powders can't come close to the nutrient density of dark green vegetables such as spinach, Romaine lettuce, kale, collard greens, mustard greens, parsley, celery, arugula, bok choi, etc.

However! Even though the real thing can't be replaced by powders, it is the **next best thing and much better than any other single vitamin or mineral you can buy**. I do recommend getting yourself a good super food raw organic powder to supplement your diet. Nobody is perfect and not everyone has the chance to eat plenty of greens through the day, so find a green powder and eat as much of it as you can.

I always recommend eating as much salad as you can, experiment with the wide variety of veggies at your disposal. Organic baby greens, romaine lettuce, red leaf lettuce, bib lettuce, cucumbers, bell peppers, dill/cilantro, kale, and others are perfect to customize your salad. Throw some nuts on top, dash some spices (experiment with different types of spices other than just salt and pepper), some sea salt, and add some flax, hemp, or olive oil and you have a wonderful meal that is going to give you everything your body needs.

Although I'm a big supporter of eating as much raw foods as possible, the change for you might be a gradual one so if you do cook greens, try to do it for as little as possible under as low temperatures as possible. Sautéed greens in some coconut oil or butter with some spices are an absolutely delicious addition to any meal. Experiment with sautéing, it usually takes about 5 minutes of prep time to cut, and 5-7 minutes to sauté. Also, **raw** greens can be thrown into pretty much any dish, when your dish is finished cooking throw some raw greens in, let it sit for a while, and there you have it, added nutrition quick and easy.

Green Smoothies

The truth is, most people do not consume even the bare minimum for green leafy vegetables. When was the last time you ate even a half cup of raw leafy greens? Chimpanzees consume more than 40% greens, that's about two bunches of greens per day from your grocery store shelf.

I used to think that a few leaves that I put into my salad was good enough. Most people think that if they eat a small salad (usually a Greek salad with useless iceberg lettuce with absolutely minimal nutritional value and practically no dark green leaves) they are good for a few days. But we don't realize that dark leafy greens are the most important and beneficial living food that we have available. Dark greens are rich in almost all essential minerals and vitamins, as well as protein!

If you look at the composition of plants, you may notice that cellulose, the main constituent of plants, has one of the strongest molecular structures on the planet. Greens possess inside them more valuable nutrients than any other food group, but all these nutrients are stored inside the cells of the plant. These cells are very tough and are made to survive on the earth. In order for the nutrients to be released, the cell wall needs to be ruptured, which is not an easy task. If you eat plenty of greens, but you do not chew them thoroughly, you are not getting the full nutritional content of the plant. The plant needs to be swallowed in a creamy consistency to ensure full benefits.

After decades of eating mostly processed and cooked food, most modern people have lost their ability to chew normally. For some, their jaw has become too narrow or their jaw muscles have become too weak to chew through rough fiber. Not even to mention that our bodies have become so unaccustomed to eating leafy greens, that for most people they are very unpalatable. These obstacles make chewing and eating enough greens to satisfy the bodies' requirement not an easy task.

Juicing or Blending?

Both options are far, far superior to any juice or commercially available vitamin mixture or powder food. I personally prefer blending because it is easier and all the fiber is retained as well as some micro nutrients found in the pulp which is usually thrown out after juicing. Blending is like eating the whole plant, in the form it was meant to be eaten, whole! Everything is eaten, in the perfect form it was meant to.

This is why blending greens in a high speed blender (especially in the high powered multi horsepower blenders) is the way to go. You can easily blend two bunches of greens with some fruits , sprouts, hemp protein, and you have yourself a **delicious vitamin, mineral, protein, and nutrient packed drink**. Drinking 2-3 cups per day is enough to satisfy your body's requirement for most nutrients and is **one of the most important dietary additions you can add to your life**.

At first start off with a 60% fresh raw fruit and 40% raw fresh greens, and as you get used to the taste and you body begins to actually crave green you can switch to a 40% fruit and 60% greens blend. Soon enough you will be drinking fully 100% green smoothies! I find apple/spinach with some honey or coconut crystals or stevia leaf is the most delicious for me. You may experiment with any type of fruit, but for greens stick to the leafy veggie powerhouses like spinach and kale.

Benefits of Green Smoothies

- Considered a super food and the most nutritious live food you can eat.
- Very easy to digest if blended well, ruptures the cell wall allowing for easy digestion and absorption.
- They are a complete food because unlike juices, they still have all the valuable fiber.
- Amongst the most palatable dishes for all people. Mixed with fruit, creates a wonderful, delicious sweet and zesty flavor. Most people are very surprised that something so green and healthy can taste so good!
- Green smoothies are chlorophyll rich. A molecule of chlorophyll closely resembles a molecule of human blood. According to Dr. Ann Wigmore, consuming chlorophyll is like receiving a healthy blood transfusion.
- They are very easy to make and cleaning up is a breeze. Consider this: spending 15 minutes making a bacon, egg and toast breakfast that has insignificant nutritional content, is full of nasty fats, and is terrible for your health, or spend 2 minutes making this amazing super-food.
- Enjoyed by people of all ages including children and babies six months or older.
- Consuming green smoothies forms a great habit for eating more greens. After a few weeks of drinking them, most people start craving and enjoying greens. Eating enough greens is often a problem for many people, and this provides a great alternative.
- Green smoothies can be consumed anywhere, just make some extra and take with you to work. They are much easier to make and much more efficient than a salad and can all fit in a small container.

Chapter 15

Healthy Sweeteners; Raw Honey, Stevia, Coconut Crystals

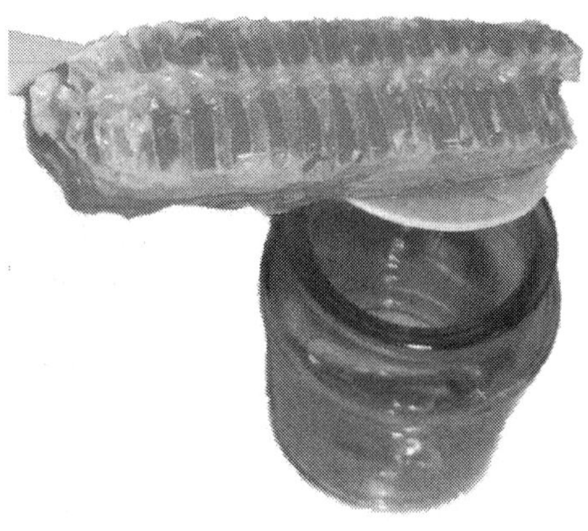

Honey is one of the oldest known sweeteners whose history spans back over 3000 years ago. In Russia, the extremely potent honey from Siberian bees was given out as a prescription for almost all ailments.

The ancient Egyptians farmed honey 3,000 years ago, and considered bees the symbol of sacred femininity. They also used honey for healing wounds and as a preservative, due to its antibacterial properties.

Honey is nature's wonder food. However, not all honey on store shelves is the same. Honey is extremely heat sensitive due to the sheer number of beneficial enzymes, vitamins, micronutrients, and minerals. Honey that has been processed in any way looses most of its benefits. Also, honey that was not properly harvested and made by bees that have been fed sugar instead of naturally collecting pollen from flowers, improper storage (left in the sun for example), all contribute to a loss in nutrients. Honey that is mass produced is just as bad as sugar.

Raw honey is the concentrated nectar of flowers that comes straight from the extractor, the bee; it is the only unheated, pure, unpasteurized, unprocessed honey. An alkaline-forming food, this type of honey contains ingredients similar to those found in fruits, which become alkaline in the digestive system. It doesn't ferment in the stomach and it can be used to counteract acid indigestion. When mixed with ginger and lemon juices, it also relieves nausea and supplies energy. Raw honey is the healthiest choice amongst the various forms of honey as it has the most nutritional value and contains amylase, an enzyme concentrated in flower pollen which helps predigest starchy foods like breads.

When it comes to honey nothing can beat power of raw honey, the elixir of life. Our ancestors had understood honey's remarkable healing ability and had used it successfully in curing many diseases. Raw honey has been reported to be good for respiratory infections, liver problems, stomach ulcers, malnutrition, digestive problems, constipation, eye diseases, infected wounds and burns, surgical wounds. It promote speedy recovery after childbirth, facilitates menstruation, it can be used against epilepsy, strengthen the immune systems, and promote general health and vitality.

Characterized by fine textured crystals, raw honey looks milkier and contains particles and flecks made of bee pollen, honeycomb bits, propolis, and broken bee wing fragments. Raw and unfiltered honey is relatively low in moisture content (14% to 18%) and has a high antioxidant level. It will usually granulate and crystallize to a margarine-like consistency after a month or two.

Processed honey will usually look much clearer and smoother which means most of the beneficial nutrients are completely gone.

I do not recommend eating maple syrup because it is boiled and looses most of its original nutritional content.

The next two sweeteners are a perfect addition to your kitchen.

Coconut Crystals

The principles of tapping the coconut tree blossoms for their sap, bears only minor resemblance to the practice of tapping maple trees for maple syrup production. Containers used to collect the sap are made out of hollow bamboo tubes that are fastened onto the thick fleshy stems covered in small flowers.

The freshly gathered coconut tree sap is oyster white in color, has a nearly neutral pH, and is already inherently sweet tasting by nature. Whereas, the sap from a maple tree (as well as the juice from an agave cactus) has very little readily available sweetness, and requires long heating times in order to produce the sweet syrup you purchase in the bottle.

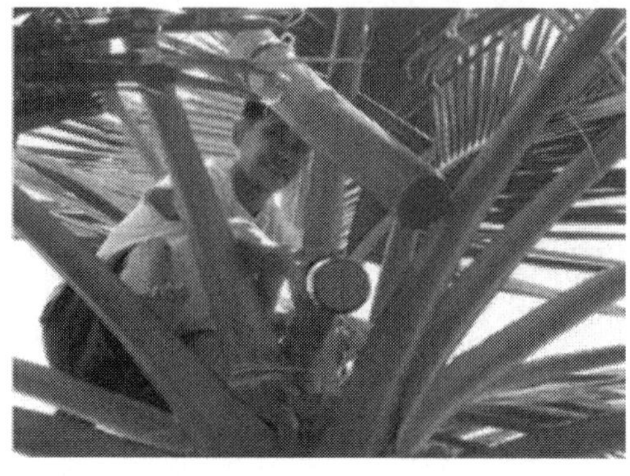

The nutrient-rich coconut sap comes right out of the tree naturally abundant in 17 Amino Acids (the building blocks of protein), broad-spectrum B Vitamins (especially rich in Inositol, known for its effectiveness on depression, high cholesterol, inflammation, and diabetes), Vitamin C, Minerals (high in Potassium, essential for electrolyte balance, regulating high blood pressure, and sugar metabolism), as well as FOS (a prebiotic that promotes digestive health).

Coconut crystals from sap is absolutely raw, unprocessed, and unheated remaining in its original and nutritious form. Not only is it sweet, but it is also nutritious!

This website has great coconut products: http://www.coconutsecret.com

Stevia

The herb, Stevia rebaudiana, has been used for centuries by the Guarani Indians of Paraguay, who had several names for the plant, several of which are Kaa'-he-E, Caa'-ehe, or Ca-a-yupe- . All referring to the sweet leaf or honey leaf. It is commonly known in South America as yerba dulce meaning sweet herb. The Guarani used stevia nutritionally and medicinally.

The plant came to the attention of the rest of the world when South American naturalist, Bertoni, "discovered" the plant in the late 1800's. After his report, the herb became widely used by herbalists in Paraguay.

Stevia's most obvious and notable characteristic is its sweet taste. However, the sweet taste is not due to carbohydrate-based molecules, but to several **non-caloric** molecules called glycosides. Individuals who cannot tolerate sugar or other sweeteners can use stevia. The first glycoside molecule was isolated from stevia in 1931 by two French chemists named Bridel and Lavieille and called stevioside.

During WWII, sugar shortages prompted England to begin investigation of stevia for use as a sweetener. Cultivation began under the direction of the Royal Botanical Gardens at Kew, but the project 'was abandoned in the aftermath of the war. Japan began cultivating stevia in hothouses in the 1950's. By the 1970's, Japan started using stevia commercially and today, they are the biggest users of the extract, which has captured 50% of Japan's sweetener industry.

Other aspects of stevia are capturing people's attention. The herb is sold in some South American countries to aid diabetics and hypoglycemics. Research has shown that a whole leaf concentrate has a regulating effect on the pancreas and **helps stabilize blood sugar levels**. Stevia is therefore useful to people with diabetes, hypoglycemia, and Candidiasis.

Other traditional uses of stevia are: lowers elevated blood pressure (hypertension), digestive aid that also reduces gas and stomach acidity, and for obesity. The herb acts as general tonic which increases energy levels and mental acuity.

The American population should have been all over this calorie-free healthy sweetener, what happened? Well, the FDA (Food and Drug Administration) banned stevia in 1991 because of heavy pressure by the sugar industry. The ban allowed it to be sold as a "dietary supplement" next to the vitamins in the health food section, but NOT in the sugar isle next to the toxic, acidifying regular sugar.

There have been absolutely no negative health consequences of Stevia, when compared with sugar which causes a whole list of health complications, and in 2008 the FDA finally allowed Stevia to be sold as a general purpose sweetener. Even Pepsi and Coca-Cola are jumping on the bandwagon with stevia sweetened drinks, but don't expect them to be out anytime soon, sugar is too cheap to be replaced by a natural healthy alternative.

You can get stevia in a whole leaf format, or in a powder/liquid that is composed of a stevia extract called Reb-A. The stevia leaves are milled, and a freshwater brewing method is used to extract the sweetness. This extract is then purified further until a very high purity Reb-A is obtained. I do recommend the whole leaf version due to other nutrients being present.

The only sweeteners I recommend are **raw unpasteurized organic honey, coconut crystals, raw agave powder, and stevia.**

Chapter 16

Bee Pollen

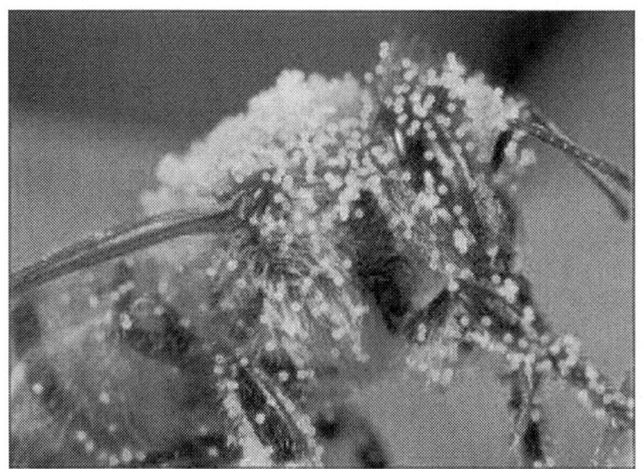

Bee pollen benefits have been used for improving health and wellness since **ancient times** and were well known to the Egyptians, Romans, and Greeks!

For **centuries** bee pollen has been consumed by many cultures not only for its numerous therapeutic properties in treating disease but as a significant source of nourishment. It's highly nutritious whole-food nature has earned it a 'super-food' status along with titles like "Food of the gods".

Bee pollen is one of the most nutritious foods on the planet!

What is pollen?

Pollen is the male seed of flowers. It is required for the fertilization of the plant. The tiny particles consist of 50/1,000-millimeter corpuscles, formed at the free end of the stamen in the heart of the blossom. Every variety of flower in the universe puts forth a dusting of pollen. Many orchard fruits and agricultural food crops do, too.

Bee pollen is the food of the young bee and it is approximately 40% protein. It is considered one of nature's most completely nourishing foods. It contains nearly all nutrients required by humans. About half of its protein is in the form of free amino acids that are ready to be sued directly by the body. Such highly assimilable protein can contribute significantly to one's protein needs.

Gathering pollen is not as easy as it sounds. Once a honeybee arrives at a flower, she settles herself in and nimbly scrapes off the powdery loose pollen from the stamen with her jaws and front legs, moistening it with a dab of the honey she brought with her from the hive. When the bee's baskets are fully loaded, the microscopic golden dust has been tamped down into a single golden grain, or granule.

One of the most interesting facts about bee pollen is that it cannot be synthesized in a laboratory. When researchers take away a bee's pollen-filled comb and feed her manmade pollen, the bee dies even though all the known nutrients are present in the lab-produced synthesized food. Many thousands of chemical analyses of bee pollen have been made with the very latest diagnostic equipment, but there are still some elements present in bee pollen that science cannot identify. The bees add some mysterious "extra" of their own. These unidentifiable elements may very well be the reason bee pollen works so spectacularly against so many diverse conditions of ill health.

Honeybees do double duty. They are programmed to gather pollen and carry it back to the hive as food for the colony. However, even more important as far as humans are concerned, they are also responsible for the pollination of more than 80 percent of green growing things. As bees buzz from blossom to blossom, microscopic pollen particles coat their stubby little bodies so densely that they sometimes look like little yellow fuzz balls. When they arrive at the next flower, a portion of the live golden dust is transferred to that blossom and pollination is accomplished.

It is important to recognize that a one teaspoon dose of pollen takes one bee working eight hours a day for one month to gather. Each bee pollen pellet, contains over two million flower pollen grains and one teaspoonful contains over 2.5 billion grains of flower pollen.

Complete Nutrition

Bee pollen contains all the essential components of life. The percentage of rejuvenating elements in bee pollen remarkably exceeds those present in brewer's yeast and wheat germ. Bee pollen corrects the deficient or unbalanced nutrition, common in the customs of our present-day civilization of consuming incomplete foods, often with added chemical ingredients, which expose us to physiological problems as various as they are numerous.

Pollen is considered an energy and nutritive tonic in Chinese medicine. Cultures throughout the world use it in a surprising number of applications: for improving endurance and vitality, extending longevity, aiding recovery from chronic illness, adding weight during convalescence, reducing cravings and addictions, regulating the intestines, building new blood, preventing infectious diseases such as the cold and flu (it has antibiotic type properties), and helping overcome retardation and other developmental problems in children. It is thought to protect against radiation and to have anti-cancer qualities.

Nutrient deficiencies and all the health problems they cause are recognized worldwide as a growing problem. Because bee pollen contains all the nutrients needed to sustain life, it is being used on an ever larger scale for human nourishment and health. Science teaches that bee pollen contains many substances that combine to make it a healthy, nutritious, complete food. There are numerous reports from medical experience that conclusively show the benefits of bee pollen exceed that of a simple food item. And the bees do most of the work.

Bee-gathered pollens are rich in proteins, free amino acids, vitamins, including B-complex, and folic acid.

According to researchers at the Institute of Apiculture, Taranov, Russia, "Honeybee pollen is the richest source of vitamins found in Nature in a single food. Even if bee pollen had none of its other vital ingredients, its content of rutin alone would justify taking at least a teaspoon daily, if for no other reason than strengthening the capillaries. Pollen is extremely rich in rutin and may have the highest content of any source, plus it provides a high content of the nucleics RNA [ribonucleic acid] and DNA [deoxyribonucleic acid]."

Bee pollen is a complete food and contains many elements that products of animal origin do not possess. Bee pollen is more rich in proteins than any animal source. It contains more amino acids than beef, eggs, or cheese of equal weight. Bee pollen is particularly concentrated in all elements necessary for life.

Since bee pollen derives from plant origin its chemical composition will vary somewhat depending on plant source, season and geographic location. The known nutrient breakdown is thought to be something around 35% protein, 55% carbohydrates, 2% fatty acids and 3% minerals and vitamins, including concentrations of B-complex vitamins, vitamins A, C, D, and E, plus beta carotene, selenium, and lecithin.

There may however still be many nutrients that so far remain scientifically undiscovered in bee pollen and these may bring about other properties and abilities in the future. Studies into the components of bee pollen therefore continue.

Pollen contains over 5,000 enzymes and co-enzymes, far more than is naturally present in any other food!

Medical Miracles

Hippocrates (460 – 377 B.C.), the first physician to concentrate on preventing disease as well as treating it, wrote of the benefits of bee pollen. Western trained doctors in Europe have, over the last century, prescribed bee pollen to treat bacterial and viral infections, along with colds and flues (due to its antibiotic properties).

Researchers have demonstrated that there is a substance in bee pollen that inhibits the development of numerous harmful bacteria. Experiments have shown bee pollen contains an antibiotic factor effective against salmonella and some strains of bacteria. On the clinical level, studies have shown that a regulatory effect on intestinal function can be attributed to bee pollen. The presence of a high proportion of cellulose and fiber in pollen, as well as the existence of antibiotic factors, all contribute to an explanation for this efficacious effect.

Working with lab animals has demonstrated that the ingestion of bee pollen has a good effect on the composition of blood. A considerable and simultaneous increase of both white and red blood cells is observed. When bee pollen is given to anemic patients, their levels of hemoglobin [oxygen-carrying red blood cells] increase considerably.

It is reported that bee pollen in the diet acts to normalize cholesterol and triglyceride levels in the blood: Upon the regular ingestion of bee pollen, a reduction of cholesterol and triglycerides was observed. High-density lipoproteins (HDL) increased, while low-density lipoproteins (LDL) decreased. A normalization of blood serum cholesterol levels is also seen.

One of the most important articles ever published on bee pollen comes from our own United States Department of Agriculture. This article, entitled "Delay in the Appearance of Palpable Mammary Tumors in C3H Mice Following the Ingestion of Pollenized Food," is the work of William Robinson of the Bureau of Entomology, Agriculture Research Administration. It was published in the Journal of the National Cancer Institute way back in October 1948, five decades ago. According to the article, Dr. Robinson started with mice that had been specially bred to develop and subsequently die from tumors. He explains, "The age at which mice of this strain developed tumors ranged from 18 to 57 weeks, with an average appearance at 33 weeks. Tumor incidence was 100 percent."

The pollen used in this study was supplied by the Division of Bee Culture and, according to the report, "was the bee-gathered type." One group of mice was fed mice chow only; another group was fed mice chow with the addition of bee pollen at a ratio of 1 part bee pollen to 10,000 parts food. Dr. Robinson's article states, "Particular attention was given to the weight of the treated animals, since underweight can in itself bring about a delay in tumor development. No decrease in weight occurred in the animals receiving the pollenized food. Instead, a slight but fairly uniform increase was noted, possibly due to a nutritional factor in pollen."

In his summary, Dr. Robinson reveals the dramatic results: "In the untreated mice [the mice not given bee pollen], mammary tumors appeared as expected at an average of 31.3 weeks. Tumor incidence was 100 percent. In the postponement series, [the mice given bee pollen], the average [onset of tumors] was 41.1 weeks, a delay of 9.8 weeks being obtained. Seven mice in this series were still tumor-free at 56 to 62 weeks of age, when the tests were terminated. I would like to emphasize that these mice were especially bred to die from cancerous tumors. Without the protection of bee pollen in their food, the mice developed tumors and died right on schedule.

Given the fact that cancer is the number-two killer in the United States (heart disease is number one), we can all certainly agree that this is an electrifying article. What happened from it? Nothing. Even the National Cancer Institute, which published it, failed to follow up on this very promising line of research. It was dropped with no explanation.

More good news comes from the University of Vienna, where Dr. Peter Hernuss and colleagues conducted a study of twenty-five women suffering from inoperable uterine cancer. Because surgery was impossible, the women were treated with chemotherapy. The lucky women given bee pollen with their food quickly exhibited a higher concentration of cancer-fighting immune-system cells, increased antibody production, and a markedly improved level of infection-fighting and oxygen carrying red blood cells (hemoglobin). These women suffered less from the awful side effects of chemotherapy as well. Bee pollen lessened the terrible nausea that commonly accompanies the treatment and helped keep hair loss to a minimum. The women also slept better at night. The control group receiving a placebo did not experience comparable relief.

A report from the Agronomic Institute, Faculty of Zootechnics, Romania, showed the immune-strengthening effects of bee pollen. According to the report, "Comparative Studies Concerning Biochemical Characteristics of Beebread as Related to the Pollen Preserved in Honey" by Drs. E. Palos, Z. Voiculescu, and C. Andrei, "An increase has been recorded in the level of blood lymphocytes, gamma globulins, and proteins in those subjects given pollen in comparison with control groups. The most significant difference occurred in lymphocytes. These results thus signify a strengthening in the resistance of the organic system."

Lymphocytes are the white blood cells that are the "soldiers" of the immune system. They are responsible for ridding the body of injurious and harmful substances, including infected or diseased cells, mutant and cancerous cells, viruses, metabolic trash, and so on. Gamma globulin is a protein formed in the blood, and our ability to resist infection is closely related to this protein's activity.

Infertility Problems

Pollen stimulates ovarian function. The best results were obtained with a pollen supplementation of 2 parts per 100 in the ration, and with the substitution of animal proteins with pollen in a proportion of 5 parts per 100. The intensity of ovulation increased. Parallel to this increase in ovulation, pollen also improves the ability of eggs to withstand the incubation period. The best results were obtained with a quantity of 4 parts per 100 of pollen added to the ration, resulting in an increase in the percentage of eggs in respect to the control group. The application of pollen is recommended whenever the end result is obtaining eggs for reproduction.

Bee Products Also Treats Allergies!

Pollen is also a remedy for hay fever and allergies. However it must be taken at least six weeks before the season begins and then continued throughout the season if it going to work.

Bee pollen has been effectively used down through the ages to rid allergy sufferers of their afflictions. This technique, called desensitization, was developed at St. Mary's Hospital Medical School in London soon after the turn of the century. The treatment consists of administering small amounts of the allergen to stimulate the patient's own immune system to produce antibodies that will eliminate the allergic reaction. It works rather like a vaccination does against childhood diseases. Desensitization is based on the premise that the administration of the allergen will cause the body to produce antibodies that will cancel out the effects of the offending substance when the patient is again exposed to it.

Leo Conway, M.D., of Denver Colorado, treated his patients with pollen. Dr. Conway reported: "All patients who had taken the antigen [pollen] for three years remained free from all allergy symptoms, no matter where they lived and regardless of diet. Control has been achieved in 100 percent of my earlier cases and the field is ever-expanding. Since oral feeding of pollen for this use was first perfected in his laboratory, astounding results were obtained. No ill consequences have resulted. Ninety-four percent of all his patients were completely free from allergy symptoms. Of the other six percent, not one followed directions, but even this small percentage were nonetheless partially relieved".

Relief of hay fever, pollen-induced asthma, with ever increasing control of bronchitis, ulcers of the digestive tract, colitis, migraine headaches, and urinary disorders were all totally successful. Unfortunately, Dr. Conway, an early pioneer in the field of allergies, is now deceased. What we did not know was just how lightning-fast it could bring relief. It actually eliminated long-standing symptoms in minutes. Everything from asthma to allergies to sinus problems cleared. These trials confirmed that bee pollen is wonderfully effective against a very wide range of respiratory distress.

The Chinese have used Bee Pollen for centuries to assist with increasing energy and libido, fighting acne, aiding in indigestion, assisting depression and helping to improve blood pressure. The list of possible benefits of this wonderful nutritious substance is growing after years of research and studies are verifying what nature has always known.

Bee Pollen Supplements may be helpful for:

- Relief for Arthritis
- Help with Prostate problems
- Improving digestion
- Skin problems such as eczema & psoriasis
- Hormonal balance, such as PMT & menopause
- Repetitive colds & flu
- Weight gain or weight loss

- Athletic performance
- Reproductive system - impotence, infertility, loss of libido etc
- Low or high blood pressure
- Nervous system problems
- Glandular problems
- Ulcers
- Hepatitis
- Bronchitis
- Chronic fatigue
- Insomnia
- Bowel problems - constipation, colitis, irritable bowel syndrome etc
- Help protect against adverse effects associated with radiation treatment
- Help prevent premature aging
- Helps eliminate toxicity from the body

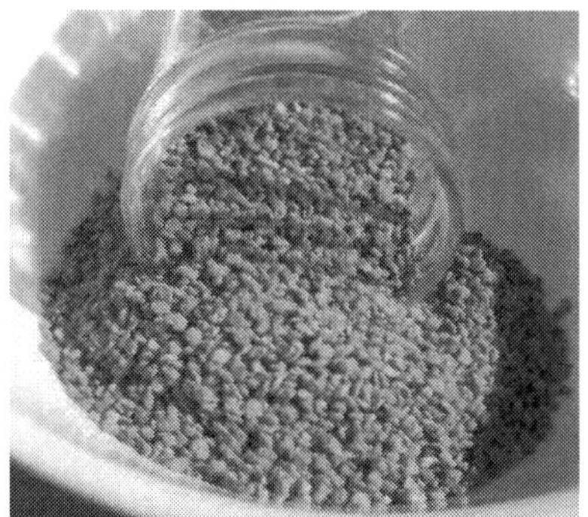

Apitherapy, a recognized form of complementary and alternative medicine, involves the use of bee products to prevent or heal medical conditions. Apitherapy recognizes all bee pollen benefits and is used in the treatment and cure of over 500 diseases and illnesses!

Chinese medicine has also recognized bee pollen benefits for **thousands of years**.

Practitioners, especially those in Europe, also prescribe bee pollen for hay fever or allergic rhinitis as well as mouth sores, rheumatism, painful urination, prostate conditions and radiation sickness.

Bee Products and Physical Activity

The British Sports Council recorded increases in strength of as high as 40 to 50 percent in those taking bee pollen regularly. Even more astounding, the British Royal Society has reported height increases in adults who take pollen. Antii Lananaki, coach of the Finnish track team that swept the Olympics in 1972, revealed, "Most of our athletes take pollen food supplements. Our studies show it significantly improves their performance. There have been no negative results since we have been supplying pollen to our athletes."

Alex Woodly, then executive director of the prestigious Education Athletic Club in Philadelphia, said, "Bee pollen works, and it works perfectly. Pollen allows super-stars to increase their strength and stamina up to 25 percent. This increase in strength and endurance may be the key to the secret regenerative power of bee pollen. Bee pollen causes a definite decrease in pulse rate. The whole beauty of bee pollen is that it's as natural as you can get. No chemicals. No steroids." Renowned German naturalist Francis Huber was a great proponent of this miraculous food from the hive. Huber called bee pollen "the greatest body builder on Earth."

Bee Pollen and Weight Control

Bee pollen works wonders in a weight-control or weight-stabilization regimen by correcting a possible chemical imbalance in body metabolism that may be involved in either abnormal weight gain or loss. The normalizing and stabilizing effects of this perfect food from the bees are phenomenal.

In weight-loss programs, bee pollen stimulates the metabolic processes. It speeds caloric burn by lighting and stoking the metabolic fires. Honeybee pollen is coming to be recognized as Nature's true weight-loss food. Bee pollen is a low-calorie food. It contains only ninety calories per ounce. (An ounce is about two heaping tablespoons.) It offers 15 percent lecithin by volume.

Lecithin is a substance that helps dissolve and flush fat from the body. This is one reason why bee pollen lowers low-density lipoproteins (LDL) surer and faster than any other food while helping increase the helpful high-density lipoproteins (HDL), which science says protect against cholesterol and heart disease.

By boosting the value of each nutrient present in the food you eat, bee pollen also eliminates cravings. Its natural phenylalanine content acts as an appetite suppressant. Phenylalanine is a natural amino acid that the body requires. It acts on your appestat, the control center that signals fullness and hunger.

Mother Nature knows what she's about. You just plain won't want to eat as much when you take bee pollen regularly. When you are overweight, phenylalanine exerts a natural appetite suppressant effect. When you need to gain weight, the phenylalanine in bee pollen works in reverse.

The chemical drug in over-the-counter weight-loss products is a manmade cousin of phenylalanine called phenylpropanolamine, which chemically depresses the appetite whether you are fat, thin, or just right. It can also give you the jitters and leave you with a drug-induced "hangover" and can be addictive. Phenylpropanolamine is a common ingredient in many decongestants, explaining why one of the side effects of these products is loss of appetite. Products that include phenylpropanolamine as an ingredient must by law carry a warning that they should not be taken by persons with certain conditions, including thyroid problems and high blood pressure.

Health and Beauty

Basic beauty begins with the glow of good health, which shines from within. A scrubbed and radiant complexion transforms any woman (or man) into a singularly attractive person. On the other hand, dull, muddy skin, often caused by poor nutrition or personal hygiene, can detract from even the most attractive. Studies have shown that unhealthy or aging skin can be dramatically improved by the consumption of honeybee pollen.

When bee pollen is included daily in the diet, it not only gives you the glow of health and aids in safe, permanent weight loss, but it can also be blended into seemingly "magic potions" to smooth, soothe, and rejuvenate every inch of the outside of your body. Several relatively inexpensive mixtures of hive products, used externally, can revitalize and rejuvenate the complexion and may even eliminate acne.

Dr. Lars-Erik Essen, a dermatologist in Halsinborg, Sweden, pioneered the use of bee products for skin conditions. He treated many of his patients successfully for acne. Dr. Essen says, "Through transcutaneous nutrition, bee pollen exerts a profound biological effect. It seems to prevent premature aging of the cells and stimulates growth of new skin tissue. It offers effective protection against dehydration and injects new life into dry cells. It smoothes away wrinkles and stimulates a life-giving blood supply to all skin cells.

The skin becomes younger looking, less vulnerable to wrinkles, smoother, and healthier with the use of honeybee pollen," Dr. Essen says. "Taken internally or used externally, bee pollen exercises a suppressive effect on facial acne. It is also an important skin rejuvenator, primarily because it contains a high concentration of the nucleic acids RNA and DNA as well as a natural antibiotic factor."

The French, long noted for their preoccupation with all things beautiful, have done a great deal of research on the use of bee pollen and other hive products in cosmetic preparations. Dr. M. Esperrois of the French Institute of Chemistry notes that honeybee pollen contains potent antibiotics that can act to reverse the effects normal aging exerts on skin, correcting darkening, wrinkles, and blemishes.

Professors N. Mankovsky and D. G. Chebotarev, two Russian scientists, confirm honeybee pollen stimulates cell renewal. They say, "The rejuvenation of skin and body cells can be encouraged by the administration of the poly-vitamins, microelements, enzymes, hormones, and amino acids present m bee pollen. These nutrients are needed by the body to form new tissue." These professors go on to praise the properties of bee pollen, calling them "vital to a form of internal and external rejuvenation at the cellular level.

Longevity and the Aging Process

According to G. Liebold, a holistic physician and psychologist of Karlsruhe, Germany, "Bee pollen is an excellent prophylaxis and therapeutic treatment against all the precocious symptoms of old age. It should be considered a universal geriatric treatment in the form of a natural remedy.

"Bee pollen causes an increase in physical and mental abilities, especially of concentration and memory ability, activates sluggish metabolic functions, and strengthens the cardiovascular and respiratory systems. This natural nutriment from the bees removes the causes of cardiovascular symptoms, such as arteriosclerosis, cerebral insufficiency, and other sequelae. It prevents nutrient deficiency during old age, gravidity [pregnancy], and the lactation [nursing] period. Bee pollen accelerates convalescence after serious illness and/or an operation, increases the body's physical defensive powers of the immune system stimulates mental and psychological resistance to stress, and creates a harmonizing of vegetative and hormonal disorders."

Dr. Nicolai Vasilievich Tsitsin, the USSR's chief biologist (and botanist) and an acknowledged expert on geriatrics, spent quite a few years pursuing the secrets of the many in what was the Soviet Union who live extraordinarily long lives. He visited the numerous small villages that dot the landscape high up in the Caucasus mountains, where the air is always clear and sweet. In summer, the breezes there are perfumed with the scent of thousands of wild flowers. The villagers work their small farms and tend their kitchen gardens without the dubious "benefits" of the space-age technologies employed by agribiz conglomerates. This is one of the few areas left in the world where the old ways still prevail.

The stalwart families who make their homes in the mountainous regions of the former Soviet Union are some of the most long-lived people in the world.

On examination, many exhibit signs of "silent" heart disease, scars of "silent" heart attacks that would have almost certainly been lethal to a modern man or woman. The hard physical work they do every day well into what some of us in the so-called civilized world consider old age plays a part in their remarkably healthy lifestyle.

Dr. Tsitsin was amazed to find more than 200 individuals over 125 years of age, all still working every day and participating actively in village life. The hard facts of their daily existence partially explained the extended life span they achieved, but Dr. Tsitsin remained puzzled. He knew there had to be some other factor entering into the equation. He set himself the task of finding the common denominator. Then he stumbled upon it.

These people kept bees. Beekeeping is a profession that in itself a historically confers some sort of "magical" life protection on its members, a fact validated by today's scientific research. Still, only very well informed, modern beekeepers are knowledgeable about the many health-promoting benefits of bee pollen and regularly serve it at table. The villagers didn't fit the profile. Dr. Tsitsin dug deeper.

He found the answer. These beekeepers, happy and fulfilled though they were with their almost idyllic pastoral existence, were very poor. Bartering among themselves to exchange homegrown or handmade products for services was the accepted way of life. They had little cash available to them, so they regularly harvested-and either sold or bartered away the pure, clear honey from the combs of their beehives. What they kept for themselves and ate regularly was the thick residue that accumulated on the bottoms of their hives.

When he was served some of the sweet, sticky stuff in the home of one of the villagers, Dr. Tsitsin realized that this was the magic elixir that contributed to the remarkable longevity. The tasty but unattractive glob was rich with golden granules of bee pollen. Dr. Tsitsin attributed the remarkable health and extended life spans of these particular Russians to the scientifically documented action of bee pollen. He concluded his report by saying, "Taken regularly and in sufficient amounts, bee pollen will prolong the life span of man for many years."

Another Russian scientist, Naum Petrovich Ioyrish, chief of the Academy of July 26, 1997 Vladivostok and author of Bees and People, agrees. In 1975, Dr. Ioyrish reported without any qualification, "Long lives are attained by bee pollen users. It is one of the original treasure houses of nutrition and medicine. **Each grain contains every important substance necessary to life**."

How to Use Bee Pollen

Each golden granule is densely packed with active enzymes, just about every nutrient that has a name, and some elements that science has not yet identified or labeled. Your digestive system may not be accustomed to such intensely rich food. If you are a beginner, introduce bee pollen into your diet slowly, a granule or two at a time. **Don't cook** with the granules or add powdered granules to anything that requires heat. Heat destroys the active enzymes and reduces the nutrient value. Otherwise, the sky's the limit.

You can: Powder an ounce or two of granules and add cinnamon to taste. Cinnamon adds a delightful spiciness and aroma to the sweetness of pollen Stir powdered granules into vegetable juices, or even into water sweetened with raw honey. Whirl the powder into salad dressings. Sprinkle whole or powdered granules on toast topped with peanut butter.

Before taking a full dose of pollen it is very important to test for a possible extreme allergic reaction by ingesting just one pellet. Then gradually build up over a week or so to the correct dose.

The optimal dose of pollen varies with individual needs. For allergy prevention all that is required is about one teaspoon per day. You should gradually increase your dose to one tablespoon. It will give about five grams of protein which is a good addtion if you already have some proteins in your meal, such as a legume dish.

Since your pollen is really a type of food and there are some fats in it. It is important to keep it refrigerated.

From a **preventative health care** perspective there is an ever increasing upward trend in the use of bee pollen for nourishment and the enhancement of overall wellness. Since bee pollen contains all the nutrients needed to sustain life, health conscious consumers have readily adopted its use as a **functional and complete food.**

Bee Pollen Tips

Of course, the quality of the Bee Pollen relies on where it is harvested. When the Bees collect the pollen, their bodies almost 'magnetize' the Pollen to them, which means the Bees are also exposed to harmful impurities found in the air as well as what they land on. These could include heavy metals like lead, airborne chemicals, toxins, and other impurities found in the environment. These are often caused by heavy population as well as heavy pollution. The soil the flowers grow in is also a factor. Most bee pollen granules in supplements are sourced from the USA and/or China. Independent laboratories frequently find traces of heavy metals present in these bee pollens as a direct result of air pollution.

So when purchasing a bee pollen supplement you need to consider the source of the pollen!

This is why a quality Bee Pollen from a healthy environment is very important. Countries such as New Zealand have a minimal population and as such have lower levels of pollution than many other countries in the world and produce one of the most nutrition dense bee products in the world. You can also go to your local farmers market to sample a variety of bee products from local bee keepers which will be far superior in quality to mass produced store varieties.

Note: Only choose semi-moist refrigerated bee pollen whenever possible. Store bought bee pollen is heated to dry the granules therefore diminishing a lot of the nutritional content. I always recommend bee pollen for everyone whether they are chronically ill, or physically active, or just wanting to stay healthy. Take a minimum one tablespoon of pollen daily up to as much pollen as you want, there is no maximum. It is so nutritious you can pretty much live off bee pollen and water if you wanted to and never get any illness as long as you live.

Chapter 17

Spirulina and Chlorella

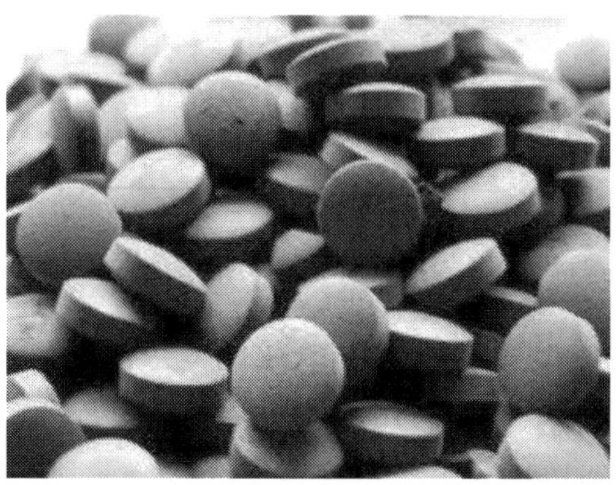

There are only a very few foods that qualify for "super foods" status, Spirulina and Chlorella fall on the list alongside superstars bee pollen, raw honey and raw milk.

What can these two superfoods really do for your health? They offer a stunning array of health benefits. Chlorella and spirulina have been shown to be effective in treating and even reversing the following conditions:

- Cancers (all types)
- Obesity
- Diabetes
- Hypoglycemia
- Arthritis
- Depression
- Severe liver damage and liver disorders
- Intestinal ulcers
- Hemorrhoids
- Asthma
- High blood pressure
- Constipation
- Bleeding gums
- Infections
- Inflammation of joints and tissues
- Body odor / breath odor
- Various degenerative diseases
- Essential fatty acid deficiencies
- Mineral deficiencies (magnesium is a common deficiency)

Both chlorella and spirulina are particularly useful for:

- People with poor digestion and assimilation (these micro-algae are easy to digest and absorb)
- People with poor vitality and anemia
- Individuals who consumer large quantities of animal protein (the micro-algae protein, in contrast, is easier to digest and offers a far healthier balance of minerals)
- People who eat refined or processed foods
- People who take prescription drugs (spirulina protects the kidneys and liver)
- People who are overweight or obese
- People who engage in physical exercise and / or strength training
- People with low energy levels (feeling depleted, exhausted, etc.)

In fact, both chlorella and spirulina have been described as "the perfect food"

Chlorella:

"Chlorella has been touted as the perfect whole food. Aside from being a complete protein and containing all the B vitamins, vitamin C, vitamin E, and the major minerals (with zinc and iron in amounts large enough to be considered supplementary), it has been found to improve the immune system, improve digestion, detoxify the body, accelerate healing, protect against radiation, aid in the prevention of degenerative diseases, help in treatment of Candida albicans, relieve arthritis pain and, because of its nutritional content, aid in the success of numerous weight loss programs."
- Earl Mindell's Vitamin Bible

Spirulina:

"Spirulina's predigested protein provides building material soon after ingestion, without the energy-draining side effects of meat protein; its mucopolysaccharides relax and strengthen connective tissue while reducing the possibility of inflammation; it's simple carbohydrates yield immediate yet sustained energy; its GLA fatty acids improve hormonal balance; and its protein-bonded vitamins and minerals, as found in all whole foods, assimilate better than the synthetic variety. Spirulina can generally be considered an appropriate food for those who exercise vigorously, as evidenced by the many world-class athletes who use it"
- Healing With Whole Foods by Paul Pitchford

Chlorella and spirulina have such strong health benefits that even well-known doctors and authors use these products and note their benefits:

“It is possible that the GLA found in spirulina and possibly these other products accounts for some of the positive effects that people experience when using them, including decreased appetite, weight loss, and improved energy levels, especially mental energy. I personally have used all of these products and must say I have experienced a subtle increase in mental clarity and alertness (not like a nervous, caffeine-type stimulation). These algae must subtly stimulate our nervous systems or release certain internal neurochemicals that create this "up" feeling.”
- Staying Healthy With Nutrition by Elson Haas, M.D.

In all, these two superfoods are effective in not just reversing a long list of serious diseases, they are powerful health enhancers that demonstrate phenomenal benefits even to people who are in "good" health!

“Both chlorella and spirulina are packed with nutrients and phytochemicals that boost health and fight disease. In this section, we'll take a closer look at their major nutritional components and see just what these superfoods have to offer.

Chlorella is a tiny, single-celled water-grown alga containing a nucleus and an enormous amount of readily available chlorophyll. It also contains protein (approximately 58 percent), carbohydrates, all of the B vitamins, vitamins C and E, amino acids, and rare trace minerals. In fact, it is virtually **a complete food**. It contains more vitamin B12 than liver does, plus a considerable amount of beta-carotene.”
- A-to-Z Guide To Supplements, James F. Balch M.D.

Scientists in China have also shown that spirulina increased the level of white cells in the blood and of nucleated cells and DNA in the bone marrow of mice that had been subjected to chemotherapy and radiation. In dogs, the spirulina extract additionally increased the level of red blood cells. The authors concluded that spirulina “has chemo-protective and radio-protective capability, and may be a potential adjunct to cancer therapy.” CancerDecisions

Protein

Other than raw milk and bee pollen, Spirulina is simply the world's most digestible natural source of high quality protein, far surpassing the protein bioavailability of even beef (which most people consider to be the #1 source of protein). The digestive absorption of each gram of protein in spirulina is four times greater than the same gram of protein in beef. And since spirulina already contains three times more protein (by weight) to begin with, the net result is that, ounce for ounce, spirulina offers **twelve times more digestible protein than beef**.

That's an astounding difference. It means that spirulina is the ideal food source for people working to get more protein into their diets:

- People who exercise vigorously or engage in strength training.
- People who are frail, who have trouble gaining weight, or who are malnourished.

In fact, there's probably no better single food source on the planet than spirulina for these people. The protein found in spirulina is also a complete protein, meaning that it contains all eight essential amino acids, unlike beans, whole grains and other plant-based foods that typically lack one or more amino acids.

Not only do these micro algae have all of the B vitamins, Vitamin C, Vitamin E, provitamin A, and so on. But what's important about these vitamins isn't just that they are present: it's the fact that they are found **in their natural forms**.

In other words, if you take cheap "bulk" vitamin supplements, you are often taking synthetic vitamins that have been manufactured in a chemical plant from ingredients that you'd never normally eat. Most synthetic vitamins may be molecularly similar to the vitamins found in plants, but clinical trial show that they aren't the same in effect. There's something almost magical about vitamins found in plants: they're simply more healthful, more absorbable, and more effective at getting the job done (the only vitamins I recommend are quality, filler free Ester Vitamin C, vitamin E, and vitamin D).

Minerals

Pretty much all Americans are deficient in most minerals including magnesium and zinc. This is due to the SAD – Standard American Diet full of nutrition-less refined foods which must be "enriched" with synthetic vitamins that are not properly absorbed or digested anyway. Virtually all low carb dieters are calcium deficient due to a lack of dietary magnesium in meats and pasteurized milk products.

These two micro algae are full of minerals your body craves. It's plants that offer the healthiest sources of the vitamins and minerals our bodies really need - in the form we need. Put simply, the minerals in micro-algae are easily absorbable by the human body. If you experienced some health benefits from taking coral calcium, you'll be stunned at the much stronger benefits from consuming micro-algae.

"The plants richest in chlorophyll—the micro-algae and cereal grasses—were cited earlier as good sources of magnesium. Green plants also have the **greatest concentration of calcium of any food**; because of their magnesium, chlorophyll, and other calcium cofactors, increasing the consumption of green plants often is a **simple solution to calcium problems**."

Essential Fatty Acids

Surprised to know that there are essential fatty acids in algae? These EFA's are the beneficial fats our bodies can't live without. Omega 3, GLA (gamma-linoleic acid), DHA (found in fish oils) are all present here!

Spirulina contains a sizable dose of GLA and omega-3 fatty acids. It is especially high in GLA, which is something that is almost universally lacking in the American diet.

Human breast milk is high in GLA, probably due to the infant child's need for brain-building fats. And since many infants never gained the important nutritional benefits of their mothers' milk, they've been GLA-deficient for their entire lives. The American diet of processed foods contains virtually no GLA whatsoever. And low-carb dieters aren't getting any either, unless they specifically supplement it. But you can get it from spirulina.

"The richest whole-food sources of GLA are mother's milk, spirulina micro-algae, and the seeds of borage, black currant, and evening primrose. GLA is important for growth and development, and is found most abundantly in mother's milk; **spirulina is the next-highest whole-food source**. We often recommend spirulina for people who were never breast-fed, in order to foster the hormonal and mental development that may never have occurred because of lack of proper nutrition in infancy. The dosage is the amount of oil that provides 150-350 mg GLA daily. A standard 10-gram dosage of spirulina provides 131 mg of GLA"
- Healing With Whole Foods by Paul Pitchford

A standard 10-gram dosage of spirulina provides 131mg of GLA! A very important thing to note here is the fact that these micro algae are **food**, they are not drugs, and many people mistakenly take far too little to have that powerful impact that it should. The more you eat the better for you, you can eat pounds of this super food only to find yourself becoming more slim and healthy. This is why you have probably never heard of these super foods, diet companies get Goosebumps just thinking about this information getting out, their whole business with their billion dollar profits depends on it!
- Healing With Whole Foods by Paul Pitchford

Chlorophyll

Chlorella is the richest source of chlorophyll on earth. What does it do? Chlorophyll is a very powerful detox agent, and people who follow standard Western diets are in desperate need of cleansing and detoxifying.

Chlorophyll helps to remove heavy metals from your body which accumulate from pesticides in the food, improper farming practices, tap water, and toxic air. If you have been eating refined non organic foods you most likely have high levels of mercury, cadmium, arsenic, lead, PCBs and other nasty contaminants floating around in your body. Chlorella and Spirulina help remove these and other toxins from your body.

Another common source for contaminants is mercury fillings used by dentists. They call them "silver fillings," actually, since they don't want to openly admit they're still putting mercury -- one of the most potent nerve toxins on the planet -- into the mouths of patients. These mercury fillings emit a steady stream of mercury vapor that gets absorbed into your body. Frequently, small bits of these mercury fillings crack, break off, and are swallowed with your food. In this way, nearly all dental patients in America and other "civilized" countries are subjected to routine mercury poisoning at the hands of their dentists.

Chlorella can help protect you against this mercury be escorting the mercury out of your body before it can do damage. If you take chlorella before and after receiving dental work, you will help protect yourself from the toxic effects of mercury fillings. This is especially important if you decide to have your mercury fillings removed, as more and more people are doing. The very process of drilling them out results in a tidal wave of mercury exposure in your body. Having a diet full chlorella offers considerable protection against the mercury bits you inevitably swallow during this procedure.

Weight Loss Benefits

In various clinical studies, micro-algae have been shown to be remarkably effective for weight loss. There are primarily two reasons for this: the correction of nutritional deficiencies, and the addition of GLA to the diet. By supplying the body with the nutrients it needs, however, those cravings can be dramatically reduced and the endocrine system can be brought back into a state of balance.

In addition to all the other dietary changes, these two super foods will do wonders for your weight loss and health!

Minimum daily dosages of Spirulina and Chlorella is 5 grams each per day. That is the minimum dose, the more you take the better for you.

Chapter 18

Sprouted Grains

The health benefits of wheat, rye, rice, quinoa, and other grains are entirely dependent on how they are eaten. Refined, processed grains are stripped of most of their nutrients, as the brain and the germ are removed. When making white flour, most of the vitamins B1, B2, B3, E, folic acid, calcium phosphorus, zinc, copper, iron, fiber and practically all other nutrients are completely lost leaving you with a useless starchy fat gainer that has a host of negative health consequences.

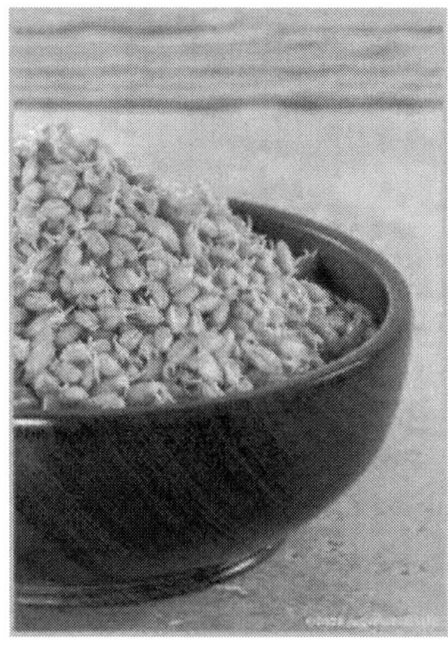

Eating refined grains has negative health effects, and they can directly contribute to problems such as obesity, high cholesterol, heart disease, stroke, hyperglycemia, and diabetes. The problems from eating refined, processed grains has only really been well documented over the past one hundred years, but people have known of the problem for thousands of years. **Traditionally, all grains and seeds, including rice, were <u>sprouted</u>**. As much as **twenty times more nutrients** are found in sprouted seeds compared to processed seeds. Wheat seeds were processed and eaten 2000 years ago but this was only during times of famine or by armies that were on the move.

Before the usage of commercial farm harvesters, grain naturally sprouted in the field before it was milled into flour. During the industrial revolution grain was quickly harvested unsprouted and moved to storage bins, casting aside the thousand year old tradition of sprouting. With this, nutrition was also set aside.

Sprouts are considered as wonder foods. They rank as the freshest and most nutritious of all vegetables available to the human diet. By a process of natural transmutation, sprouted food acquires vastly improved digestibility and nutritional qualities when compared to non-sprouted embryo from which it derives. Sprouted foods have been part of the diet of many ancient races for thousands of years. Even to this day, the Chinese retain their fame for delicious mung bean sprouts.

Sprouts provide all the essential vitamins and minerals, they are a natural multivitamin. They should form a vital component of our diet. Sprouting requires no constant care but only an occasional sprinkling of water.

All edible grains, seeds and legumes can be sprouted, if it is possible try to find ones that are organic and not genetically modified. Even if you are unable to acquire organic ones, they will still bring a ton of benefits.

Generally the following are used for sprouting :

Grains : Wheat, spelt, rye, millet, oat, amaranth, rice, quinoa, kamut, buckwheat, maize, ragi, bajra and barley.
Seeds : Alfalfa seeds, radish seeds, fenugreek seeds, carrot seeds, coriander seeds,
pumpkin seeds and muskmelon seeds.
Legumes : Mung, Bengal gram, lentils, groundnut and peas.

Alfalfa, as the name in Arabic signifies, is the king of all sprouts. Grown as a plant, its roots are known to burrow as much as 12 meters into the subsoil to bring up valuable trace minerals of which manganese is especially important to health and digestion ; it is a vital component of human insulin. Apart from minerals, alfalfa is also a rich source of vitamins A,B,C,E and K and amino acids. Sesame seeds are another good source of nourishment. They contain all the essential amino acids in their 20 per cent protein content, and higher concentration of calcium than milk. They are high in lecithin, unsaturated fats, vitamin E and vitamin B complex, besides other live nutrients.

The Benefits of Sprouted Flour:

- **Easier to Digest** – Sprouting breaks down the starches in grains into simple sugars so your body can digest them like a vegetable.
- **Increased Vitamin C** – Sprouting produces vitamin C.
- **Increased Vitamin B** – Sprouting increases the vitamin B content (B2, B5, and B6).
- **Increased Carotene** – Sprouting increases the carotene up to eight times.
- **Increased Enzymes** – enzymes are actually produced during sprouting.

- **Reduction of Anti-nutrients** – Sprouting neutralizes enzyme inhibitors and phytic acid, which is a substance present in the bran of all grains that inhibits absorption of calcium, magnesium, iron, copper and zinc.

Sprouted grain breads are significantly higher in protein, vitamins and enzymes and the complex starches are converted into natural sugars. They are also low GI, so they are digested more slowly by the body, keeping the blood sugar levels stable for longer, making people feel more satisfied. This leads to snacking less. It is interesting to note that the more highly processed a food is, the higher GI it is. A loaf of white bread is significantly higher GI than a loaf of sprouted grain bread.

Those who have any allergies or intolerances to wheat or grains in general may find that they have absolutely no negative health reactions to sprouted grains. We should **ONLY eat sprouted grains** as they are a perfect fit for our digestion and proper absorption.

Organic sprouted whole grains or flour made from sprouted grains is available here: http://www.organicsproutedflour.net/

I only know of one company that produces bread and cereals from sprouted grains, I eat them sometimes and they are absolutely delicious. The company is called “Food For Life Ezekiel 4:9” and they produce delicious breads and cereals which should be available in major grocery stores or natural food markets.

Make Your Own Sprouts

Making your own sprouts is very easy. Simply take some organic grains/seeds/nuts/legumes, spread them out on a plate or dish, pour some water but don’t cover the seeds in water, and wait a day or so until the sprouts are about a few millimeters in length. Change the water once or twice and you will have your own home made sprouts, give it a shot!

You can make your own sprouts or buy them from a store, the benefits will astound you. You can eat them just on their own with some spices and oil, sprinkled on salads, sandwiches, soups, or pretty much any other dish.

Chapter 19

Organic Vs. Natural – What's The Difference?

Although the terms "**natural**" and "**organic**" are often used together or interchangeable it's actually very different.

In the food industry today, there's **NO** official definition of "**all natural.**" It means whatever the food companies want it to mean. It can mean, for example, that all the chemicals found in the product simply aren't listed on the label. (There's **no requirement** for food companies to list chemical contaminants found in their foods.)

A food labeled "**all natural**" can contain:

- pesticides
- herbicides
- toxic heavy metals
- trace amounts of PCBs
- toxic fluoride
- hidden MSG
- high-temperature cooking by-products
- synthetic chemical vitamins
- other non-natural substances

According to the FDA – their definition of "natural"

Natural foods are processed without preservatives or additives, but may have been grown **with** the use of pesticides or other conventional methods. The Food and Drug Administration (FDA) regulates the term 'natural' **only as it applies** to added color, synthetic substances, and flavors. The term 'natural' can include free-range and hormone-free, and it can mean that a product contains no synthetic ingredients or color additives. The key word here "can" but it doesn't have to!

Marketing experts know that, for many consumers, natural equals healthy, and "healthy" <u>sells</u>.

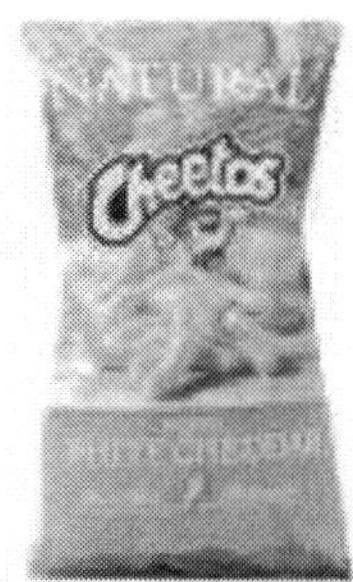

In fact, the word **"natural"** on a food package may mean next to nothing because unlike "organic," "natural" **has no meaning in law or regulation**. For these reasons, the use of "natural" on food products all too often distracts attention from more important issues.

Makers of potato chips--and corn chips, pancake mixes, frozen waffles, frosted breakfast cereals, ice cream and other taste tempters want you to think **"natural"** is good for you or at least you not feeding your family junk. That's why the word **"natural"** appears so frequently on food packages these days.

"Natural" is very misleading if it implies that a product is free of chemical additives (often not the case) or that competitors' products are "unnatural and therefore bad for you.

The production of organic foods helps to honor the balance of nature through "old fashioned" farming methods. Conventional pesticides, synthetic fertilizers, antibiotics and growth hormones are almost never used on organic farms (with exceptions). Instead, they use renewable resources and focus on soil and water conservation to help preserve the environment for future generations.

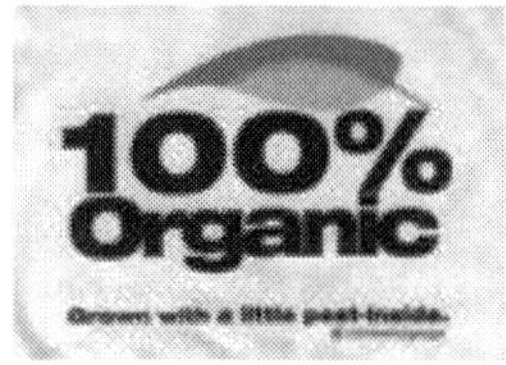

Organic farming is also regulated by the country where you are located (for example the United States Department of Agriculture –USDA - which abides to strict quality standards for growing and handling). To locate Certified Organic products in the store, look for a label or seal with the words "Organic" which ensures the product is 95-100% organic.

Nonetheless, ALWAYS read the label and don't settle for any labels or claims on the package!

The greedy giant corporations have taken advantage of the gullible consumer and have really mastered the art of selling junk and making people believe that it is actually good for them. These days I do my best to buy local products by small "mom and pop" companies produced by people who actually **care** about others. Let's stop giving our money to giant, greedy, lying companies selling us junk and making us sick. We are the ones that keep them in business, we are the ones supporting their unfair, toxic, and wasteful practices. I say we put an end to this and vote with our wallets.

UPC Codes on Produce

Do you know what it all means?

Have you ever noticed the food labels on your produce – fruit and vegetables? Produce now carry a sticker called "price look-up codes (PLUs). This tells the clerk the price, but not only that, it can help YOU. These stickers tell you how fruits and vegetables were grown. There are more than 1,300 PLU codes currently assigned to produce. Here is what they mean:

You would have either a 4 or 5 digit codes. Below is a chart that will help you identify how produce is grown.

Organically	Conventionally	Genetically Modified
5 digits	4 digits	5 digits
Starting w/ no. 9	Starting w/ no. 3 or 4	Starting w/ no. 8

A conventionally grown banana has a PLU of 4011, an organic banana is 94011 and GM banana is 84011.

To see a database of PLU codes, go to www.plucodes.com.

Chapter 20

Putting It All Together

These next steps are what make winners, what make the success stories, and what will actually **change your life**. If what you learn doesn't get put into practice, then it's useless knowledge. So let's put some of the things we have just learned into practice. But remember, these things are a lot easier than you expect, and with a bit of patience will make your life happier and healthier!

The main thing to remember is that the more natural and raw food you eat, the faster and easier you will lower your risk of countless diseases and regain your health. There is nothing you need to "do," your body will do it all for you, you just have to turn the right key and the door will open by itself. Your "open sesame," your secret password, your master key is just eating and living the way your body was made to.

Get rid of all the empty calories, the processed garbage food and replace them with nutrient dense fruits, vegetables, nuts, sprouted grains, and super foods mentioned above. Give your body the nutrition it craves and it will naturally lose weight and cure itself from all nasty ailments.

The golden rule is eat as much raw as possible, stay away from processed foods and gravitate towards natural, whole, nutrient dense alternatives. If you have a craving for some junk, always give yourself an alternative and allow the gradual change to take effect. Take healthy snacks with you, make you own lunch, and get rid of all the temptations at home; throw away or donate all the junk food you have at home! And if you go to restaurants, find some local vegetarian ones, and taste for yourself how delicious and filling the meals can be.

And remember, if you happen to slip, don't worry, just get right back up and continue. Allow yourself **once in a while** to indulge on something less than perfect. Start shopping at whole food stores and farmers markets, get into the "scene" and open a whole new world for yourself. It is easier than it sounds; all it takes is the first few steps to begin the path.

First Steps

So, you open up your fridge and notice a lot of things that you now know are putting the "stick in the wheel" of your weight loss and health. If you want to keep being fat, sick, and tired, then by all means leave everything as it is, but if you have decided to change your life, then I will recommend that you definitely change what's in your fridge and pantry.

Step 1 – Take a big garbage bag.
Step 2 – Go to your fridge and pantry.
Step 3 – Notice the Cookies? Cakes? Pastries? Chips? Chocolate bars? Frozen dinners?

Take all that and place everything gently in the garbage bag which you will later throw out or donate. Check your drawers and fridge for any of these fat stimulating and unhealthy things:

- Slim shakes or protein shakes that are loaded with sugars, flavour enhancers, high fructose corn syrup, hydrogenated oils, sugars, and many more nasty ingredients slowing down your weight loss and actually **causing** health problems.

- Protein/energy bars are mostly refined sugars, starches, poorly digestible soy protein, mucous causing whey protein, artificial flavours and preservatives and have no beneficial fibre.

- Rice cakes (fat free or regular) are really just high refined starches with no fibre breaking down immediately into simple sugars raising insulin and promoting fat storage in your body.

- Cookies, pastries, or low sugar/low fat desserts are stock full of artificial sweeteners (fooling your brain into releasing insulin because it senses a lot of sugar when it is not, which stimulates hunger due to all that insulin floating around unused), preservatives, artificial colors, white flour (devoid of all minerals and nutrients which digests into sugars and gets stored as fat), and a host of fat storing chemicals you would rather avoid all together.

- Soft drinks, especially diet soda, are loaded with sugars or artificial sweeteners like NutraSweet or Splenda which fool your brain into releasing huge loads of insulin promoting more hunger, and having huge impacts on your nervous system.

Aspartame releases aspartate during digestion which is an excitatory neurotransmitter used by the brain. Neurotransmitters are amino acids or proteins, and when normal neurotransmitters such as aspartate and glutamate cross this barrier **in excess** such as when one drinks or eats anything with these artificial sweeteners, they will cause poisoning and lead to the death of the nerve cells within the brain and spinal cord. This is because the blood-brain barrier cannot discern the amount that is needed from too much leading to various neurological disorders.

- Refined vegetable oils like canola, corn, soybean, sunflower, safflower or fake oils like Crisco or margarine which stimulate heavy inflammatory responses in the body leading to heart disease, plaque, diabetes, and many more nasty issues (not to mention they are all genetically modified leading to DNA damage).

- Regular or whole grain cereals are touted as healthy breakfast meals when in fact they are sugar bombs filled with inflammatory oils, colors, and artificial flavours leading to fat loss sabotage and disease.

Step 4 – Go to your favorite grocery store and begin your learning process! Go though the fresh food isles on the outside of the store, and avoid the inside of the store, where all the junk is. You now you have the power and freedom of educated choice!

Most Important Steps:

1. Processed foods and additives are your TRUE enemy and are much more important to look out for rather than calories/fats/or carbs. Get rid of as many artificial foods and additives as you can.
2. Eat as much raw food and as little animal food as possible to regain your digestive function, stimulate toxin removal, increase your metabolic rate, improve all organ function, activate fat burning, and begin curing all your so called "incurable" diseases and ailments.
3. Drink a minimum 1.5-2 litres of clean filtered water EVERY DAY to guarantee a smooth and easy way for all your toxins to leave your body ensuring a lightning fast path towards weight loss and health.

4. Supplement with bee pollen, raw milk, raw honey, spirulina/chlorella, raw superfood green powders, and a few good quality vitamins so that your body has all the required nutrients to keep itself healthy (vitamin C, E, D).
5. If your budget allows, try to get as much of your food organic - I know how expensive it can be, but sometimes organic is even cheaper than regular produce. For example in my local grocery store, organic and regular apples cost exactly the same, so I of course grab the organic ones, while some berries are nearly double the price, so I settle for regular non-organic ones. As long as you eat more raw fruits and veggies, be they organic or non-organic, you will have better health.

Superfoods that you absolutely must have in your kitchen.

Bee pollen
Raw milk
Raw butter
Spirulina/Chlorella
Hemp oil/hemp protein/hemp seeds
Spinach/Kale
Coconut Oil
Stevia leaf
Whole food green powder

Many people ask me what I eat, so here is the breakdown of my **very simple** diet.

Breakfast
For breakfast I make myself a large green smoothie with spinach, apple, bee pollen, hemp protein, and some coconut crystals or honey.

Snacks
I snack on all sorts of organic fruits and raw nuts throughout the day without limiting myself or counting calories, fats, carbs or any other nonsense. Apples, bananas, pears, mangoes, papayas, grapes as well as raw almonds, walnuts, pecans etc. and I drink a liter or so of raw organic milk depending on my preference that day.

Lunch
I will make myself a sprouted grain mix with whatever sprouted grains I have. I'll eat this with a large salad full of leafy greens with some hemp oil, hemp seeds, and spices for flavor.

Dinner
A big salad and another green smoothie tops off my dinner.

I also make sure I drink 1.5-2 Liters of water daily, get about 20-30 grams of spirulina and chlorella, 5 grams of vitamin C (regular vitamin C not the Ester C kind), 400-800 IU of vitamin E, and 4000 IU of vitamin D. And I don't eat like this because I have to or force myself to do this; my body has adjusted so that I get all my nutrients without cravings from other foods.

This is a very basic meal plan, but a raw food diet is extremely diverse, you can search on Google for raw food or vegetarian recipes and you will be amazed at the possibilities.

Easy Dietary Additions

These tips are easy additions to your diet, if you get rid of all the junk and start your new diet with these items, you will see changes within your body within the first few days.

- ***50% of your meals have to be raw***. Meaning a salad with all meals and raw unprocessed nuts/fruits/dried fruits/raw food bars as snacks.
- Drink 2 green smoothies daily with hemp protein and a scoop of a whole food green powder.
- In the morning take a teaspoon of **bee pollen** under the tongue and let dissolve, then swallow. Or add it to your smoothies, shakes or salads.
- Drink at least 1.5-2 Litres of **clean filtered water daily** (drink 500 ml or 16oz of water as soon as you wake up).
- Supplement with **minimum** 5-10 grams of spirulina and chlorella each per day, as well as 5 grams of vitamin C (L-ascorbate), 800 IU of vitamin E, and 6000 IU of vitamin D.
- Take a 15 minute walk every day, rain or shine.

7 Steps to Health

Part 2: Illness and Disease Prevention

Introduction

The huge rise of the pharmaceutical industry seen in the last couple of decades should be followed by the reduction of diseases right? Since there are thousands upon thousands of drugs for every possible disease or illness, people should be feeling better, healthier, more vibrant and full of energy, right? You would think so. But the fact is, EVERY SINGLE disease is on the rise EVERY SINGLE year!

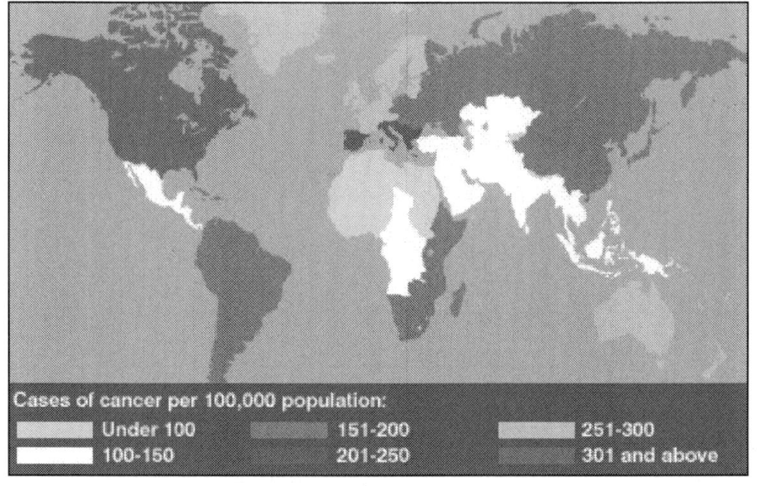

Why do first world countries have the most cancer? Aren't we supposed to have the "best" medical system, the best drugs, and the most advanced surgical procedures?

CHART 1.1: CANCER DEATH RATES (PER 100,000 PEOPLE)[1]

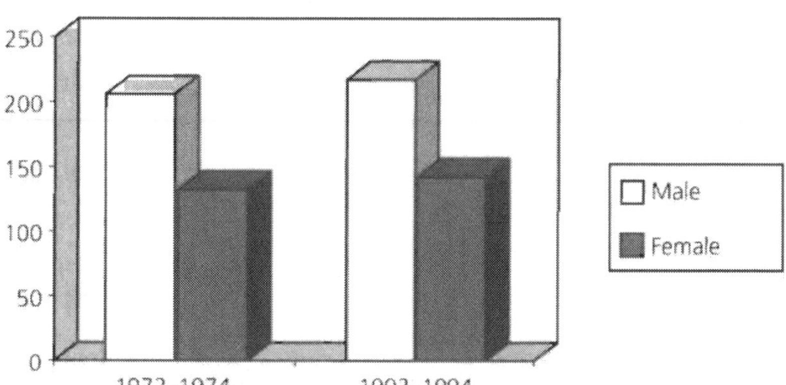

"Nearly half of Americans suffer at least one chronic disease, everything from allergies to heart disease - 20 million more than doctors had anticipated this year, researchers say. "

"In 1947, there were an estimated 600,000 cases of diabetes in the United States.....Today the Metropolitan Life Insurance Co.'s quarterly Statistical Bulletin estimates that diabetics make up 5 percent of the US population, or 13 million persons.......So, while the US population has approximately doubled since the 1940's, the number of diabetics has risen more than 20 times."-- Harris Coulter

These statistics are frightening. We are made to believe that our health care is perfect, that we are curing disease, and that people are becoming healthier. This is a lie. Statistics show a completely different picture; we are very sick and all our advancements in healthcare have absolutely nothing to show for, except for a **rise in every single disease** and even larger increases in drug company profits.

This is not a healthcare system, it is a sick care system. Pharmaceutical companies would hate for you to learn the truth that nearly all of these diseases can be totally reversed and even cured just by diet alone!

Let me remind you that from physician error, medication error, and adverse events from drugs and surgery kill *225,400 people per year*. That makes the ***health care system the third leading cause of death in the United States***, behind only cancer and heart disease.

Leading Causes of Death

Cause of Death	Deaths
Diseases of the Heart	710,760
Cancer (Malignant Neoplasms)	553,091
Medical Care[11]	225,400
Stroke (Cerebrovascular Diseases)	167,661
Chronic Lower Respiratory Diseases	122,009
Accidents	97,900
Diabetes Mellitus	69,301
Influenza and Pneumonia	65,313
Alzheimer's Disease	49,558

Death by Health Care

Number of Americans Per Year Who Die From:	
Medication Errors[13]	7,400
Unnecessary Surgery[14]	12,000
Other Preventable Errors in Hospitals[11]	20,000
Hospital Borne Infections[11]	80,000
Adverse Drug Effects[15]	106,000

The last and largest category of "Adverse Drug Effects" are people who die from unintended and undesired effects of a drug, ***at normal doses.*** Even with the use of approved medication and correct procedures, over one hundred thousand people die every year from the medication that is supposed to be making them healthier. More than 33000 soldiers have died in the war in Iraq since 2003, that means <u>every single year three times more people die from prescription medication than all the American casualties in the Iraqi war</u>. There is a war happening on our own soil.

So why are people becoming sicker and sicker, even with the advancements in healthcare? You must understand that the whole idea of disease eradication is by its very nature incompatible with, and completely opposed to the interests of the pharmaceutical investment industry. The elimination of diseases will eliminate the multibillion dollar profits, and thus destroy the whole industry. Most pharmaceutical companies are publicly traded corporations whose ONLY object is to increase profits. Their sole interest is selling you drugs for your symptoms, so you keep on coming back for more. “Don’t worry, you keep on hitting your finger with that hammer and we’ll keep on selling you more drugs.” They take advantage of peoples’ vulnerabilities and sell you ineffective drugs with so many side effects that you will need a few more kidneys and livers just to deal with these toxic poisons. At best, most drugs just suppress the symptoms of diseases only for a short while. However, because they are making the body do something unnatural, and because they are made from highly poisonous chemicals, they cause other bodily systems to fail causing a snowball effect where more drugs are needed to cope with the side effects of previous drugs and so on.

"*The doctor of the future will give no medicine, but will interest his patients in the care of the human frame, in diet and in the cause and prevention of disease.*"
- Thomas Edison

If you are taking non-prescription over the counter or prescription drugs on a regular basis, and you are under the age of 60, it is a well known fact that these drugs WILL cause you serious medical conditions later on in life. Just read the complications and side effects printout with your medication.

This might seem irresponsible or shocking, but my policy is “just say no” to drugs, the legal and the illegal kind ☺ Let me explain. People around the world believe the myth as told so by the governments and the drug companies’ story tellers that people will be healthier if they take more drugs. As if a correlation exists between health and the amount of drugs that one takes. I don’t remember the last time I took a drug, and I also don’t remember the last time I was sick, for anything. And if I did get sick it would be a fraction of the time most people experience. Am I a good customer for the drug companies? Will you be a good customer if you are healthy, happy, and full of energy? This is why they spend millions upon millions of dollars spreading massive smear campaigns on natural remedies, vitamins, minerals, and the such, that cut into their greedy profits.

"...he cited a rural Maryland physician's lament about his diabetic patient, an overweight farmer whose insurance pays for a 20-minute visit, just enough time to test his blood sugar and adjust medication. The doctor says helping the man lose weight would do more good, but **he is not paid to do that**." *Chronic Illness Burden Rising Faster Than Expected,* The Associated Press

Doctors are trained to treat symptoms of disease, not the disease itself. Here is something to think about; there has not been a pharmaceutical drug that has ever cured a disease (cured meaning it is gone forever, forgotten, and nobody needs to take any drugs or have surgery for that disease ever again).Can you find one?

"The top 10 drug companies are reported to have profits averaging about 30 percent of revenues-a stunning margin. Over the past few years, the pharmaceutical industry as a whole has been by far the most profitable industry in the United States."
-Angell M, "The Pharmaceutical Industry-To Whom Is It Accountable?" New England Journal of Medicine, June 22, 2000.

"In every year since 1982, the drug industry has been the most profitable in the United States, according to Fortune magazine's rankings. During this time, the drug industry's returns on revenue (profit as a percent of sales) have averaged about three times the average for all other industries represented in the Fortune 500."
-Public Citizen Report, "Rx R&D Myths: The Case Against the Drug Industry's R&D 'Scare Card," July 23, 2001.

"Put together, the market capitalization of the four largest [pharmaceutical] companies is more than the economy of India." David Earnshaw, formerly director of European government affairs for SmithKline Beecham, now leader of Oxfam's campaign on access to medicines.
-Quoted in Roger Dobson, "Drug Company lobbyist joins Oxfam's cheap drugs campaign," BMJ, 322, April 28, 2001, p. 1011.

Legendary economist Paul Zane Pilzer has written, "What we call the 'health care' business is really the sickness business. The $1.4 trillion we spend on medical care is concerned with treating the symptoms of sickness. It has very little to do with being stronger or healthier." Pilzer predicts that wellness is destined to become a trillion dollar industry.

Think about it, if your doctor has, let's say, 300 patients, and they all become healthy – nobody is coming into his office anymore, his is broke! What incentive does he have to keep you healthy? None! This may sound a little harsh but even the hands of the good doctors are tied, because even if they do know some alternative treatment, they can only prescribe drugs and surgery or risk losing their license, being sued, ridiculed, or thrown out of high job positions, as many honest doctors already have been.

A *cured* patient is a lost source of income. A sick patient who is marginally "improved" is a *manageable* patient.

"This guy's doctor told him he had six months to live. The guy said he couldn't pay his bill. The doctor gave him another six months."

- Henry Youngman

Managing patients means routine office visits and renewing of drug prescriptions. Therefore, a manageable patient is a continuing source of income; a cash cow if you will. Multiply that by a few hundred million people and you get an idea why this deceit is being put upon you. The profits from the so called "health-care" industry are staggering!

The thrust of the orthodox pharmaceutical agenda is to provide **temporary relief**, while never addressing the **cause** of the disease condition. This agenda insures regular visits to the doctor's office and requires the patient to routinely return to the pharmacy to refill his prescriptions. This is what the game is all about folks, plain and simple. Deny it, or understand how the system works and get healthy, it's your choice.

Medical Mafia

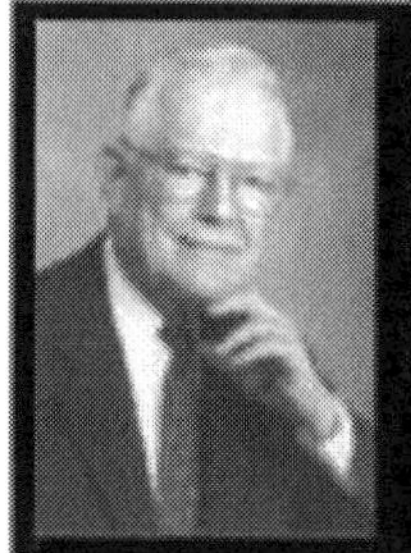

"We have a multi-billion dollar industry that is killing people, right and left, just for financial gain. Their idea of research is to see whether two doses of this poison is better than three doses of that poison."

Glenn A. Warner, M.D.

"People think the FDA is protecting them. It isn't. What the FDA is doing and what the public thinks it's doing are as different as night and day."
Former commissioner of the FDA, Dr Herbert Ley, in testimony before a US Senate hearing. (This doesn't just apply to the United States; the multi-billion dollar drug companies have their grasp on every country in the world)

A large part of this medical disaster that the United States currently experiences is due to the way our medical community is organized. Basically it is not organized to heal and to cure disease; the medical community, particularly at its upper levels, is a commercial venture organized to make money for its practitioners. The Cardiac surgeon, for example, does nothing whatsoever to cure cardiac disease. Three to five percent of the heart surgery patients die on the operating table. **Cardiac surgery provides no better three year survival rate than no treatment at all.** ***A Harvard survival study of 200,000 patients revealed that the long term survival rate of patients subjected to surgery was no better than the survival rate of those that had no surgery.*** --- GANGSTERS IN MEDICINE By Thomas Smith

"We've got a network of evil in this country that we can't hide from any longer."

Dr. John Yiamouyiannis
(Fluoride the Aging Factor)

Dangers of Pharmaceutical Drugs

"Modern medicine is not a science and modern clinicians and medical researchers are not scientists. Modern clinicians may use scientific techniques but in the way that they treat their patients they are still quacks......Medicine is no longer an independent profession. Doctors have become nothing more than a link connecting the pharmaceutical industry to the consumer."

Dr Vernon Coleman

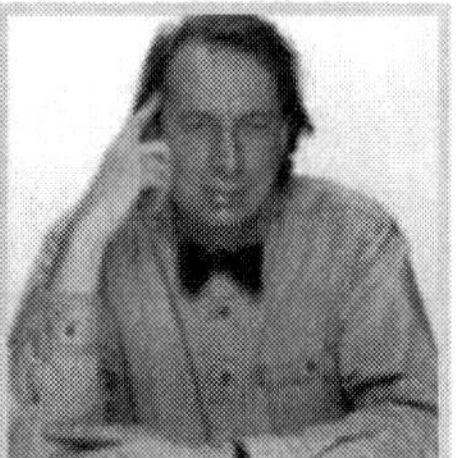

"They are running a monopoly and they will lie, cheat and steal to keep it that way."
--- Dr Eva Snead

Did You Know?

"Pfizer Pays $2.3 Billion to Settle Marketing Case - WASHINGTON — The pharmaceutical giant Pfizer agreed to pay $2.3 billion to settle civil and criminal allegations that it had illegally marketed its painkiller Bextra, which has been withdrawn. It was the largest health care fraud settlement and the **largest criminal fine of any kind, ever**." – New York Times, September 2, 2009

'The whole culture of Pfizer is driven by sales, and if you didn't sell drugs illegally, you were not seen as a team player,' said Mr. Kopchinski. Also, per ABC News, 'At Pfizer, I was expected to increase profits at all costs, even when sales meant endangering lives,' Kopchinski said, in a statement. 'I couldn't do that.'

"Statistics prove prescription drugs are 16,400% more deadly than terrorists"

A tragedy happened on September 11th which will be remembered for the time to come. 2996 people lost their lives and thousands more injured as four commercial airlines crashed that day. But what if six jumbo jets crashed every single day for a year totaling 783,936 deaths every year in the United States? Wouldn't that be a cause for concern, some grounds on which to look over the airline industry, a valid reason to inspect airplanes or maybe totally get rid of them?

Well, according to the groundbreaking 2003 medical report Death by Medicine, by Drs. Gary Null, Carolyn Dean, Martin Feldman, Debora Rasio and Dorothy Smith, 783,936 people in the United States die every year from conventional medicine mistakes. 106,000 of those are from properly prescribed prescription drugs, according to Death by Medicine. That also is a conservative number. Some experts estimate it should be more like 200,000 because of unreported cases of adverse drug reactions. That's three times deadlier than automobile fatalities.

This makes prescription drug death the fourth leading killer after heart disease, cancer and stroke. Look at these numbers more carefully, that's about 300 deaths **per day** from regular prescription drugs, yet when an airplane crashes it gets more media attention and governmental scrutiny than the 300 medication-related deaths which occurred not only on the same day as the airline crash, but also every day before and after for decades.

"Prescription drugs...account for more deaths each year than all murders, auto accidents and airplane crashes combined. It is estimated that 100,000 people die every year from the adverse effects of prescription drugs, and 1 million are injured so severely they require hospitalization." **Thomas Moore**, "*Prescription drug risks are too high*" The Miami Herald, April 12, 1998, p. 6L.

"It has been estimated that fatalities directly attributable to adverse drug reactions are the fourth to sixth leading cause of death in US hospitals, exceeding deaths caused by pneumonia and diabetes. The economic burden resulting from drug-related morbidity and mortality is equally significant and has been conservatively estimated at $US30 billion dollars annually, and could exceed $US130 billion in a worst-case scenario." **White TJ, Araakelian A, Rho JP**, "*Counting the costs of drug-related adverse events*" Pharmacoeconomics, 15(5): 445-58, May 1999.

"David Lawrence, CEO of Kaiser Permanente, the nation's oldest HMO, calls medication errors 'the number one public health risk in the United States, ahead of tobacco, alcohol, [illegal] drugs, or guns." **Ted Sandoval**, "*Cutting Medication Errors Requires Proactive Steps*" Web MD, Medcast, June 20, 2000.

All drugs have negative side effects, even aspirin. However, prescription drugs have far more potentially dangerous side effects than do over-the-counter medications. Most people who take these drugs according to their physicians' directions do not experience serious side effects, but some do. Some people have severe allergic reactions, some suffer heart attacks or seizures, and some experience organ damage because of the prescription drugs they take. One of the most common serious drug problems is liver damage because most medicines taken by mouth are ultimately processed through the liver.

In addition to the negative side effects induced by individual drugs, some drugs interact negatively with certain foods or with other drugs.

"With so many people on so many pills, small wonder that part of the increase in healthcare costs is illness caused by drug interactions. A Queen's University study of seniors' medication released in January, for example, found that in 96% of cases studied, doctors' knowledge of their patients' medication use was inaccurate. On average, the patients had a daily dose of seven medications." **Candis McLean**, "*The real drug pushers*," Report Newsmagazine, March 19, 2001.

Another factor involved in the large number of people killed or made ill by prescription drugs are medication errors, and the primary reason for medication errors can be traced to the sheer number of prescription drugs on the market.

"There are currently more than 17,000 trade and generic names for drugs in the United States, according to the Institute for Safe Medication Practices in Huntingdon Valley, Pa. The organization also estimates that the number of drugs on the U.S. market has grown 500% in the last decade." Braus P, "*Want to avoid drug errors? New software can help*," **American College of Physicians-American Society of Internal Medicine Observer**, April 2001.

"Baycol is the 12th prescription drug to have been taken off the U.S. market because of dangerous side effects since 1997. Some critics said many of those bans happened because the FDA, under political pressure, had sped up drug approvals during the 1990s. Baycol was not a 'fast-track' drug: The agency spent 11 months reviewing it before approving it in 1997." "*Bayer Pharmaceutical's Cholesterol-Lowering Drug Baycol Linked to Deaths, Pulled Off Market,*" **AP**, Aug. 8, 2001. One of the statin drugs, Baycol destroyed muscle tissue and was linked to 31 deaths in the U.S. and 9 abroad.

"Rezulin [a diabetes drug] was taken out of pharmacies and off the market. But by then it was linked to 63 deaths from liver failure." "*FDA: Guardian Or Rubber Stamp?*" **CBS Evening News**, July 12, 2001.

After FDA approval, it was discovered that Glaxo Wellcome's flu medication Zanamivir could be dangerous for patients with underlying respiratory diseases such as asthma or other chronic pulmonary illness. After some deaths were reported, the FDA issued a warning and required labeling changes for the drug.

The Food and Drug Administration (FDA) estimates that Vioxx may have contributed to 27,785 heart attacks and sudden cardiac deaths between 1999 and 2003. Merck pulled Vioxx, a popular pain reliever widely used by arthritis patients, off the market, saying it was "putting patient safety first" but the Wall Street Journal reported earlier that company officials had **fought for years to protect the highly profitable drug and to keep news of the health risks quiet**. Vioxx was a big moneymaker for Merck, generating about $2.5 billion in yearly sales. That's 2.6 times more deaths in half the time than soldier casualties in the whole 8 years of the war in Iraq.

The reported adverse effects of drugs are only the tip of the iceberg. Consider 'Digoxin', the best-selling heart drug. According to an article in JAMA, the Food and Drug Administration (FDA) receives about 82 reports each year involving Digoxin, yet a systematic study of Medicare records reveals 202,211 hospitalizations for Digoxin adverse effects in a 7-year period (Moore, "Time to act on drug safety," p. 57). That's more than 28,000 reactions per year, 82 of which the Food and Drug Administration (FDA) hears about.

As bad as some of the manipulations of clinical trials and study data and published clinical reports are, none approach the sheer immorality of some of the drug companies' clinical trials conducted in developing countries. Test subjects in developed countries today are legally protected against abuse, but protective laws in some poorer countries are more lax and are not as rigidly enforced.

"An investigation into corporate drug experiments in Africa, Asia, Eastern Europe and Latin America reveals a booming, poorly regulated system in which experiments involving risky drugs proceed with little independent oversight, and impoverished, poorly educated patients are sometimes tested without understanding that they are guinea pigs. These foreign trials speed new drugs to the marketplace-where they are often sold mainly to patients in wealthy countries." Joe Stephens, "Testing drugs: Overseas trials lack oversight: Companies target patients in poor nations," The Miami Herald, Jan 7, 2001, p. 1L.

"'We're colonizing a region for clinical trials' declared Juan Pablo Guzman, who has worked on clinical trials in Latin America for Searle and Pharmacia, at June's annual meeting of the Drug Information Association in San Diego. 'We have to believe there is gold at the end of the journey.'" "*Latin America is fertile ground for experiments*," **The Miami Herald**, Jan 7, 2001, p. 3L.

In one such instance, researchers for Pfizer clinically tested what the company believed to be a promising new antibiotic on Nigerian children who had fallen victim to the country's meningitis epidemic. Among the 200 test subjects, 11 died and others suffered meningitis-related symptoms such as seizures, blindness, deafness, and lameness. The drug being tested, orally-administered Trovan, had never been approved or tested for use with children, and chemically similar drugs had caused joint damage in animal experiments. According to an article in the Miami Herald, Pfizer's own internal report showed children died shortly after taking oral Trovan.

"The experiment's final report concluded that Trovan and the comparison drug were equally safe and effective." Joe Stephens, "Testing drugs: Overseas trials lack oversight," The Miami Herald, Jan. 7, 2001. But of course many of the sick and dying in these countries will never be able to afford treatment with the successful drugs once they are approved as safe and efficacious by the FDA.

10 prescription drugs withdrawn from the market since 1997

These drugs were taken off the market because of serious, often lethal side effects.

Rezulin: Given fast-track approval by the Food and Drug Administration (FDA), Rezulin was linked to 63 confirmed deaths and probably hundreds more. "We have real trouble," a Food and Drug Administration (FDA) physician wrote in 1997, just a few months after Rezulin's approval. The drug wasn't taken off the market until 2000.

Lotronex: Against concerns of one of its own officers, the Food and Drug Administration (FDA) approved Lotronex in February 2000. By the time it was withdrawn 9 months later, the Food and Drug Administration (FDA) had received reports of 93 hospitalizations, multiple emergency bowel surgeries, and 5 deaths.

Propulsid: A top-selling drug for many years, this drug was linked to hundreds of cases of heart arrhythmias and over 100 deaths.

Redux: Taken by millions of people for weight loss after its approval in April 1996, Redux was soon linked to heart valve damage and a disabling, often lethal pulmonary disorder. Taken off the market in September 1997.

Pondimin: A component of Fen-Phen, the diet fad drug. Approved in 1973, Pondimin's link to heart valve damage and a lethal pulmonary disorder wasn't recognized until shortly before its withdrawal in 1997.

Duract: This painkiller was taken off the market when it was linked to severe, sometimes fatal liver failure.

Seldane: America's and the world's top-selling antihistamine for a decade, it took the Food and Drug Administration (FDA) 5 years to recognize that Seldane was causing cardiac arrhythmias, blackouts, hospitalizations, and deaths, and another 8 years to take it off the market.

Hismanal: Approved in 1988 and soon known to cause cardiac arrhythmias, the drug was finally taken off the market in 1999.

Posicor: Used to treat hypertension, the drug was linked to life-threatening drug interactions and more than 100 deaths.

Raxar: Linked to cardiac toxicities and deaths.

"1935 The Pellagra Incident. After millions of individuals die from Pellagra over a span of two decades, the U.S. Public Health Service finally acts to stem the disease. The director of the agency admits it had known for at least 20 years that Pellagra is caused by a niacin deficiency but failed to act since most of the deaths occured within poverty-stricken black populations."---A History Of US Secret Human Experimentation

A Bit of History

This process is nothing new. Former FDA Commissioner James L. Goddard, in a **1966** speech before the Pharmaceutical Manufacturers Association, expressed concern about **dishonesty in testing** new drugs. He said:

"I have been shocked at the materials that come in. In addition to the problem of quality, there is the problem of dishonesty in the investigational new drug usage. I will admit there are gray areas in the IND [Investigation of New Drug] situation, but the conscious withholding of unfavorable animal clinical data is not a gray area. The deliberate choice of clinical investigators known to be more concerned about industry friendships than in developing good data is not a gray area."

Goddard's successor at the FDA was Dr. Herbert Ley. In 1969, he testified before the Senate committee and described several cases of **blatant dishonesty** in drug testing. One case involved an assistant professor of medicine who had tested **24 drugs for 9 different companies**. Dr. Ley said:

"Patients who died while on clinical trials were not reported to the sponsor... Dead people were listed as subjects of testing. Your Guide to Gentle, Non-toxic Healing People reported as subjects of testing were not in the hospital at the time of the tests. Patient consent forms bore dates indicating they were signed after the subjects died."

Another case involved a **commercial drug-testing firm** that had worked on 82 drugs from 28 companies. Dr. Ley continued:

"Patients who died, left the hospital, or dropped out of the study were replaced by other patients in the tests without notification in the records. Forty-one patients reported as participating in studies were dead or not in the hospital during the studies... Record-keeping, supervision and observation of the patients in general were grossly inadequate."

Maintaining the High Cost of Medicines

It is evident that giant multinational pharmaceutical companies are doing everything in their power to maintain the high costs of their products, even when those costs mean that essential drugs will not be available to the poor or the elderly with low incomes.

"Using big money, creative court challenges and a regulatory system prone to delays, the nation's leading manufacturers of brand-name drugs are fighting harder than ever to keep cheaper generic imitations off the market.... Generic drug makers have at times enriched themselves by keeping their products off the market, deliberately, in exchange for payments from patented drug companies." Greg Fields, "Brand-name drug makers' tactics slow generics," The Miami Herald, Aug. 17, 2000, p. A1.

According to Public Citizen Magazine, the big drug companies are charging these seniors twice as much on average as the companies charge their most favored customers such as HMOs and the Departments of Veterans Affairs and Defense. Public Citizen claims that the mark-up for Medicare outpatients for Merck's high cholesterol drug Zocor is 144%. The organization says that the mark-up for Pharmacia's diabetes medication Micronase is a whopping 363%, and that Abbot Laboratories' hormone treatment Synthroid is even worse at an incredible 1,446%.

The current belief in the United States is that taxpayers have to assume some of the burden of drugs. Through the government health programs your tax dollars pay for some of the drugs. However, the taxpayers **have already paid for the basic research to develop many of these drugs and have even paid for some of the clinical trials!** Remember folks, it is us who pays for the research and development of the drugs (not the cures, but patentable medication from which a profit can be made), then pays for the clinical trials, and then pays for the drug itself! Absurdity beyond belief. These "institutes" which collect donations to find "cures" for heart disease, diabetes, cancer etc. have no other goal but to find a patentable drug which they can market and make huge profits.

Sharon Davis and Mary Palmer of the US Department of Commerce did some research on the actual cost of drugs. They looked at offshore chemical synthesizers that supply the active ingredients found in drugs approved by the FDA. As they have revealed, a significant percentage of drugs sold in the United State contain active ingredients made in other countries.

They obtained the actual price of active ingredients used in some of the most popular drugs sold in America. The chart below speaks for itself.

Celebrex 100 mg
Consumer price (100 tablets): $130.27
Cost of general active ingredients: $0.60
Percent markup: 21,712%

Claritin 10 mg
Consumer Price (100 tablets): $215.17
Cost of general active ingredients: $0.71
Percent markup: 30,306%

Keflex 250 mg
Consumer Price (100 tablets): $157.39
Cost of general active ingredients: $1.88
Percent markup: 8,372%

Lipitor 20 mg
Consumer Price (100 tablets): $272.37
Cost of general active ingredients: $5.80
Percent markup: 4,696%

Norvasec 10 mg
Consumer price (100 tablets): $188.29
Cost of general active ingredients: $0.14
Percent markup: **134,493%**

Paxil 20 mg
Consumer price (100 tablets): $220.27
Cost of general active ingredients: $7.60
Percent markup: 2,898%

Prevacid 30 mg
Consumer price (100 tablets): $44.77
Cost of general active ingredients: $1.01
Percent markup: 34,136%

Prilosec 20 mg
Consumer price (100 tablets): $360.97
Cost of general active ingredients $0.52
Percent markup: 69,417%

Tenormin 50 mg
Consumer price (100 tablets): $104.47
Cost of general active ingredients: $0.13
Percent markup: 80,362%

Vasotec 10 mg
Consumer price (100 tablets): $102.37
Cost of general active ingredients: $0.20
Percent markup: 51,185%

Xanax 1 mg
Consumer price (100 tablets) : $136.79
Cost of general active ingredients: $0.024
Percent markup: 569,958%

Zestril 20 mg
Consumer price (100 tablets) $89.89
Cost of general active ingredients $3.20
Percent markup: 2,809%

Zithromax 600 mg
Consumer price (100 tablets): $1,482.19
Cost of general active ingredients: $18.78
Percent markup: 7,892%

Zocor 40 mg
Consumer price (100 tablets): $350.27
Cost of general active ingredients: $8.63
Percent markup: 4,059%

Zoloft 50 mg
Consumer price: $206.87
Cost of general active ingredients: $1.75
Percent markup: 11,821%

Prozac 20 mg
Consumer price (100 tablets) : $247.47
Cost of general active ingredients: $0.11
Percent markup: 224,973%

This is extortion folks.

Clinical Trials

Let's look at these so called "scientific studies" which drug companies use to push their drugs or discredit natural remedies. The fact is that studies are funded by someone, and are commissioned for a specific reason. They are either requested to prove something works or to prove that something doesn't work. Studies are never commissioned to find the truth. They are paid for to give a specific and preplanned result. Drug companies have specific ways in which they organize studies.

First, they produce secret studies to get some preliminary information on how to conduct the final study that will give them the required result. These preliminary studies are never released to the public and are only done to find the best way to organize the final study to give the drug companies the desired end result. Drug companies fund 99% of all studies, directly or indirectly. To hide the fact that a drug company is funding a particular study, sometimes the funding is 10 times removed! By channeling money through smaller companies, groups, foundations, and institutes the study seems like it is honest and truthful. These studies that produce results and supposedly "prove" that a particular drug is safe and effective are completely false and misleading!

For example, first they run studies to find out what kind of person has the least adverse reaction to their new drug, or no reaction at all. Then they test various doses of the drug to figure out one that has the least side effects. Let's say they find that 45 year old physically fit healthy females are the least prone to side effects. In their final study they then recruit only 45 year old physically fit healthy females, and get their desired end result.

If you were a dishonest crook whose only motive was money, and you were funding a study to prove the effectiveness of your product. Wouldn't you try absolutely everything to get the desired results? Especially if billions of dollars were at stake?

"I always use one thing that really points out the fact, which is that, once the FDA approves the medication or a drug for use by the general public, they know less than half of the serious adverse drug reactions when that drug is released. It is just impossible to know them all. Well, they find out, and the next question should be, "How do they find out the others?" Well, it's owing to you, the public, or what is called, "the great clinical trial." It is you who finds out. You are the guinea pig.

You might be wondering why such a small amount of drugs get taken off the market even though there are so many deaths.

“It is a voluntary reporting system. Less than one percent of these adverse drug reactions are really reported back to the FDA, because doctors and hospitals are not required to report them back. It is voluntary. Then, it is reported to a committee in the FDA that has no authority. Once enough of these red flags come in on a drug, then they'll send it back to the original committee that approved the drug in the first place. I do not feel that they have an unbiased representation when they look at this. That’s why over 99 percent of the time all that happens is a change to the drug label or what we call a package insert. This usually goes unnoticed even if they send out a "dear doctor" letter warning doctors about these drugs, and that they better be careful here. There have been studies that show doctors don’t pay much attention to that. So it’s not a very good system.”
Dr. Ray Strand

This means that a small fraction of the side effects ever get reported and if they do, not much actually happens. It takes a few severe drug reactions or deaths to raise any concerns. And if any serious reactions do get noticed, all that happens is a change in the drug label, with a few more side effects added to the list.

Remember the fact that drug companies routinely and frequently fund studies to prove that their competing products are ineffective and unsafe. Drug companies, directly or indirectly, fund hundreds of secret preliminary studies on natural remedies to organize a “final study” that proves a particular remedy is unsafe and/or ineffective. The public never hears about these preliminary studies and most of the time does not know that the funding comes directly from the drug companies themselves! Then you see a news report stating that a certain remedy has been scientifically “proven” to be unsafe and ineffective and that is a blatant lie, a deception and falsehood. The few genuine independent real studies or observations and experiences from doctors and patients around the world are completely ignored.

The final studies are usually done on healthy individuals and many times not even in the age category the drug is marketed for! For example, a clinical trial might over-select young, healthy subjects when the drug being tested is intended for use primarily on older patients.

"Rochon et al. found that only 2.1 percent of subjects in trials of nonsteroidal anti-inflammatory drugs were 65 years of age or older, even though these drugs are more commonly used and have a higher incidence of side effects in the elderly." Bodenheimer T, "Uneasy Alliance-Clinical Investigators and the Pharmaceutical Industry," New England Journal of Medicine, 342(20), May 18, 2000.

Critics of the FDA point out the agency's close ties to the big drug companies as one of the problems in the drug approval process. A USA Today report found that more than half the advisors to the FDA have "financial relationships" with drug companies that have an interest in FDA decisions (De Angelis C, "Conflict of Interest and the Public Trust," JAMA, Nov 1, 2000). But even if panel members involved in approving a drug are scrupulously honest, they still depend on data from that company's clinical trials to approve the drug as safe and efficacious, and the data can be misleading.

"Efforts by drug companies to suppress, spin, and obfuscate findings that do not suit their commercial purposes were first revealed to their full, lethal extent during the thalidomide tragedy. Although government drug regulation schemes around the world are now in place, the insidious tactics of Big Pharma have changed little." "The Tightening Grip of Big Pharmaceutical Companies," Editorial, The Lancet, April 14, 2001.

In comparison trials, the drug being tested might show that it is more effective than the drug it is being compared with simply because higher dosages of the new drug were administered. And, since the data from the trials are generally housed and often analyzed by the drug companies themselves, unfavorable results can be suppressed or long-term data showing negative effects might be removed completely.

The highly advertised (and expensive) anti-inflammatory drug Celebrex was hailed by an article in the Journal of the American Medical Association as vastly superior to existing (and far less expensive) anti-inflammatory drugs such as aspirin and Ibuprofen (Motrin and Advil) because it eliminated the problem of gastric bleeding associated with these drugs. However, researchers at the Therapeutics Initiative in Canada discovered that the study's authors had cut the trial data off at six months. The longer-term results showed that Celebrex was also associated with gastric bleeding, but that it just took longer for these side effects to manifest themselves. The FDA had concluded that there were no major differences between Celebrex and the existing medications, but the published study in JAMA left out the longer-term data.

"Perhaps even more importantly, the [Therapeutics Initiative] report suggests significant safety concerns. 'Any benefit in serious gastrointestinal side effects appear to be cancelled by increased cardiovascular events, including heart attacks, clotting, hypertension and heart failure,' Dr. Wright [director of TI] declares. Celebrex may be 'trading off a decreased chance of stomach ache and ulcer for potentially serious cardiovascular problems.'" Candis McLean, "The real drug pushers," Report Newsmagazine, March 19, 2001.

Given so many potential hazards-from prescription errors to life-threatening side effects, it is clear that pharmaceutical products can kill. Nevertheless, most people naïvely continue to believe that FDA approval means a drug has been thoroughly tested and is safe for them to use.

A study published in the Journal of the American Medical Association (January 22, 2003;289:454-465) found that scientific studies funded by an industry-related source are close to **four** times more likely to yield results that favor the industry than those sponsored by independent sources. Researchers analyzed data from eight individual articles that had addressed the association between industry sponsorship and research outcome. They combined data from these studies, which together amounted to 1,140 original studies, in order to reach a conclusion that may be more reliable than the original studies alone.

Unwanted Results are not Published

Results showed that industry-sponsored studies were **3.6** times more likely to have results that favored the industry than studies with no financial ties to the industry. Drug companies *publish* only a fraction of the studies they fund -- the ones that *promote their drugs*. If a study does not have findings that are favorable to its product, it is unlikely it will ever make it into a journal for publication.

There are simply thousands of scientific studies out there that have never been seen by you or your physician because they have been screened out by editors and reviewers who are being paid to uphold an industry agenda.

Published studies overwhelmingly favor the funding company's drug. Whichever drug is manufactured by the study sponsor is the drug that comes out on top, *90 percent of the time!*

Selectively omitting negative results from clinical trials can actually be deadly to your health. Merck & Co. proved this statement when during clinical trials of their Vioxx drug they concealed the fact that three patients suffered heart attacks. They conveniently omitted this data (along with other relevant findings) from the copy of the study they submitted to the *New England Journal of Medicine* for publication. The omissions were uncovered years later during the 7,000 Vioxx lawsuit litigations.

Favorable Studies Submitted Multiple Times

If a clinical study shows positive results it is often submitted multiple times in such a way that the reader doesn't realize it's the same study, hidden by different authors and details. Analyzers have had to look very carefully to determine which studies are actually duplicates because they are so cleverly disguised.

Trials that showed greater treatment effectiveness were significantly more likely to be duplicated. In one analysis of published reports about ondansetron (an anti-nausea drug), the same study was published 5 times. This duplication of data led to a 23 percent overestimation of ondansetron's effectiveness when a meta-analysis was performed!

In addition, the editorials that follow a study are submitted by so-called "unbiased" experts and then published in reputable journals. Contrary to popular belief they are often done by non-neutral parties who have a financial tie to the drug maker.

Dr. Golomb, a professor at UC San Diego, gives an example of a trial on calcium channel blockers (a type of heart medication). The connection between authors declaring their support for calcium channel blockers and those not in support of them was highly statistically tied to their relationship with the drug manufacturer - in fact, the odds that their opinion was NOT due to their affiliation was more than 1,000:1. In other words, if the author of a drug study is on the drug manufacturers payroll then they are 1000 times more likely to praise the drug than someone who is not paid by the drug manufacturer. And here we are thinking all these scientists are unbiased and have the good of the people at heart.

Ghostwriting

What you are about to read is quite sobering. Many of the articles that you may find in medical journals supposedly written by well-known academics are actually written by unacknowledged ghostwriters on Big Pharma's payroll. Ghostwriters are paid individuals who sign their name while having no actual relation to that document which they sign.

Writing in the UK Guardian on Thursday, 7th February, 2002, senior health editor Sarah Bosely reports that: *"Scientists are accepting large sums of money from drug companies to put their names to articles endorsing new medicines that they have not written - a growing practice that some fear is putting scientific integrity in jeopardy."*
Consider the example of Parke-Davis and their drug Neurontin. Parke-Davis contracted with a "medical education communication company," or MECC, which is a company paid almost exclusively by pharmaceutical companies to write articles, reviews, and letters to editors of medical journals to cast their products in a favorable light.

In this case, MECC was paid $13,000 to $18,000 per article. In turn, MECC paid $1,000 each to friendly physicians and pharmacists to sign off as authors of the articles, *making the material appear independent.*

"The medical journals have enormous influence on which drugs doctors prescribe and the treatment hospitals provide. It has been revealed that hundreds of journals were never written by doctors but by ghostwriters, who the pharmaceutical companies hire.

By lending their name and reputation on the journals, the doctors can get paid a well-off amount of money while the ghostwriters remain hidden."
The Guardian, December, 7 2003

This strategy was used by Pfizer for marketing Zoloft. A document was written that included 81 different articles promoting Zoloft's usefulness for everything from panic disorder to pedophilia.

There was a problem however, for some of those articles the name of the author was listed as "to be determined," even though the article was listed as already completed. The truth was that Pfizer wrote the article, and then shopped around for scientists willing to claim authorship, to give it an image of credibility. These big corporations do whatever they want and sell you whatever they want; nobody is looking out for you, you MUST take care of *yourself.*

In 2004, Dr. Richard Horton, editor of *the Lancet*, wrote, "Journals have devolved into information-laundering operations for the pharmaceutical industry." Three editors, who agreed to discuss finances only if they remained anonymous, said a few journals that previously measured annual profits in the tens of thousands of dollars now make millions annually. Merck also went as far as publish a completely fake journal in 2003. (Merck paid medical journal publisher company Elsevier [whose CEO Sir Crispin Davis sits on GlaxoSmithKline's board] to publish a fake medical journal with articles favorable to Merck's drugs: [Bob Grant - The Scientist - 30th April 2009])

Drug maker Wyeth flooded medical journals with some 40 ghostwritten articles authored by prominent physicians who sold their name for cash, in an all-out effort to offset the scientific evidence linking its female hormone replacement drug, Prempro, to breast cancer.

"LITTLE ROCK, Ark. (AP) — A federal judge has ordered the unsealing of thousands of pages of documents pertaining to the ghostwriting practices of Wyeth Pharmaceuticals, which is being sued over hormone replacement drugs." -July 25, 2009 By The Associated Press

The structures goes something like this; studies are financed by Big Pharma (sometimes even by you when you donate your hard earned savings to some corrupt medical organization that is supposedly still looking for "the cure"), trials are carried out by Big Pharma, results are manipulated by Big Pharma, studies published in journals are funded by Big Pharma thus showing only the results they want, doctors are brainwashed into prescribing drugs sold by Big Pharma, then you pay for these poisons, and in the end everyone is left feeling sicker and unhealthier. If this isn't insanity then I don't know what is.

These supposed guardians of our health are being paid what to say. One physician said, *"What day is it today? I'm just working out what drug I'm supporting today."* From top to bottom, the delivery system of 21st century conventional healthcare is being bought out.

And so it goes on. And all the while, the mortality statistics worsen. Yet still, the money - your money - just keeps filling the pockets of Big Pharma. On that note, The Campaign Against Fraudulent Medical Research states: *"The next time you are asked to donate to a cancer organization, bear in mind that your money will be used to sustain an industry which has been deemed by many eminent scientists as a qualified failure and by others, as a complete fraud."*

What Happens to Those Who Speak Out?

Intimidating phone calls, direct threats, loss of funding, bans from organizations, loss of licenses, ridicule etc.

In one case, Dr. Buse, an endocrinologist who is the incoming president of the American Diabetes Association, presented data in 1999 about his concerns about the risks of Avandia. Dr. Buse was intimidated with multiple phone calls by drug company officials. They suggested he could be financially liable to the company for $4 billion in lost revenues due to his "unscrupulous remarks."

Court evidence now available on-line at the University of California library shows drug giant Merck systematically targeted "hit-lists" of doctors in order to discredit, neutralize, ridicule, or destroy the critics who spoke out against the safety and effectiveness of Merck's drugs.

The methods used to do this included threatening to cut research funding and attempting to block academic appointments. Remember, drug companies do not want to save lives and will do anything to stop a whistleblower from telling the truth, even if it's a doctor or scientist.

One memo from a drug company stated: "we may need to seek them out and destroy them where they live…."

Dr Andrew Wakefield said when interviewed by CBS:- *"This is not conspiracy. This is corporate policy."* – [CBS News – Research Links Kids Vaccines & Brain Damage - October 9, 2009 childhealthsafety].

Loss of jobs and reputation, even death threats are a normal occurrence to truth seekers and whistleblowers. They don't want anyone messing

"Since the 1920s, virtually all continuing medical and public health education is funded by pharmaceutical companies. In fact, today, the FDA can't even tell health scientists the truth about vaccine contaminants and their likely effects. **The agency is bound and gagged by proprietary laws and non-disclosure agreements forced upon them by the pharmaceutical industry**. Let us not forget that the pharmaceutical industry, as a special interest group, is the number one contributor to politicians on Capital Hill."--Leonard Horowitz

"Since vaccine development information is considered proprietary (protected by nondisclosure policies) government officials and researchers must **shield potential safety issues from public scrutiny**. This censorship is rationalized by the all too persuasive argument that vaccines cannot be criticized lest the public become non-compliant in taking them. Finally, this silence is buttressed by the small number of people capable of critically evaluating vaccine manufacturing and safety testing procedures. In essence, health care professionals and the general public know little about the possible dangers of live viral vaccines."--Dr Martin

Too Big to Nail

Drug companies these days are almost completely safe from any prosecution for their crimes or wrongdoings. A CNN report from April 2, 2010 reveals the truth about how shielded these huge drug companies really are.

For example, the world's largest pharmaceutical company Pfizer engaged in illegal promotion of their drug Bextra for off-label use, even though they knew it was associated with an increased risk of stroke and heart attacks. In 2005 it was pulled from the market but not before many people were damaged by its use.

Federal prosecutors quickly realized that convicting Pfizer would be a corporate death sentence since any company convicted of major health care fraud is excluded from Medicare and Medicaid. So they cut Pfizer a deal. Just as the big banks on Wall Street were deemed "too big to fail," Pfizer was deemed "too big to nail."

Prosecutors claimed the financial losses to shareholders and job losses by Pfizer would be too great from being excluded from the Medicare/Medicaid programs. Prosecutors then went ahead and charged a Pfizer subsidiary Pharmacia & Upjohn Co. instead (this company was incorporated the very same day its lawyers filed a guilty plea, kind of like a sacrificial lamb created specifically for this purpose).

In the end, all Pfizer lost was about three month's profit, but all contracts, including those with Medicaid and Medicare, were spared.

There are hundreds of examples like these, and the moral of the story is; governments or giant corporations don't give a hoot about you or your health.

Censorship

Between 1992 and 1996, FDA prohibited companies that sell folic acid from telling women of childbearing age that .4 mg of folic acid daily before pregnancy could reduce the incidence of neural tube defects (including spina bifida and encephaly) by 40%. **FDA's censorship contributed to a preventable 10,000 neural tube defect births.**

Between 1994 to 2000, FDA prohibited companies that sell omega-3 fatty acids from telling Americans that those fatty acids found in flax and hemp oil could reduce the risk of coronary heart disease by as much as 50%. **FDA's censorship contributed to a preventable 1.8 million sudden death heart attacks.**

Between 2000 and the present, FDA prohibits companies that sell saw palmetto extract (the fruit of the dwarf American palm tree) from telling Americans that saw palmetto reduces enlarged prostates and relieves related symptoms. Approximately 50% of all men age 50 and older suffer from enlarged prostates and are denied access to this information.

Between 2000 and the present, FDA prohibits companies that sell glucosamine and chondroitin sulfate from telling Americans that those dietary ingredients treat osteoarthritis and relieve osteoarthritic pain and stiffness. **Approximately 20 million Americans suffer needlessly from osteoarthritis.**
StopFDACensorship.org - FDA and Health Freedom Protection Act

"FDA censors every claim that a dietary ingredient treats disease, regardless of the proof in support of the claim. FDA only allows drug companies to make claims of treatment. It protects a monopoly for those companies at the expense of the health and freedom of the American people. The FDA's unconstitutional system of speech censorship and monopoly protection has got to come to an end."

So What?

Where does all this leave you, the patient or caregiver? Well, hopefully, it leaves you **somewhat skeptical** about claims by the cancer "industry" that all therapies not sold by BristolMyers-Squibb or Merck or Abbott Labs or whoever are "**unproven**" and therefore pure "**quackery**."

As a bare minimum, to avoid being damaged by this system, you **must** educate yourself. You must be prepared to get more than one opinion. Then, when you've found the doctor (or homeopath or naturopath) that you trust, you **must be prepared to co doctor** with him or her throughout your treatment. Better yet, get the knowledge you need and heal yourself.

This book is designed to end your **blind** faith and trust in our system of cancer "therapy" and arm you with the power to search beyond it and heal yourself. Faith is fine, if it derives from the power of knowledge.

You Have The Power -- Use It

We're going to arm you with **information** -- from books, the Internet, newsletters, magazines and any other source. You will be able to **take charge** of your health. We are hoping you will not be satisfied with **treating symptoms**. You will want to **treat causes**.

But before you can treat causes, you need to understand them.

Bill Henderson, the author of "*Cancer Free*" says "Twenty years ago, one of my wife's cancer surgeons told me, '*80% of it is still mystery to us.*' At the time, I didn't know what he meant. Now, I think I do."

What he meant was that what happens in your body **at the cellular level** is indeed mystery to almost all doctors.

- Interactions between your **brain** and your **immune system**.
- What emotional and other **stress** does to your immune system.
- How **your teeth and jaws** can affect the rest of your body.
- Exactly what **chemotherapy** does to your immune system.
- How the side effects of chemo can be **offset with natural substances**.
- What the **long term** effects of chemotherapy are.
- What other treatments are available to **recover from cancer**.
- How **non-toxic substances** can boost your immune system.
- What organs are affected by **nutritional** deficiencies.
- How **cells react** to food and medicine.
- How exercise and nutrition affect diseases like **diabetes**.
- What **"free radicals"** do to your health.

Your Guide to Gentle, Non-toxic Healing

- Which **antioxidants** are the most effective against free radicals.
- What **natural substances** provide your body with antioxidants.
- ...**and many, many more.**

You **must not trust** everything you are told by a person with M.D. after their name. You must **monitor** everything that is done to your loved one in a hospital. That means spending the night in their hospital room with him/her. We have found that it is very hard to convince many people of those **two simple facts**. If you have had that same frustrating experience, here are a few statistics that might help you next time.

Doctors are officially the third leading cause of death in the United States. In causing the death of their patients, they trail only cancer and heart disease. There are currently more than (probably **much** more than) 250,000 deaths per year from **iatrogenic** causes in the U.S. That strange word means "**induced in a patient by a physician's words or actions.**" Here's the published breakdown for 1999:

12,000 Unnecessary surgery
7,000 Medication errors in hospitals
20,000 Other errors in hospitals
80,000 Infections in hospitals
106,000 Non-error, negative effects of drugs

This information is from an article by Dr. Barbara Starfield of the John Hopkins School of Hygiene and Public Health in the *Journal of the American Medical Association* (JAMA Vol 284, July 26, 2000). The above statistics come from the review process that happens after every death in a hospital to determine the true cause of each death for insurance purposes and to get **smarter about treatment**.

The truth is drug companies have become the largest sponsors of medical research. They are *selling* a product.

The bottom line is the drug companies aren't going to protect you.
The government won't protect you.

The American Medical Association won't protect you (or any other corrupt medical organization or association for that matter).

And it is highly unlikely that your physician can protect you either -- even a well-meaning one -- when he or she is operating within a system that has become RIGGED for Big Pharma profit.

Only YOU can protect yourself.

Don't Believe What You Hear

PR (public relations) was created to manipulate public opinion. More and more of what we hear, see and read as "news" is actually PR content. On any given day much of what the media broadcasts or news print is provided by the PR industry. There are two kinds of "experts" we're dealing with -- the PR spin doctors behind the scenes and the "independent" experts paraded before the public, scientists who have been hand-picked, cultivated, and paid handsomely to promote the views of corporations which are involved in controversial actions.

While drug companies must submit direct-to-consumer advertisements to the U.S. Food and Drug Administration (FDA), the agency's review of drug ads is often not completed until after the ad has been widely circulated. What does this mean for consumers? Advertised drugs are not necessarily safe, and drug advertisements should be looked at with discretion.

If the FDA finds a drug ad to be false or misleading, it will issue a regulatory letter to the manufacturer. In the late 1990s, the FDA issued more than 100 such letters per year, but as of November 2002, only 24 had been issued for the year. The decrease, thought to be the result of a new legal review of proposed regulatory letters, has raised concerns that potentially misleading drug advertisements may be gaining public exposure.

This sharp rise in deaths from pharmaceutical drugs coincides with the direct marketing of prescription medication to the public. Prescription drug sales have soared nearly 500 percent since 1990. Since 1997, when the FDA relaxed television and radio advertising restrictions for prescription drugs, the big pharmaceutical companies have increasingly turned to direct-to-consumer (DTC) marketing to increase their profits.

According to a Consumer Reports analysis of Food and Drug Administration (FDA) regulatory letters from 1997 to 2002, the Food and Drug Administration (FDA) charged drug companies with a variety of violations including omitting or minimizing drug risks, exaggerating the effectiveness of a drug, promoting unapproved uses for a drug, making false claims that a drug is superior to another, promoting drugs which are still experimental, using inconsistent or incorrect labeling information, and giving misleading or false information to doctors. These are not "minute abs," or "instant muscle" fitness machines they are selling, these are not recipe books that they are promoting; they are selling toxic chemicals that people will have serious health complication from, and are getting away with false advertising.

"Last year pharmaceutical companies spent $1.8 billion on 'direct to consumer' advertising, mostly on television. Advertising expenditure in 1999 rose by 38.5% from the $1.3 bn spent in 1998, and was 33 times the amount spent on media advertisements in 1991." Fred Charatan, "Prescription drug sales boosted by advertising," BMJ, 321, Sept. 30, 2000, p. 783.

And it appears to be working. As the big drug companies have poured more and more money into DTC television ads, drug spending has risen enormously, and the bulk of the rise was accounted for by increased sales of the most heavily advertised prescription drugs.

"Doctors wrote 34.2% more prescriptions in 1999 than in 1998 for the 25 drugs promoted direct to consumers that contributed most to overall drug spending. Doctors wrote only 5.1% more prescriptions for all other prescription drugs." Charatan, BMJ, Sept. 30, 2000, p. 783.

However, some physicians and industry watchdog organizations are becoming increasingly alarmed by the influence of the drug companies' direct-to-consumer advertising tactics. They point out that not only do all drugs-especially prescription drugs-have negative side effects, but that such continual bombardment by drug ads "normalizes" taking drugs. It is forming a belief that taking drugs is as normal as breathing, that taking medication is perfectly ok. They have done a good job making us believe that only medication can cure anything. This couldn't be farther from the truth!

"It's insidious; companies want you to think there's something wrong with you. It's saying in effect, 'If you've got a problem, the way to deal with it is through pills.' It's also 'medicalizing' a problem which may not be a problem you need to deal with, like male pattern baldness or shyness. Once you have a drug, it becomes a medical problem." Dr. Joel Lexchin, a Toronto physician and member of Medical Reform Group. Quoted in Candis McLean, "The real drug pushers," Report Newsmagazine, Mar 19, 2001.

In addition to increasing numbers of these highly profitable "lifestyle" drugs, the pharmaceutical industry has capitalized on the current medical focus on prevention by turning out more and more medications designed to prevent disease, such as drugs to lower cholesterol and blood pressure levels.

Even such toxic and costly pharmaceuticals as chemotherapy drugs are sometimes used without sufficient justification, despite their serious side-effects.

"Many patients with cancer receive chemotherapy at the end of life, even if their kind of cancer is known to be unresponsive to the drugs, according to a study reported at the recent annual meeting of the American Society of Clinical Oncologists held in San Francisco." Gottlieb S, "Chemotherapy may be overused at the end of life," BMJ, 322, May 26, 2001, p. 1267.

Dr. Ezekiel Emanuel, lead author of the study, also noted that chemotherapy is very expensive, $38,308 for treatment of a patient in the final year of life as compared to $27,567 for a patient not in the final year of life.

While treating cancers known to be unresponsive to chemotherapy with these drugs may do nothing to help suffering patients, it certainly benefits the pharmaceutical companies providing the drugs. The fact is that all drugs, not just chemotherapy drugs, have potentially serious side effects, and no drug should be prescribed unless it is truly necessary to the health and well-being of a patient. Not even if the patient insists on having it because he or she has seen an upbeat television ad and is convinced that the advertised wonder drug will cure all of life's pains and anxieties.

Does anyone out there really believe that Americans are getting 1/2 a trillion dollars of benefits from these drugs? Drug companies are smart. They have been able to change the rules so that they can now market to consumers directly. Is it any wonder why 2/3 of doctor visits result in a drug prescription?

Media, under the influence of the pharmaceutical companies, (we may go as far as to say they are run by the same people) has cleverly steered public belief into a very dangerous direction. Through clever marketing ploys pharmaceutical companies devise advertisements, pay scientists who have been hand-picked, cultivated, and paid handsomely to promote the views of corporations which are involved in controversial actions. It is false conventional wisdom that for example;

"The cure for cancer is near"
"Pharmaceuticals restore health"
"America has the best health care in the world"
"Vaccination brings immunity"
"When a child is sick, he/she needs immediate antibiotics"
"When a child has a fever he/she needs Tylenol"

Etc. etc. etc.

In "Trust Us We're Experts", Stauber and Rampton point to some convincing data describing the science of creating public opinion in the U.S. and abroad. They trace modern public influence back to the early part of the 1900's, highlighting the work of people like Edward L. Bernays, the "Father of Spin". Edward Bernays laid the groundwork for the growing public relations industry in the 1920s to the power it holds over public policy today. Edward L. Bernays took the ideas of his famous uncle Sigmund Freud himself, and applied them to the emerging science of mass persuasion.

In his book "Propaganda", Bernays argued that scientific manipulation of public opinion is key. "A relatively small number of persons," he wrote, "pull the wires which control the public mind." Bernays believed that "somebody interested in leading the crowd needs to appeal not to logic but to unconscious motivation." Bernays dominated the PR industry until the 1940s, and was a significant force for another 40 years following that. During that time, Bernays took on hundreds various assignments to create a public perception about some product or idea.

For example, as a new member on the Committee on Public Information, one of Bernays' first assignments was to help **sell** the First World War to the American public with the idea to "Make the World Safe for Democracy." Notice he was selling the war like a product, a product which was completely useless yet brought billions into the pockets of weapons manufacturing corporations and other companies that profited from the war.

A few years later, Bernays helped popularize the notion of women smoking cigarettes, by organizing the Torches of Liberty Brigade in which suffragettes marched in the parade smoking cigarettes as a mark of women's liberation. Always up for a challenge, Bernays set up the advertising format, along with the AMA, which lasted for almost 50 years proving that cigarettes are beneficial to health. Bernays also popularized the idea of bacon for breakfast.

Bernay's job was to reframe an issue, to create a certain image which would put a particular concept or product in a desirable light. Bernays described the public as a 'herd that needed to be led.' And this herdlike thinking makes people "susceptible to leadership." Bernays never strayed from his fundamental axiom to "control the masses without their knowing it." The best PR takes places when the people are unaware that they are being manipulated. It's easier to control those who don't know they are being controlled. A slave that knows he is a slave will always have the desire to escape, but a slave that does not know he is a slave will continue to be a slave and be very happy being so.

Stauber describes Bernays' rationale like this: "the scientific manipulation of public opinion was necessary to overcome chaos and conflict in a democratic society."

Once these marketing ploys were uncovered and psychology as a means to instill belief began to be used in selling products, Bernays's list of clients grew like a well watered rose, pretty on the outside but full of thorns on the inside. Global corporations eagerly jumped on the opportunity to create an image for their products and sell to the susceptible public whatever they wanted, be it a product or a belief.

"Those who manipulate the unseen mechanism of society constitute an invisible government which is the true ruling power of our country. We are governed, our minds molded, our tastes formed, our ideas suggested largely by men we have never heard of.

This is a logical result of the way in which our democratic society is organized. Vast numbers of human beings must cooperate in this manner if they are to live together as a smoothly functioning society.

In almost every act of our lives whether in the sphere of politics or business in our social conduct or our ethical thinking, we are dominated by the relatively small number of persons who understand the mental processes and social patterns of the masses. It is they who pull the wires that control the public mind." A paragraph from Bernlays' book Propaganda.

For decades they have created the opinions that most of us were raised with, on virtually any issue which has the remotest commercial value, including:

pharmaceutical drugs	vaccines
medicine as a profession	alternative medicine
fluoridation of city water	chlorine
household cleaning products	tobacco
dioxin	global warming
leaded gasoline	cancer research and treatment
pollution of the oceans	forests and lumber

images of celebrities, including damage control	crisis and disaster management
genetically modified foods	aspartame
food additives; processed foods	dental amalgams

Bernays learned early that the most effective way to create credibility for a product or image is through "independent third party" endorsements. For example if GM was to come out and say that global warming was a hoax thought up by some tree hugging liberals, people would suspect GM's motives since they make their fortunes selling automobiles.

But if some third party organization or institute with a credible sounding name like the Global Climate Coalition comes out with a scientific report that global warming is actually fiction, then people will begin to think and doubt the original issue.

So that's exactly what Bernays did. He set up "more institutes and foundations than Rockefeller and Carnegie combined." (Stauber p 45)

Silently financed by the industries whose products were being evaluated, these "independent" research agencies would churn out "scientific" studies and press materials that could **create any image their buyers wanted**. Such front groups are given credible-sounding names like:

Temperature Research Foundation	Manhattan Institute
International Food Information Council	Center for Produce Quality
Consumer Alert	Tobacco Institute Research Council
The Advancement of Sound Science Coalition	Cato Institute
Air Hygiene Foundation	American Council on Science and Health
Industrial Health Federation	Global Climate Coalition
International Food Information	Alliance for Better Foods

They sound pretty legit don't they?

Canned News

These organizations and hundreds of others like them are front groups whose sole mission is to advance the image of the global corporations who fund them. This image is partly accomplished by an endless stream of "press releases" which announce "breakthroughs" in research to every radio station and newspaper in the nation. Most of these canned reports read just like a news report, and that is because they have been carefully structured in the news format.

When a journalist looks at the report, they don't even have to do any research or changes. Entire sections of the release or in the case of video news releases, the whole thing can just be used as it was written and voila! Instant news – copy and paste edition, written by corporate PR firms, without a smidgeon of scientific evidence.

Does this actually happen? Every single day since the 1920s, when the whole idea of the News Release was invented by Ivy Lee. Sometimes half the stories appearing in an issue of the Wall St. Journal are based exclusively on these press releases from drug companies. Medical breakthroughs or creatively written lies?

Propaganda Tactics

As the science of mass control evolved, public relation firms developed further guidelines for effective presentation. Here are some of the most important tactics they use:

- Dehumanize the attacked party by labeling and name calling (Bill O'Reilly uses this tactic superbly on his show, when loosing an argument he childishly reverts to name calling)
- Speak in glittering generalities using emotionally positive words like "freedom" or "change" etc. (listen to a speech by any prominent politician since they use masterfully created speeches)
- When covering something up, don't use plain English; stall for time; distract
- Get endorsements from celebrities, churches, sports figures, street people - anyone who has no expertise in the subject at hand (we

unconsciously believe someone we recognize and trust, like a celebrity)

- The 'plain folks' ruse: us billionaires are just like you
- When minimizing outrage, don't say anything memorable, point out the benefits of what just happened, and avoid moral issues

Keep this list. Start watching for these techniques. Not hard to find - look at today's paper or tonight's TV news. See what they're doing; these guys are good!

Great PR

We can now see how much of an effect great PR can have. Let's look at an example of truly great PR; how leaded gas came into the picture.

In 1922, General Motors discovered that adding lead to gasoline gave cars more horsepower. Some concern arose about safety, so GM paid the Bureau of Mines to do some fake "testing" and publish false research that supposedly "proved" that lead inhalation was not harmful. Enter Charles Kettering.

Charles Kettering, founder of the world famous Sloan-Kettering Memorial Institute for medical research, also happened to be an executive with GM. Oh what a coincidence. Then we have this worldly institute issuing reports stating that lead is a naturally occurring substance in our bodies and our bodies have ways of eliminating this toxin at low levels. Cigarettes were considered safe in the 1950s and were smoked by doctors in commercials and print advertising.

Sloane Kettering opposed all anti-lead research for years and without any real scientific opposition for the next 60 years gasoline became increasingly leaded until the late 1970s when 90% of gasoline was leaded. This trend finally came to a halt when it was just too obvious to hide that lead was a major carcinogen and began to be phased out in the late 80s. So throughout those 60 years, 30 million tons of lead was released in vapor form onto your streets, your carefully mowed lawn, and of course your lungs. **30 million tons**.

Now that's what I call great marketing!

Science these days has turned into another commodity that is bought and sold. And the marketplace is your television, your newspaper or your magazines. Yet when you go to this marketplace, the sellers don't ask you what you want or whether you need it at all, they just go ahead and place whatever they want in our slowly shrinking minds (Three fourths of California high school seniors can't read well enough to pass their exit exams. [SJ Mercury 20 Jul 01]).

As you have seen above, just because you have seen it on TV, newspaper, or radio doesn't mean it's true. Guard your minds from the onslaught of these ridiculous clowns dancing in front of you trying to make you believe these things. Always ask, what are they selling here, and who's selling it? Mass media is like a repetitive puppet show showing the same thing over and over and over again, day by day.

Think about the news of the past couple of years for a minute. Do you really suppose the major stories that have dominated headlines and TV news have been "what is actually going on in the world?" Do you actually think there's been nothing going on besides the artificial financial slump, the contrived power shortages, the re-filtered accounts of foreign violence and disaster, and all the other non-stories that the puppeteers dangle before us every day?

The sole purpose of news is to **keep the public in a state of fear and uncertainty** so that they'll watch again tomorrow and be subjected to the same thing. Simple? Yes, that's the mass media mastery – simplicity, the invisible hand. Like Edward Bernays said, "the people must be controlled without them knowing it."

Do you need someone to spoon-feed you your values or ideas?
Are those shows really amusing, or just a necessary distraction to keep you from looking at reality, or trying to figure things out yourself by doing a little independent reading?

Stop subjecting yourself to this insanity, to the lies and deception. Turn off your TV's and spend more time with your family, go outside, visit your friends, play a board game with your children, become the smart, powerful, free individual that you ALREADY are! They can do whatever they want, but if we don't buy their fake merchandise they have nobody to sell it to. If you stop the demand, there will be no supply. The only reason they can do this is because we let them. Real knowledge takes a little effort and at least one level above what everyone knows, real knowledge will bring you more happiness, love, and change your life for the better.

Together we can spread real knowledge.

The Truth

Bang for Your Buck

Americans pay more for health care than any other country in the world. So does paying more for healthcare give you better health and longer life expectancy? No. The following graphs show that in 1996, average life expectancy in the US was 18th of all countries, being 5 years lower than Canada and behind the UK. But Americans were paying US$1000 or over per person, 33% more than Canadians and nearly 66% more than the British. Now take a look at the graph and see what Americans were (and are) getting for their money?

Notice Singapore and Greece. Even though America is the highest spender, there are still millions of people without access to basic care.

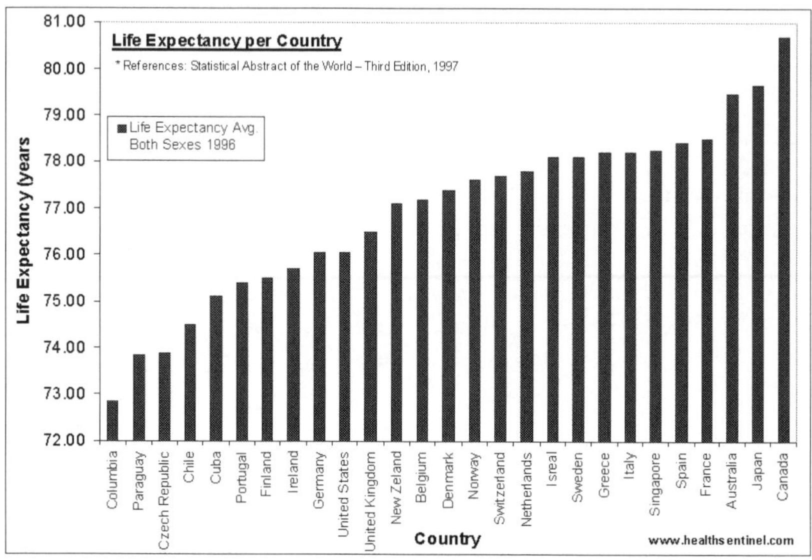
Life Expectancy per Country
* References: Statistical Abstract of the World – Third Edition, 1997
Life Expectancy Avg. Both Sexes 1996
Life Expectancy (years
81.00
80.00
79.00
78.00
77.00
76.00
75.00
74.00
73.00
72.00
Columbia
Paraguay
Czech Republic
Chile
Cuba
Portugal
Finland
Ireland
Germany
United States
United Kingdom
New Zeland
Belgium
Denmark
Norway
Switzerland
Netherlands
Isreal
Sweden
Greece
Italy
Singapore
Spain
France
Australia
Japan
Canada
Country
www.healthsentinel.com

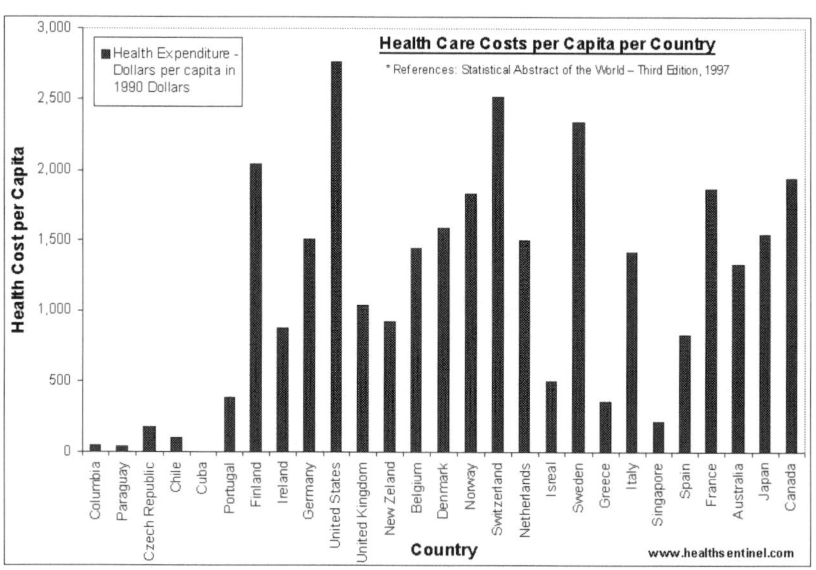
Health Care Costs per Capita per Country
* References: Statistical Abstract of the World – Third Edition, 1997
Health Expenditure - Dollars per capita in 1990 Dollars
Health Cost per Capita
3,000
2,500
2,000
1,500
1,000
500
0
Columbia
Paraguay
Czech Republic
Chile
Cuba
Portugal
Finland
Ireland
Germany
United States
United Kingdom
New Zeland
Belgium
Denmark
Norway
Switzerland
Netherlands
Isreal
Sweden
Greece
Italy
Singapore
Spain
France
Australia
Japan
Canada
Country
www.healthsentinel.com

Why Does a Salad Cost More Than a Burger?

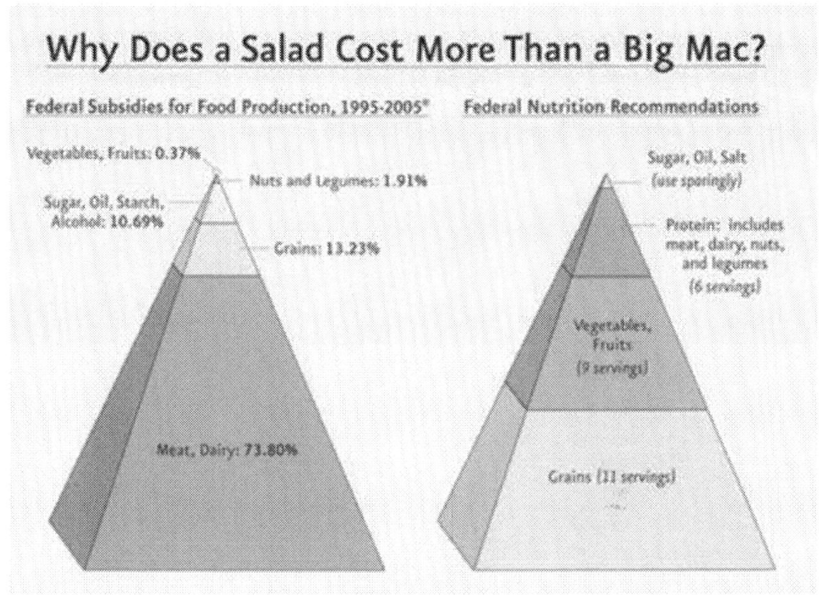

"The Farm Bill, a massive piece of federal legislation making its way through Congress, governs what children are fed in schools and what food assistance programs can distribute to recipients. The bill provides billions of dollars in subsidies, much of which goes to huge agribusinesses producing feed crops, such as corn and soy, which are then fed to animals. By funding these crops, the government supports the production of meat and dairy products—the same products that contribute to our growing rates of obesity and chronic disease. Fruit and vegetable farmers, on the other hand, receive less than 1 percent of government subsidies.

The government also purchases surplus foods like cheese, milk, pork, and beef for distribution to food assistance programs—including school lunches. The government is not required to purchase nutritious foods." (http://www.pcrm.org/magazine/gm07autumn/health_pork.html)

Basically, governments get more money from lobbying firms of giant corporations that sell meat products/dairy so they subsidize those farmers and leave the green producing ones fending for themselves. That means your fatty burger will cost you less than healthy greens. If you are healthy you are not profitable, so go on eating your burgers with cola. After all the CEO's have high electric bills on their mansions and gas prices are pretty high on their Ferraris.

When you eat this cheap, nutrient lacking food, you get fat! And it's highly profitable to keep you fat, because when you are fat you are sick, and when you are sick you need all sorts of pills, drugs, and surgery. You turn into a walking money machine for these greedy heartless corporations.

Natural Cures

"If we all worked on the assumption that what is accepted as true really is true, there would be little hope of advance."
Orville Wright

"Most secrets of knowledge have been discovered by plain and neglected men than by men of popular fame. And this is so with good reason. For the men of popular fame are busy on popular matters."
Roger Bacon (c. 1220 – 1292), English philosopher and scientist

The following section deals with some of the most important things regarding your health. I highly urge you to read carefully through it and analyze the information.

Have you ever asked yourself what happened to the act of actually curing diseases?

The patient's immune system, and the immune system alone, is responsible for healing and recovery from ill health. **The use of drugs and vaccines represents an assault on the immune system**. In some cases, the use of a particular drug might be a wise choice to speed healing and recovery for the patient, but the use of natural, orthomolecular (substances normally found in Nature) therapies and substances that can more effectively address the cause of the disease should be **considered first** because natural substances work in *harmony with Nature.* They aid and stimulate the body to truly cure itself, without the terrible millstone of drug side-effects.

The human body is predisposed to heal itself and to exist as a healthy, thriving organism. We inhibit that process by ingesting unhealthy foods, fouling our inner environment with toxins, and relying upon poisonous substances to treat disease conditions.

The next section is an overview of some alternative therapies that have demonstrated themselves to be effective and readily obtainable, usually at a low to modest cost. This list is far from complete.

There is a HUGE amount of evidence and proof from around the world that natural remedies are effective and safe in treating countless ailments. But because of drug lobbyists, suppression, ridicule, fake studies, and other cover ups, you have never heard of them.

For it is a sad fact that, these days, that the discoveries of "unknown" things, instead of being welcomed with excitement, is often criticized as illusory, or tabooed as "fantasy." Nowhere are these taboos more prevalent than in the field of the biomedical sciences and the multibillion-dollar pharmaceutical industry with which it interacts.

The fact is that there are hundreds upon hundreds of genuine, kindhearted, truth seeking doctors and scientist around the world who are not concerned about money but want to get the truth out and help the people. Unfortunately those are the people we rarely hear about, and I am just another reporter bringing you the truth!

Most people are under the influence from the drug companies that “cures” must be bought in the form of some treatment or pill that they sell. I’m sure you knew that they lobbied government to pass a law that states only a drug or an approved medical device can prevent, cure, or treat a disease. And if someone, regardless who, stands up and says to all “Hey, eat this orange and you it will cure your scurvy, mate!” He will go to jail. That’s right, if someone has (and they have) found a natural cure for a particular disease and claims that it will cure your disease, even if it has ample evidence, you will get sued and probably get sent to jail (for example over 35 years ago when some of the world's top scientists claimed that when vitamin B17 is consumed from apricot seeds or such, the components of the seed make it 100% impossible to develop cancer and will kill existing cancer in most cases, the FDA and the pharmaceutical industry began a massive smear campaign to get it off the market as soon as possible, and that’s why you probably have never heard of this miracle vitamin).

Why? Because “big-pharma” can’t patent an orange and charge you a thousand dollars per slice, because they can’t patent a leaf and make billions of dollars, because they can’t make money from natural remedies that are freely available to all. It doesn’t even matter if medical scientists around the world agree that most diseases are caused by nutritional deficiencies.

NOTHING ON PLANET EARTH CAN CURE, PREVENT, OR TREAT A DISEASE, except drugs, surgical procedures, or medical treatments. That is the current ridiculous law.

In order to break free from this notion that drugs are the only answer, people must stop thinking of bodily systems as individual entities that are neatly divided, and think of the whole body as a system that is infinitely interconnected within itself, as well as to all matter on earth — living or otherwise.

Everything is connected within our bodies; if we have some pain, some discomfort, some symptom, then it is not due to a lack of drugs or surgery. It is something a lot more complex, something that is due to a variety of factors. In most cases, taking drugs for some symptom is like trying to fix your bathroom door when you left the tap on and the water is overflowing. Treating the SYMPTOM is not treating the CAUSE. We need to treat the CAUSE, not the SYMPTOM.

Only the body can cure and heal itself, everything else we put into it either suppresses the symptoms by making the body do something unnatural or, as in natural remedies, help the body heal itself by eliminating nutritional deficiencies, eliminating toxins, and bringing the body back into a state of balance. It is not normal for you to be sick, our bodies are always supposed to be in a state of balance and health.

Legendary economist Zane Pilzer writes, “I define ‘wellness’ as money spent to make you feel healthier, even when you’re not ‘sick’ by any standard medical terms ... As much as we focus on the financial and lifestyle benefits of the business, the real benefit is what you can do to change a life -- and the lives of all people who are touched by that life.”

What about the so called "vitamin toxicity"? There is not even one death per year from vitamins, yet some think they are dangerous. There are over 100000 deaths per year from properly prescribed medication, yet everyone thinks they are safe. I think it is time we change our views on vitamins and minerals, don’t you?

“Nature cures, not the physician”
- Hippocrates

We all know the phrase; you are what you eat.

In an interview with Aaron Russo, an entertainment businessman, filmmaker, libertarian political activist, who spent the later part of his life spreading the truth, talked about in one of his interviews about his meetings with Kevin Rockefeller. The Rockefeller family is one of the richest families in the world making their riches from the oil industry back in the 19 hundreds. The family has close financial ties to many of the world's biggest corporations such as Chase Bank, JP Morgan, and is involved with the world's biggest institutions.

When discussions turned to global control, and Aaron Russo would say that their views differed on the government agendas and such, Aaron said the following regarding the type of reply he would get from Kevin Rockefeller "It was like, what do you care about them? What do you care about those people? What difference does it make to you? Take care of you own life, do the best you can for you and your family, what are the rest of the people… they don't mean anything to you, they're just **serfs**, they're just people…"

You are just a piece of meat in the grinder to the giant corporations, you mean nothing to them, absolutely nothing. They think they can do whatever they want with you, I think otherwise. Get informed and change your life, because nobody else will do it for you.

Diet

People's interest in nutrition is very strong; everywhere you look there is something about how to eat, what to eat, when to eat, even what the movie stars eat. Diet books are best sellers year after year promoting new fad diets, on the front page of almost every single health magazine is some "new" nutrition advice, newspapers run articles and TV and radio programs constantly discuss diet and health.

With this massive barrage of information, you would think people would be skinny and healthy, yet the opposite is true. Are you confident that you know the truth regarding your health and wellness? Are vitamins good for you and how much is good enough? Should I be drinking water or have more fiber? Are carbohydrates the ones making me fat? Are environmental effects the cause of cancer? Or is it my predisposition to cancer? Are unhealthy fats the cause of my diabetes?

I'm going to guess that you don't really know the answer to these questions, and if that is the case, you are definitely not alone. Opinion and information on this subject is beyond ridiculous, everyone seems to have some sort of method, some sort of diet, some weird set of things that one must do. But even then, *very few people truly know what they should be doing to be healthy, vibrant, and absolutely free of disease.*

This isn't because the science hasn't been done. We are all familiar with the vast amount of information, studies, and links proving the relationship between nutrition and health. The reason is because the *real* science, the *genuine* information that is **actually** important has been buried beneath the giant heap of irrelevant, useless, and harmful information; the junk science, fad diets, and food industry propaganda. These days it is very difficult to find information that is actually going to help you.

I want to change that. I want to give you a framework, a base for understanding nutrition and health that will eliminate confusion, misunderstanding, and give you all the necessary tools that you can use to lose weight, cure and prevent disease, and live a healthy and more fulfilling life as a result.

I think you deserve to know the truth regarding our medical system, food and drug system, and health policy. I think you deserve to know what is being done and not being done to keep you sick and unhappy, and I want to shed some light on what is *actually* important and what *actually* matters. And I think you deserve to know that the most common notions you have been told about the food you eat, and about health and disease are wrong:

- Chemicals in the environment, as bad as they might be, as well as your "predisposition" to cancer are not the main causes of this serious disease.
- Your genes that you inherit from your parents are not the most important factors that will determine whether you will suffer from any one of the ten diseases on the list.
- Hoping that drug manufacturers or genetic research is eventually going to discover the miracle pill to "cure" any disease is ignoring the decades of scientific studies and research that prove diseases can be cured with diet alone.
- Controlling any one aspect of your diet, for example carbohydrates, fats, protein, or any one nutrient is not going to lead to any strong improvement in your health.
- Drugs and surgery DO NOT cure the diseases that kill most people today.
- Most likely you doctor does not know what you need to do to be the healthiest that you can be.

The research is out there; the studies, findings, and evidence all show that we need to redefine how modern medicine goes about treating and curing disease. What you will also realize as you read on, is that the medical establishment is not actually interested in making you healthy and does everything in their power to keep it that way. The only person who is going to make you healthy is **you**.

Some of the findings published in the most reputable scientific journals, show that;

- Dietary change can enable diabetic patients to go off their medication.
- Heart disease can be reversed with diet alone.
- Cancer can be reversed with diet alone.
- Consuming store bought pasteurized dairy foods can increase the risk of prostate cancer and other types of cancer (raw dairy products on the other hand are very beneficial for health and can be consumed).
- Kidney stones, diabetes, headaches, migranes, Lupus, and many other diseases can be reversed by diet alone.

- Type 1 diabetes, one of the most devastating diseases that can fall upon a child is convincingly linked to infant feeding practices.

All these findings demonstrate that a proper diet is the most powerful weapon we have against disease and illness. An understanding of this scientific evidence is not just important to keep you healthy; it also has profound consequences for our *entire society*. We must understand why such a gross misunderstanding dominates our society, why we have been so greatly mistaken in our understanding of diet and disease, and what exactly we must do to promote health and treat disease.

We all know how fat and sick our nation is, there is no need for me to tell you that. We all know that every single disease including cancer, heart disease, diabetes, infectious diseases, degenerative diseases etc, are all on the rise and that half of Americans have a health problem that requires taking a prescription drug every week. We all know that depression is on the rise, psychotic disorders are on the rise, people are feeling unhappy, and the overall quality of life is decreasing.

I'm not going to bore you with numbers or complex figures on each vitamin and each mineral, that information is everywhere. The topic of diet seems very complex, and if you want to make it complex you can, but it can be very simple if you know the basics. What I'm going to do is give you a much bigger picture, a totally different perspective on diet and nutrition which you probably have not heard before. I will give you principles, not confusing numbers. Guidelines which will give you a solid foundation with which you can customize your own diet to fit you own needs. It will be simple, but might not be easy!

The most important idea to understand is that there is really only ONE disease; the malfunction of our cells. A cell malfunction can be traced to two causes; deficiency and toxicity. By addressing these two causes through nutrition (and stress reduction) almost all disease can be cured and reversed. The most important aspect is *nutrition*. It all comes down to three things; breakfast, lunch and dinner.

I can remember when I was young, and how and what my family would eat. We never really gave much thought to which foods we were eating, which foods were best, or which foods should be avoided; we pretty much just ate what everyone else did. Nobody really told us what foods were good, we just ate what was available, what was tasty or convenient, or what our parents taught us to eat. Most of us live within strong cultural and societal boundaries which define the way we eat, our preferences and habits. It is not until only until some years ago that diet became a hot topic, and then all the confusion began!

Most people that I question have quite a few diet tips, advice, or guidelines. They think they know what to eat and strongly believe that they know what should be done. Yet, the more I listened, the more I understood just how much confusion, junk-science, and "fads" have overtaken peoples' minds. So what do you say we put an end to all the confusion? Lets crack open the fresh new understanding that will lead you on a road full of discoveries, smiles, and happiness!

What are the biggest diet beliefs that we have today? Well, we must eat plenty of meat, milk, and eggs for the protein of course! Universities and governments around the world have been working very hard since around the 1970's to ensure the whole world has a "proper" intake of animal-based protein especially trying to ensure a "protein-gap" in the developing worlds.

For ten years Dr. Colin Campbell (author of *The China Study*) and his team worked in China and the Philippines, with the goal of improving childhood nutrition among the poor (a project funded by the U.S. Agency for International Development). The aim of the project was very simple; to make sure that children were receiving as much protein as possible. It was thought that much of childhood malnutrition in the third world was caused by a lack of protein, especially from animal-based foods.

It was at that time that Dr. Campbell discovered a dark secret. Children who ate the highest protein diets were most likely to get liver cancer! They were children from the wealthiest families; families that could afford more meat.

In another research study from India, the findings were very interesting indeed. Two groups of rats were administered a very strong cancer causing agent aflatoxin. Then, one group was fed a diet composed of 20% protein, a number very close to what many of us in the West consume, and the second group was fed 5% protein. Amazingly, every single rat that was fed 20% protein developed liver cancer, and every single rat that was fed 5% animal protein lived on without any cancers whatsoever. It was a very convincing 100 to 0 score showing how nutrition had a much greater effect than chemical carcinogens.

To say that protein is unhealthy, let alone that it causes cancer, one will probably get labelled as a heretic and be hung by his peers, even if it is "good science." Dr. Campbell recites his story of how he made the discoveries for himself regarding protein and nutrition, and became very interested in this dangerous topic (speaking against a popular belief was like shooting yourself in the foot in regards to your career a few decades ago, and today the trend has not changed; saying anything against orthodox beliefs is a very dangerous career move for most scientists and doctors).

Dr. Campbell needed to know more, so he started an in-depth laboratory program investigating the effects of protein on health. They were very cautious and conservative with their hypothesis and interpretations in fear of saying something too radical. He was studying the effects of protein on cancer and other diseases. Eventually, his research went on to be funded by some of the biggest institutes (NIH, American Cancer Society, American Institute for Cancer Research, etc.) for *27 years*, and his results published in many of the best scientific journals.

His findings were nothing less than shocking; it did not matter how much cancer causing chemicals you gave the animals, if they did not eat animal protein, they did not develop cancer! Low protein diets also dramatically blocked subsequent cancer growth. This protein-cancer connection was in fact so strong that *they could turn cancer growth on and off simply by changing the amount of animal protein consumed.* Now that is one powerful statement that should have been on the front pages of newspapers and medical journals.

There were a few other very interesting findings; the protein that had the strongest cancer causing effect was casein which makes up 87% of cow's milk and promoted all stages of the cancer process. The proteins that did not promote cancer at all, even at very high levels, and even reversed cancer growth were ***plant based*** proteins. This is quite shattering for most peoples' nutritional views and beliefs.

The interesting thing to consider is that the studies did not end there. They went on to direct the *largest and most comprehensive study of diet, lifestyle, and disease with humans in the* ***history of biomedical research***. The biggest health study that you probably never heard about. It was a massive research task that involved Cornell University, Oxford University and the Chinese Academy of Preventive Medicine. The New York Times called it the "Grand Prix of Epidemiology." This project studied a huge range of diseases and diet and lifestyle factors in rural China and Taiwan. It is known as the China Study and produced more than 8000 statistically significant associations between various dietary factors and disease. Comparing that to regular studies, the results are absolutely mindboggling.

The most remarkable findings from this study were that among the many associations between nutrition and disease, *people who ate the most animal based protein got the most chronic diseases*! Even relatively small intakes of animal based foods were associated with adverse effects. However, people who ate the most plant based foods were the healthiest and tended to avoid chronic disease. From study to study, these findings were very consistent; *eating animal based protein was always linked to higher incidence of disease and illness*, and eating more plant based foods linked to better health and lower incidence of disease.

Dr. Campbell did not end there, even at his monumental and impressive research findings he continued on. Along with the experience of many other doctors, he showed that heart disease, diabetes, and obesity can be reversed by a healthy diet. Those are very conservative statements, the truth is; *almost every single chronic disease can be reversed by diet alone.* Various cancers, autoimmune diseases, bone health, organ health, brain disorders (Alzheimer's), ADHD in children, hormonal misbalances (emotional), and many other diseases are very strongly influenced by diet. Time after time, research showed that a plant based diet reversed diseases and promoted optimal health. *The results are consistent.*

Even with this monumental research activity, at the shocking facts and proof, people are still very confused, and this information still has not reached mass media. People are being led down a road of illness, disease, pain and suffering in the name of profits. These very simple cures are not talked about, and very heavily suppressed. I will repeat this many many times, the only person who can cure you of your diseases, restore you to optimal health, and make your life happier is YOU! Almost *every single choric disease and illness that plagues our society today is curable and preventable*, quite easily! It all comes down to what we put in our mouths; it's as simple as that.

Simplifying Nutrition

Many of us think that we are well informed about nutrition, although in most cases we are not. We either jump on the no fat or high protein or low carb wagon, then embrace vitamin E or calcium supplements, and usually focus on one nutrient or extremely small aspect of nutrition thinking that we have unlocked the secret of good health. In recent years people have fallen for fad diet after fad diet, the Dr. Atkins or Protein Power craze, the low fat diets, and countless other diets. But in reality there is increasing evidence that these modern diet fads especially the high protein diets continue to inflict a variety of dangerous health disorders. Most times, not knowing and not understanding nutrition can hurt us.

So why all this confusion? Well, far too often science tends to focus on very specific details while completely ignoring the whole or the larger picture. They put all their effort into one box, one specific nutrient or one very small aspect of the whole, whether it be vitamin E to treat heart disease or vitamin A to prevent cancer isolating specific biological parts of food trying to reach broad conclusions about diet and health. This can lead to contradictory results which confuse scientists and policy makers and end up in a very confused public.

The story goes much deeper than that, the confusion is purposefully created by the people who stand to profit from the confused public. You might be familiar with some of the "health" books on the shelves of your nearby bookstore; Dr. Atkins' New Diet Revolution, The South Beach Diet, Sugar Busters, The Zone, and many others. What these books have done is made nutrition even more confusing, more difficult to understand and ultimately much more elusive.

What's the problem anyway? Is it fats? Is it the carbohydrates? Is it the protein? How many calories should I be eating? What's the ratio of nutrients that will make me lose weight fast? What vegetables should I be eating for my blood type? Am I eating the right supplements? If you are not exhausted, starving, or constipated from these ridiculous plans then you are probably having a major headache trying to count and measure the fats, carbs, protein, and calories.

This is not health, these are fad diets that are only meant to capitalize on your confusion and make billions of dollars. They are nothing but the worst of science and medicine. If you are looking for a quick fix, or some gimmicky monthly eating plan then maybe this book is not for you. I'm here to give you a much deeper understanding of your body and your health. There is a much easier and simpler way that will bring you more benefit than any fad diet, eating plan, drug or surgery ever can, without any side effects.

The evidence can no longer be ignored. The people in science or medicine who choose to turn the other way are being more than stubborn, they are being irresponsible. It is now known that even genetic predisposition is no match for diet. With proper nutrition, we can avoid these "genetic" diseases even though we may have a gene responsible for that disease. Cancer, diabetes, heart disease, Alzheimer's and many others all can be reversed with proper nutrition.

The Protein Mystery

The story of protein these days has a kind of "mythological" air about it. It is as if protein is some miraculous nutrient that has a death grip upon the body; breakfast, lunch, and dinner and if, god forbid, one meal doesn't have some sort of animal based foods then it's not considered a proper meal, and worse yet, terrible health consequences are *bound* to follow. As they say of course. As Goethe said: "We are best at hiding those things which are in plain sight." Nothing has been so well hidden as the untold story of protein. Everywhere you look, it's all about the protein, almost every thought in biomedical research deals with protein.

Since the days of the Dutch chemist Gerhard Mulder who discovered this nitrogen containing chemical, protein regarded as the most sacred of all nutrients. Even the word itself comes from the Greek word *proteios*, which means "of prime importance." And since the nineteenth century, protein was quite firmly established with meat, and this connection has stayed with us for more than one hundred years. The first thing that might come to mind when I say protein is beef, and if that's the case, you are not alone.

There is great confusion about some basic questions regarding protein:

- What are good sources of protein?
- How much protein should one consume?
- Is plant protein as good as animal protein?
- Is it necessary to combine certain plant foods in a meal to get complete proteins?
- Is it advisable to take protein powders or amino acid supplements, especially for someone who does vigorous exercise or plays sports?
- Should one take protein supplements to build muscle?
- Some protein is considered high quality, some low quality, what does this mean?
- Where do vegetarians get protein?
- Can vegetarian children grow properly without animal protein?

The most fundamental belief regarding protein is that protein is meat and meat is protein. This is because most of the animal based foods are pretty much composed entirely of protein; remove the protein from a beef steak and you will have a puddle of water, fat, and some trace vitamins and minerals. Protein is the core of animal based foods. Early scientists of our day like Carl Voit (1831-1908) were big promoters of protein. Voit found that a person only needed 48.5 grams per day, but recommended 118 due to the cultural bias at the time. As he said, "a large protein allowance is the right of a civilized man." Protein equalled meat and meat at that time was a sign of wealth, prosperity, and class, and he figured that you can't really get too much of a good thing.

The cultural bias was firmly rooted. If you ate plenty of protein, meaning meat, you were civilized and rich, and if you were poor you ate staple plant foods like potatoes and bread. The lower classes were considered lazy and stupid as a result of not eating enough meat, or protein. Elitism and arrogance dominated the field of nutrition in the nineteenth century bringing forth concepts that more protein is better, more civilized, and even more spiritual.

Protein, carbohydrates, and fat are the main building blocks of our body, they are the *macro*nutrients. The remaining parts are *micro*nutrients; all the vitamins and minerals. The combination of these parts is what makes the whole function. Proteins are long chains constructed from hundreds of thousands of amino acids, like a bracelet of beads, and each functions as enzymes, hormones, structural tissue or transport molecules. As protein is broken down and worn out by our bodies, it must be replaced by the food we eat. There are eight amino acids ("colored beads") that can only be provided from the food we eat, the are called "essential." The difference between protein quality is how well they supply all the necessary amino acids to replace the ones that were worn out or broken down. In other words, it is the ability of the food proteins to provide the right kinds and amounts of amino acids to make new proteins. If a food provides all the necessary amino acids and all 8 "essential" amino acids upon digestion, then it will be considered a high quality protein.

What food do you think we would have to eat that that would provide our body with all the necessary amino acids? Human flesh. It has just the right amount of all the needed amino acids our body would need. While humans are not on the menu in most parts of the world, we eat the next so called "best" protein of other animals. They are considered high quality because they contain most or all of the "essential" and "non-essential" amino acids. While the "lower quality" protein of plants may lack a few of the amino acids, as a *group* they do contain all of them.

There is something misleading about the term "quality" which does not necessarily mean health. It is referring to how efficiently food proteins are used to promote growth. Basically, it says if growth occurs quicker with a type of protein then it is high quality, but again, that does not mean it is healthy. There are giant heaps of evidence that show that the so called "low quality" plant protein allow for slow but steady synthesis of new proteins, and are the *healthiest* types of protein. Remember the phrase "slow and steady wins the race?"

We all know that plants have plenty of protein, but people will still ask sometimes, "Where do I get my protein?" There is still concern about the perceived poor quality of plant protein, which has led people to believe that they must carefully combine proteins from different plant sources during each meal so that they can compensate for the amino acid deficit. In reality this is not necessary; we now know that through very complex metabolic processes, the human body can get all the essential amino acids from the natural variety of plant proteins we encounter every day. This means we don't have to meticulously plan out each meal to get the required amino acids, regular plant based food along with our liver work perfectly fine together to ensure our body has all the required amino acids.

Since the 1970's universities, institutes, and government agencies have been seriously concerned with the world's "high quality" protein intake, mostly from livestock. We were so concerned with this aspect of nutrition that we set up many high scale projects to get protein to starving children across the world.

To address this dire problem:

- MIT was developing a protein-rich food supplement called INCA-PARINA.
- Purdue University was breeding corn to contain more lysine, the "deficient" amino acid in corn protein.
- The U.S. government was subsidizing the production of dried milk powder to provide high quality protein for the world's poor.
- Cornell University was providing a wealth of talent to the Philip-pines to help develop both a high-protein rice variety and a live- stock industry.
- Auburn University and MIT were grinding up fish to produce "fish protein concentrate" to feed the world's poor.

And this is only a few examples. Our tax dollars were subsidizing farms and food producers to make more protein; we thought it was a worldwide crisis that people were not getting enough protein. The Food and Agriculture Organization of the United Nations declared in 1970 that "...by and large, the lack of protein is without question the most serious qualitative deficiency in the nutrition of developing countries. The great mass of the population of these countries subsists mainly on foods derived from plants frequently deficient in protein, which results in poor health and low productivity per man."

Bruce Stillings at the University of Maryland and the U.S. Department of Commerce, another proponent of consuming animal-based diets, admitted in 1973 that "although there is no requirement for animal protein in the diet per se, the quantity of dietary protein from animal sources is usually accepted as being indicative of the overall protein quality of the diet." He went on to say that the " ... supply of adequate quantities of animal products is generally recognized as being an ideal way to improve world protein nutrition."

Of course, it is correct to say that a supply of protein can help to improve nutrition in the third world. But what kind of protein? Animal based protein is not the only answer; it is actually a very poor answer in terms of human health, finances, sustainability, energy use, and agricultural yields.

The truth is people who do not consume meat aren't in any way more protein-starved than their meat-eating counterparts. According to a paper published in 2002, John McDougall, MD, concluded that "it is impossible to design an amino acid–deficient diet based on the amounts of unprocessed starches and vegetables sufficient to meet the calorie needs of humans."

The story of Dr. Campbell's protein research in the Philippines is quite interesting. His team went there to try and bring an end to child malnutrition. In the urban areas of some of the big cities, as many as 15-20% of the children aged three to six years were judged to be third degree malnourished which meant near starvation. That is a huge number. Teams from many universities went to the Philippines, Haiti, and other underdeveloped countries to try and educate the population about nutrition and proper protein intake because they thought proper protein intake was the key element that was missing from their diets. They also noticed a very high incidence of liver cancer, and thought it was because of the very potent cancer causing toxin called aflatoxin which was primarily in peanuts and corn, two very popular and widely consumed foods in the big cities in the Philippines. Two areas with the highest incidences of liver cancer were Manila and Cebu, the biggest cities in the Philippines, and they were also areas with the most aflatoxin consumed.

But as it turned out the story was much deeper than that. Dr. Campbell made acquaintance with Dr. Jose Caedo, an advisor to President Marcos. He was told that the liver cancer problem in the Philippines was very serious and was claiming the lives of children before the age of ten. When in the West, this disease mostly strikes people only after forty years of age. Dr. Caedo even recited stories of operating on children younger than four years old for liver cancer!

In itself this was shocking enough, but what he heard next was even more striking. The children who got the most liver cancer were from the best fed and most affluent families. The families who he thought ate the healthiest diets similar to our own meaty diets and had the most money were the most disease stricken. They consumed more "high quality" animal protein than anyone else in the country, and yet they were the ones getting liver cancer.

It didn't make any sense, how could this be happening? Worldwide, countries with the highest incidence of liver cancer were the ones with the lowest average protein intake so it was believed that a deficiency in protein lead to liver cancer. Further, it was the reason Dr. Campbell and his team went to the Philippines; to increase the protein consumption in as many malnourished children as possible. But now he was hearing that the best fed children had the highest incidence of liver cancer. At first, this made no sense to him, but over time his own information increasingly confirmed these observations.

It was at that time that he discovered the research paper from India that experimented on rats that were fed aflatoxin and then put on a 20% and 5% protein diet. The group that was put on the 5% protein diet got no liver cancer despite the aflatoxin. The 100 to 0 score was very convincing and was very consistent with his previous observations for the Philippine children. Those who were most vulnerable to liver cancer were those who consumed diets higher in animal protein.

During his early research, Dr Campbell had some close family members die from cancer and he promised himself that he would go wherever his research led him to try and understand this horrible disease, and do everything he can to try and cure it. His personal experiences taught him that even if some research went against his or the beliefs of his peers he would not turn his back on it just because it was "uncomfortable" or "provocative" as many of his peers did. From his early thoughts and personal experience, the idea that cancer was strongly linked with nutrition fuelled his desire to try and find the cause between this link. He began doing fundamental research to see not only if, but also how, consuming more protein leads to more cancer. His research led him farther than he could have imagined; the findings that he and his colleagues and students generated just might make you think twice about your current diet. But even more than that, his findings lead to bigger questions, questions that would lead to cracks in the very foundation of nutrition and health.

Proof, or Is It?

When we say science "proves something," that is a very elusive statement. Even more that in the "core" sciences like biology, chemistry, and physics, establishing *absolute* proof in medicine and health is close to impossible. The primary objective in research is figuring out what is only *likely* to happen under specific circumstances. This is because research in medicine and health is inherently statistical. If you jump up in the air, will you come back down? Yes, that is physics. If you smoke 4 packs a day, will you get lung cancer? The answer is maybe. Medicine can tell you that you odds of getting lung cancer will be higher, but nobody can tell you with full certainty that you will get lung cancer.

The reason for such difficulties in nutrition research is the vast amount of differences in each individual. We live all sorts of ways, what we eat, what we do, where we go, our genetic background. The fact that we live all sorts of different ways makes proving any one factor and any one disease is nearly impossible, even if you had the perfect set of subjects, unlimited funds and time. What usually happens is *observation* of what occurs under specific conditions and sometimes intentionally *intervene* with a hypothetical treatment to see what happens. It is really observational and interventional research, nothing ever is proven with complete accuracy or certainty. And as the mass of findings come in, researchers weigh the evidence for or against a certain hypothesis. When the weight of the evidence favours an idea so strongly that it can no longer be plausibly denied, they advance the idea as likely truth.

It is in this way that many scientists, researchers, and doctors around the world, including Dr. Campbell, are advancing an argument for a whole food, vitamin rich plant based diet, and those seeking truth regarding diet and health by weighing the evidence from a variety of available studies will be amazed and enlightened by the astonishing health benefits of such a diet.

Big Fear

Cancer is probably the most feared disease in the world. Slowly and painfully being consumed for months or even years before passing away is a horrific thought to say the least. So when the media reports on a newly found chemical carcinogen, the public reacts quickly. Some reports even cause panic which was the case with Alar, a chemical that was sprayed on apples as a growth regulator. Shortly after, a report from the Natural Resources Defense Council (NRDC) titled "Intolerable Risk: Pesticides in Our Children's Food", the television program 60 Minutes aired a segment on Alar. In February 1989 a representative of NRDC said on CBS's 60 Minutes that the apple industry chemical was "the most potent carcinogen in the food supply.

Public reaction was swift. One woman even called to police to chase down a school bus to confiscate her child's apple. School boards across the country even stopped serving apples and after this hot topic the U.S. Apple Association lost over $250 million. Finally in response to the public outcry, the production and use of Alar came to a full stop in 1989.

Stories like Alar are not uncommon. Over the past several decades, many chemicals have been identified in the popular press as cancer causing agents. You may have heard of some:

• Aminotriazole (herbicide used on cranberry crops, causing the "cranberry scare" of 1959)
• DDT (widely known after Rachel Carson's book, Silent Spring)
• Nitrites (a meat preservative and color and flavor enhancer used in hot dogs and bacon)
• Red Dye Number 2
• Artificial sweeteners (including cyclamates and saccharin)
• Dioxin (a contaminant of industrial processes and of Agent Or- ange, a defoliant used during the Vietnam War)
• Aflatoxin (a fungal toxin found in moldy peanuts and corn)

All these chemicals have a similar story in regards to cancer. In each case the chemical was found to increase cancer rates in experimental animals and public as well as government reaction was very quick and strong. For example; when nitrosamines (a scary family of chemicals that are added to meat to kill bacteria and add a pink color and desirable taste to hot dogs, bacon, canned meat, and even fresh meat on grocery store shelves) were "reasonably anticipated to be human carcinogens" by the U.S. National Toxicology Program they were quickly pounced on.

That is not the whole story by the way. These scares came from an animal study that divided twenty rats into two groups each exposed to a different level of NSAR (N-nitrososarcosine). The high dose rats were given twice the amount that the low dose rats received. Of rats given the low dose of NSAR, just over 35% of them died of throat cancer. Of rats given the higher levels, 100% died of cancer during the second year of experiment. But how much NSAR did the rats get? In the low dose, to give you an example, to get the same amount of NSAR you would have to eat 270 000 sandwiches each with one pound of bologna on them every day for thirty years. If you do this, you would have about as much exposure to NSAR (per body weight) as the rats in the "low dose" group.

Because higher cancer rates were seen in rats and mice using a variety of methods of exposure, NSAR was "reasonably anticipated" to be a human carcinogen. And since the animal dosages were so astronomical nobody really knows what the real danger level is for humans, and it is quite impossible to find out. Nonetheless animal experiments alone were considered enough to conclude that NSAR is "reasonably anticipated" to be a human carcinogen.

In 1970, when an article in the prestigious journal Nature concluded that nitrites help to form nitrosamines in the body, thereby implying that they help to cause cancer, people became very concerned. The official phrase was; "Reduction of human exposure to nitrites and certain secondary amines, particularly in foods, may result in a decrease in the incidence of human cancer. All of a sudden, nitrites were seen as a potential killer and many products came under fire. Ralph Nader had called hot dogs "among America's deadliest missiles." Some consumer advocacy groups were calling for a nitrite additive ban, and government officials began a serious review of nitrite's potential health problems.

The issue jolted forward again in 1978, when a study at the Massachusetts Institute of Technology (MIT) found that nitrite increased lymphatic cancer in rats. The study, as reported in a 1979 issue of Science, 15 found that, on average, rats fed nitrite got lymphatic cancer 10.2% of the time, while animals not fed nitrite got cancer only 5.4% of the time. This finding was enough to create a public uproar. Fierce debate ensued in the government, industry and research communities. When the dust settled, expert panels made recommendations, industry cut back on ni- trite usage and the issue fell out of the spotlight.

The moral of the story is that scientific results can make a very big stir in the public when it comes to cancer causing or very dangerous chemicals. A rise in cancer incidence from 5% to 10% in rat studies by nitrites caused an explosion of controversy and millions of dollars in spending. Nobody is denying the fact that these additives are very dangerous and may cause serious health concerns, it is the mere possibility, however unlikely that it may be, that it could cause cancer that alarms the public and brings along such a huge government and research community uproar and media coverage.

But what if research has produced considerably more impressive scientific results which were far more substantial? What if there was a chemical that could turn cancer on and off in **100% of the test animals**? Furthermore what if this chemical could do all this in routine levels of intake and not the colossal levels used in the NSAR experiments? Finding such a chemical would be the holy grail of cancer research and the implication towards human health would be enormous. We would assume that such a chemical would be of much more concern than nitrites, or Alar, or even aflatoxin.

This is exactly what the research on protein shows. From his early studies to the work in the Philippines, to the Indian research paper, and all the way into the China study and all the following studies and anecdotal evidence from his peers and doctors from all across the world, time and time again research shows that animal protein intake is a huge link to cancer and nearly every other "western" disease our society is plagued with.

Scientists are a very sceptical bunch, and upon discovering the link between protein and cancer Dr. Campbell had to conduct his studies extremely thoroughly, he had nothing to gain and everything to lose. If he openly said that protein was responsible for cancer he might have been labelled a heretic and cast out like many other truth seeking individuals. For more than 25 years he received funding from the NIH and other top research agencies like the American Cancer Society, the American Institute for Cancer Research, and the Cancer Research Foundation of America) which led to more than 100 scientific papers published in some of the best journals on the topic.

The Link

At the start of their research many question arose. The biggest one being; “why does protein affect the cancer process and what are the mechanisms?” So their first step was to figure out whether protein intake affected the enzyme principally responsible for aflatoxin metabolism, called the mixed function oxidase (MFO). This enzyme being studied is very complex because it also metabolizes pharmaceuticals and other chemicals and both detoxifies and activates aflatoxin.

The first hypothesis they made was that the proteins we consume alters tumor growth by changing how aflatoxin is detoxified by the enzymes present in the liver. Then they questioned whether the amount of protein that we eat could change the enzyme activity. After a series of experiments it was quite clear that *enzyme activity could in fact be easily modified simply by changing the level of protein intake.*

Dr. Campbell's research supported the earlier research in India that decreasing protein intake (20% to 5%) not only greatly decreased harmful enzyme activity but did so very quickly. This means less toxic by-products had the potential to bind to and mutate the DNA. They tested this implication of whether a low protein diet actually decreased the binding of aflatoxin product to DNA and showed exactly that. Evidence showed that a low protein diet decreases enzyme activity and prevents dangerous carcinogen binding to DNA. These were very impressive findings, enough to show how eating less animal protein leads to less cancer. But they wanted to know more and continued their research.

As they continued on they came upon some remarkable discoveries about low animal protein diets and their effects:

- Less aflatoxin entered the cell
- Cells multiplied more slowly
- Multiple changes occurred within the enzyme complex to reduce its activity
- The quantity of critical components of the relevant enzymes was reduced
- Less aflatoxin-DNA connections were formed

Their research added a great deal of weight to the Indian studies showing more than one way or mechanism that low protein diets work. From their extensive research one idea seemed very clear: *lower protein intake dramatically decreased tumor initiation or formation.* This finding, even though well proven, is enormously provocative for many people.

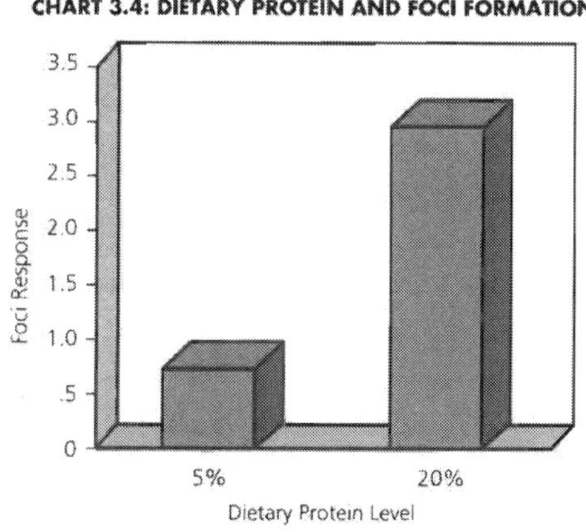

That was an incredible finding, but they decided to do more experiments. They asked questions like: what happens during the promotion stage of cancer, the all-important reversible stage? Would the benefits of low protein intake achieved during initiation continue through promotion? Due to the difficult nature of studying this stage of cancer which requires rats to live until they develop full tumors, the expenses, and long time they decided to look at little microscopic cell clusters which were called foci.

Foci are precursor clusters of cells that grow into tumors and they appear right after initiation is complete (initiation can be explained in the example of a seed going into the ground, the seed representing cancer). And although most foci do not become full blown tumor cells, they are predictive of tumor development.

They came upon some remarkable findings. *Foci development was almost entirely dependent on how much protein was consumed, regardless of how much aflatoxin was consumed!* After initiation with aflatoxin, foci grew far more with the 20% animal protein diet and than with the 5% protein diet.

Then they tested whether different protein diets had any affect on varied doses of aflatoxin. They wondered whether the animals that start with lots of cancerous seeds are able to overcome their situation by eating a low animal protein diet. One group was administered a high dose of aflatoxin and fed a low protein diet, the other group was administered a low dose of aflatoxin and fed a high protein diet.

The results once again shocked the team. Animals starting with the most cancer initiation (high-aflatoxin dose) developed substantially less foci when fed the 5% protein diet. In contrast, animals initiated with a low-aflatoxin dose actually produced substantially more foci when subsequently fed the 20% protein diet. A principle was being established. Foci development, initially determined by the amount of the carcinogen exposure, is actually controlled far more by dietary protein consumed during promotion. Animal protein during promotion trumps the carcinogen, regardless of initial exposure.

Dr. Campbell's own account: "Here is a step-by-step sequence of experiments, carried out by my graduate student Linda Youngman. All animals were dosed with the same amount of carcinogen, then alternately fed either 5% or 20% dietary protein during the twelve-week promotion stage. We divided this twelve-week promotion stage into four periods of three weeks each. Period 1 represents weeks one to three, period 2 represents weeks four to six, and so on.

When animals were fed the 20% protein diet during periods 1 and 2 (20-20), foci continued to enlarge, as expected. But when animals were switched to the low-protein diet at the beginning of period 3 (20-20-5), there was a sharp decrease in foci development. And, when animals were subsequently switched back to the 20% protein diet during period 4 (20-20-5-20), foci development was turned on once again. In another experiment, in animals fed 20% dietary protein during period 1 but switched to 5% dietary protein during period 2 (20-5), foci development was sharply decreased. But when these animals were returned to 20% dietary protein during period 3 (20-5-20), we again saw the dramatic power of dietary protein to promote foci development.

These several experiments, taken together, were quite profound. Foci growth could be reversed, up and down, by switching the amount of protein being consumed, and at all stages of foci development."

Basically, the results showed that no matter how much cancer causing chemical was used, diet had a much stronger effect on whether or not foci (precursors to tumors) developed. More *animal protein intake always equalled cancer growth and formation while less animal protein equalled a reduction in cancer growth and formation.*

Their experiments also demonstrated that the body can "remember" early toxin insults, even though they may lie dormant for years with low protein intake. "That is, exposure to aflatoxin left a genetic "imprint" that remained dormant with 5% dietary protein until nine weeks later when this imprint reawakened to form foci with 20% dietary protein. In simple terms, the body holds a grudge. It suggests that if we are exposed in the past to a carcinogen that initiates a bit of cancer that remains dormant, this cancer can still be "reawakened" by bad nutrition some time later."

What the studies show is that cancer is strongly modified even by relatively small protein consumption. They investigated a range of 4-24% dietary protein and found that up to about 10% foci did not develop. Beyond 10% foci development increased dramatically with increases in dietary protein.

CHART 3.6: FOCI PROMOTION BY DIETARY PROTEIN

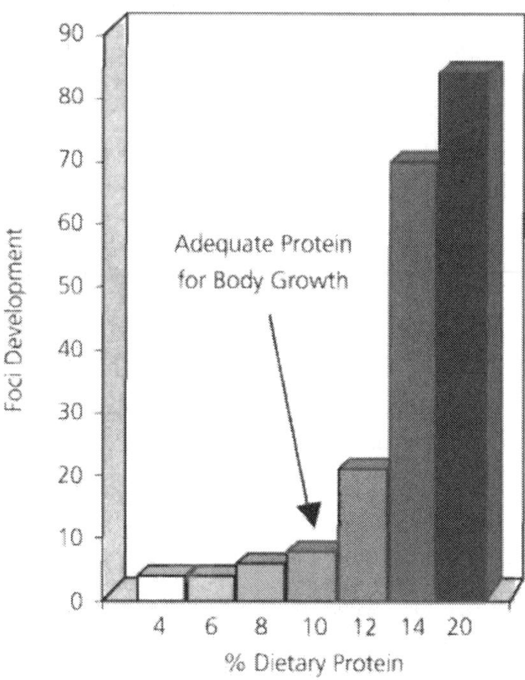

What is very interesting is that they found that foci developed only when the animals met or exceeded the amount of dietary protein required for body growth and development (12%). In other words, if this amount was exceeded, disease began. The other interesting fact is that the percentage of necessary protein intake between rats and humans is remarkably similar. The recommended daily allowance (RDA) for protein is 10%, meaning we should be getting 10% of our energy from protein. Actually this number is much higher than what is required by the body, but since there is so much variation from individual to individual, 10% is recommended to ensure a proper amount for all people. The national average for protein intake is about 15-16% meaning 70-100 grams while 10% is about 50-60 grams depending on body weight and calorie intake. Does this mean we are at greater risk for getting cancer? Studies definitely point at that.

Another experiment was set up to explain if much higher doses of aflatoxin would have an effect between the low and high protein diets. This is what they found: in the group of rats fed 20% protein, the foci increased in number and size as the dose increased, as was expected. But in the 5% protein group, there was no difference between the amount of aflatoxin administered, *there was absolutely no foci response even when maximally tolerated aflatoxin doses were given.*

CHART 3.7: AFLATOXIN DOSE—FOCI RESPONSE

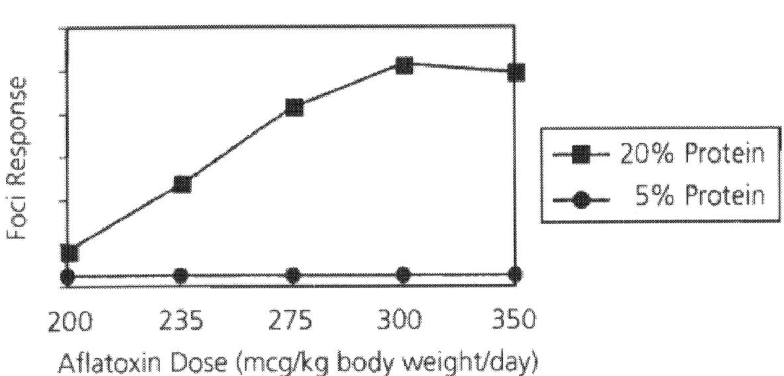

No matter how much cancer causing chemicals were administered, the low protein 5% group saw absolutely no change in cancer growth or formation. Is it possible that chemical carcinogens, in general, do not cause cancer unless the nutritional conditions are "right"? Is it possible that, for much of our lives, we are being exposed to varying amounts of cancer causing chemicals, but cancer does not develop unless we consume foods that promote and nurture tumor development? It is quite clear; *we can control cancer through nutrition.*

Are All Proteins Alike?

What you have read so far is quite stunning and the findings are very provocative. The ability to control cancer through nutrition is still a very radical idea, and if that's not enough, would the *type* of protein make a difference? For the previous experiments casein was used (treated and processed casein isolate, NOT raw milk), which makes up 87% of cow's milk protein. So they decided to test whether or not plant protein would have the same effect on cancer growth. The answer they found was a resounding "NO." In further experimentation, ***plant protein did not promote cancer growth, even at very high levels of intake***. For example, *gluten*, the protein of wheat, *did not promote the same results as casein, even when fed the same 20% level.*

CHART 3.8: PROTEIN TYPE AND FOCI RESPONSE

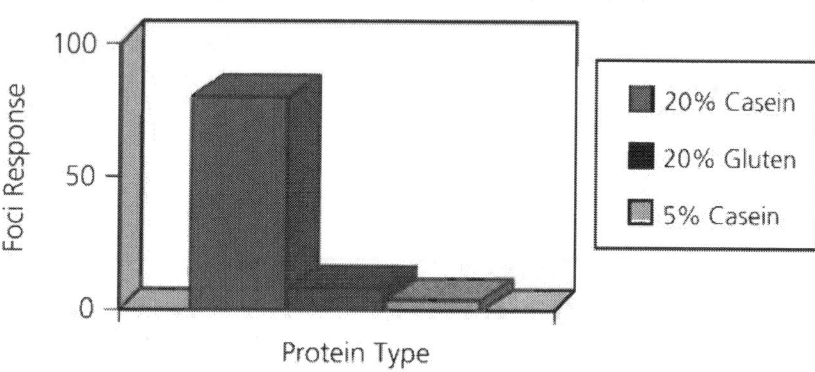

Soy protein also had *no effect*. Casein, the protein in milk and milk products, was not looking so good after these findings. But it's important to say that pasteurized (boiled) and homogenized (filtered through tiny membranes to break apart fat clusters) milk, which in other words is store bought milk, is completely different than raw milk straight from the udders of a cow that is raised in a natural environment, feeds on grass rather than corn/soy/various animal parts, and has had no toxic vaccinations. Raw milk is a completely different product compared to boiled milk where all the proteins have coagulated or fused together, and where almost all the nutrients are rendered useless. Raw milk, and raw milk products (yes it's possible to make cottage cheese without heating up milk) are one of the most beneficial products on the face of the earth (by the way, you might have heard that milk and milk products cause the formation of mucous in our bodies, if you drink milk at night and in the morning hot, no mucous will form, try it!).

These experiments showed that just like a light switch, they could control cancer growth just by changing the protein intake, regardless of initial carcinogen exposure.

Up to this point in their experiments Dr. Campbell and his team relied on the early indicators of tumor development by looking at the early cancer like foci cells. It was then they decided to do the grand finale, the big study where they would measure complete tumor formation. They organized a large study of a few hundred rats and examined tumor formation over their entire lifetimes. What they found was nothing less than astonishing.

Since rats live for around two years, the study length was 100 weeks. All the animals that were administered aflatoxin and fed the 20% protein diet were dead or near death from liver tumors at 100 weeks. All the animals that were administered aflatoxin and then fed the low 5% protein diet were alive, active, healthy, and with a sleek coat at 100 weeks. This was a virtual 100 to 0 score, which is something almost never seen in research, and almost identical to the similar Indian research.

In the same experiment they switched the diets of some rats at either forty or sixty weeks, to see whether they could reverse or promote cancer growth. Animals switched to a high protein diet from a low protein diet had significantly less tumor growth (35%-40% less!) than animals fed a high protein diet. Animals switched from a low protein diet to a high protein diet halfway through their lifetime started growing tumor again. These findings again confirmed their earlier studies using foci. It all comes down to the fact that ***nutrition can turn cancer "on" and "off."***

CHART 3.9A: TUMOR DEVELOPMENT AT 100 WEEKS

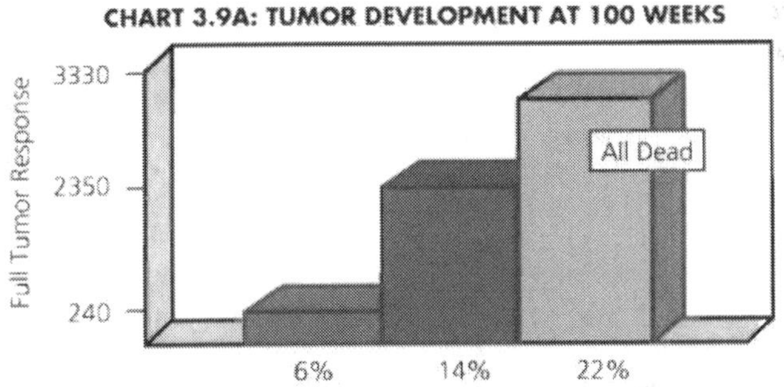

CHART 3.9B: EARLY FOCI, "LIFETIME"

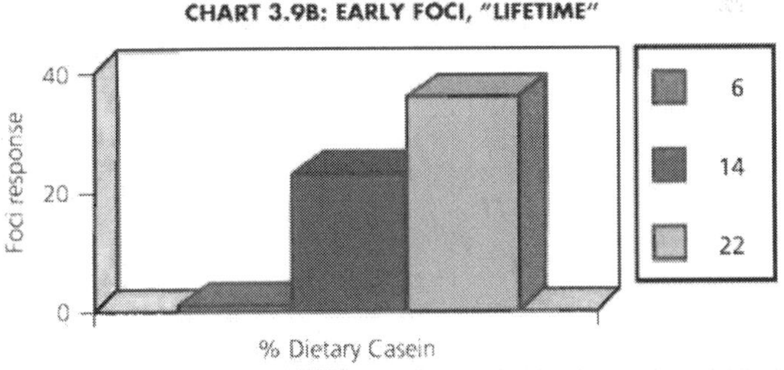

Dr. Campbell writes; "How much more did we need to find out? I would never have dreamed that our results up to this point would be so

incredibly consistent, biologically plausible, and statistically significant. We had fully confirmed the original work from India and had done it in exceptional depth."

Other Cancers, Other Carcinogens

So how does this apply to human health and liver cancer in particular? They decided once again that one way to investigate this question is to research other species, other carcinogens and other organs. If such effects are brought by casein, then humans better take note. So their research took on a bigger scope to see whether their discoveries would hold up.

During the time their rat studies were underway; other studies were published claiming that chronic infection with hepatitis B virus was the major risk factor for human liver cancer. They claimed that people who remained chronically infected with this virus had twenty to forty times the risk of getting liver cancer. There was quite a lot of research on this subject but it was all focused on the mechanism by which HBV works, with absolutely no attention given to the effects of nutrition on tumor development. Dr Campbell writes that he was quite amused watching for several years how one community of researchers argued for aflatoxin as the key cause of human liver cancer and another community argued for HBV, but nobody dared to suggest that nutrition played any role in cancer.

They decided to figure this out as well, and see whether casein had any effect on HBV induced liver cancer in mice. This went much further, now they were dealing with much more than just aflatoxin. They began by setting up a group of transgenic mice (DNA was infected with HBV), and after much difficulty finally secured funding for research (the reviewers did not take kindly the notion that protein could have such an effect on cancer, and it was showing that he experiments were quite explicit in questioning the mythical health value of protein). What did their research show? *They got essentially the same results as in their previous studies.*

CHART 3.10: DIETARY PROTEIN EFFECT ON GENETICALLY-BASED (HBV) LIVER CANCER (MICE)

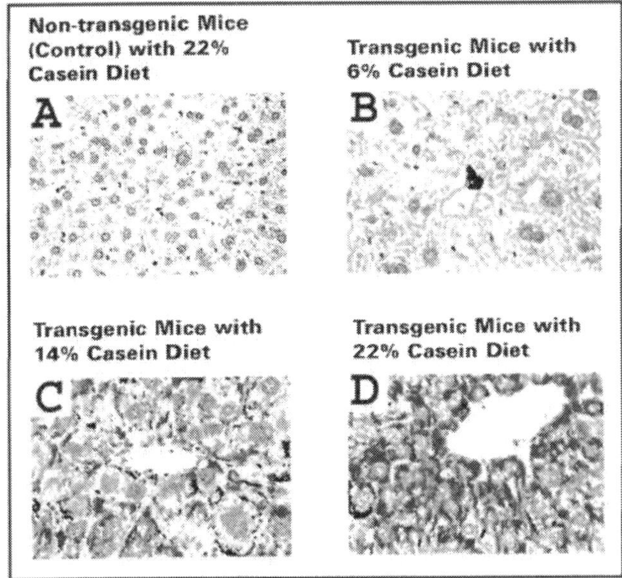

This chart shows the difference in cancer growth with different protein intakes. The darker color material is indicative of cancer development. There is intense early cancer formation in the 22% casein group (D), much less in the 14% casein group (C), and none in the 6% casein group (B), picture (A) is the control with no virus gene.

So far, they concluded that it doesn't matter whether it is a carcinogen aflatoxin, or mice infected with HBV, casein promotes liver cancer in both.

Next question they asked was: "can we generalize these findings to other cancers and to other carcinogens?" At the University of Illinois Medical Center in Chicago, another research group was working with mammary (breast) cancer in rats. This research showed that increasing intakes of ca- sein promoted the development of mammary (breast) cancer. They found that higher casein intake:

- promotes breast cancer in rats dosed with two experimental carcinogens (7,12 dimethybenz(a)anthracene (DBMA) and N-nitroso-methylurea (NMU))
- operates through a network of reactions that combine to increase cancer

- operates through the same female hormone system that operates in humans

It was a one-two knockout punch. An impressively consistent pattern emerged that casein is the "switch" that controls cancer growth no matter what organ or carcinogen present. The only question that has not been answered is; "why is this information still not widely known?"

Even though Dr. Campbell reached very impressive results that could just as well be used as they are, he continued on! He wanted to broaden his evidence, and find out what effect other nutrients have on cancer, and how they interact with different carcinogens and different organs. They began other studies with fish protein, dietary fat, and some antioxidants. *The results of these studies, and many others, showed that nutrition is much more important in controlling cancer promotion than the dose of initiating carcinogen*. The *Journal of the National Cancer Institute* even featured some of his studies.

It was quite clear, from all the research a pattern emerged; ***nutrients from animal based foods increase tumor development while nutrients from plant based foods decrease tumor development***. The pattern was consistent no matter what carcinogen was used, what organ was studied, or what nutrient was looked at, from one mechanism to another, from one stage to another, the pattern was exactly the same; animal based foods promote cancer formation.

These results were indeed spectacular, even the researchers could never have imagined these findings. At the same time one thought bothered Dr. Campbell as he writes "all this evidence was gathered in experimental animal studies...In other words, are these principles regarding animal protein and cancer critically important for all humans in all situations, or are they merely marginally important for a minority of people in fairly unique situations?" Ideally, he thought, this evidence would be gathered with rigorous methodology, and would investigate dietary patterns comprehensively using large numbers of people who had similar lifestyles, similar genetic backgrounds, and at the same time had widely varying incidence of disease.

The ability to conduct such as study was at best, extremely rare. But during the year of 1980, Dr. Campbell had just the opportunity to conduct such a massive and detailed study. It was a once in a lifetime opportunity. He was given a chance to do a human study that would take all those principles they began to uncover in the lab to the next level. They were on to study the role of nutrition, lifestyle and disease in *the most comprehensive manner ever undertaken in the history of medicine*. They were on to...

The China Study

It all started very quickly. Early in the year 1980, a very distinguished senior scientist from China, Dr. Junshi Chen, came to Cornell to work in Dr. Campbell's lab. Just to clarify this situation, Dr. Chen was only one of the first handful of Chinese scholars to visit the U.S. following the relationship between those two countries.

During the early 1970's, the premier of China, Chou EnLai, was dying of cancer. He then initiated a nationwide survey to collect information about a disease that was not very well understood. What followed was a monumental survey of death rates for twelve kinds of cancer for more than 2400 Chinese counties and 880 million (96%) of their citizens. It was quite a feat, with 650000 workers, becoming the most ambitious biomedical research project ever undertaken. The result was a color coded atlas showing where certain types of cancer were high and where they were nonexistent.

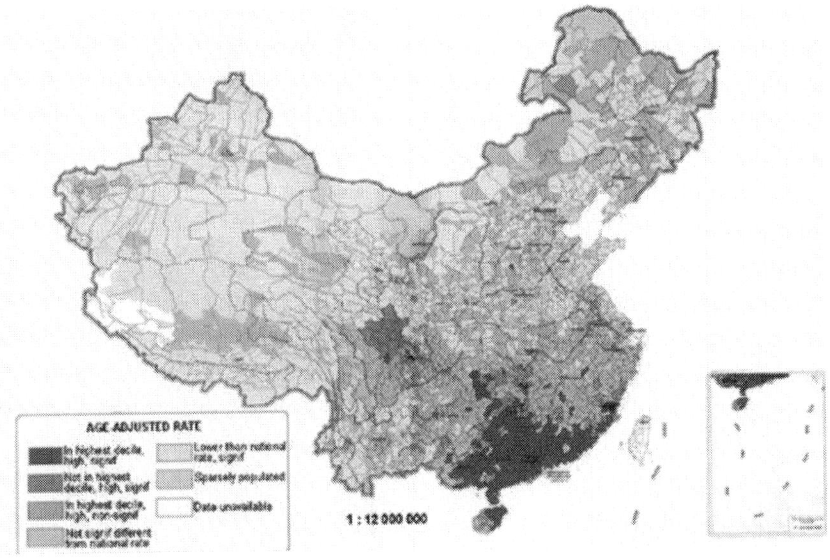

This atlas showed that cancer in China was very geographically localized with some cancers more common in some places than others. The data was quite remarkable because it included a population that was of the same ethnic group and similar genetic backgrounds but had astoundingly large geographic variations in cancer rates; counties with higher cancer rates were up to 100 times greater than counties with lower cancer rates! So why were there such great differences in cancer rates? A few prominent scientists had already reached that conclusion. The authors of a major review on diet and cancer, prepared for the U.S. Congress in 1981, estimated that genetics only determines about *2-3% of the total cancer risk.*

By the way, the U.S. population sees at most, two to three times the cancer rates from one part of the country to another. In fact, very small differences can stir up a big fuss. Two counties in Long Island had rates of breast cancer only 10-20% higher than the state average. This difference was enough to bring it to front page news, raise a huge scare in people, and move politicians to action. Contrast this with the 100 times (10,000%) difference that some counties in China had.

Since China was such a genetically homogenous population, these stark differences had to be explained another way; primarily by environmental causes. The researchers had to figure out why there was such great difference between counties, why some counties had such high incidences of cancer, and why, overall, China was less cancer stricken than the U.S.

After some discussion and the timely "coming together" of science, politics, and financing Dr. Chen and Dr. Campbell decided it was time to conduct the most comprehensive study of diet, lifestyle, and disease every taken. After assembling a world class scientific team, it was the first major research project between China and the U.S.

As Dr. Campbell recites: "We decided to make the study as comprehensive as possible. From the Cancer Atlas, we had access to disease mortality rates on more than four dozen different kinds of disease, including individual cancers, heart diseases and infectious diseases. We gathered data on 367 variables and then compared each variable with every other variable. We went into sixty-five counties across China and administered questionnaires and blood tests on 6,500 adults. We took urine samples, directly measured everything families ate over a three-day period and analyzed food samples from marketplaces around the country.

The sixty-five counties selected for the study were located in rural to semi-rural parts of China. This was intentionally done because we wanted to study people who mostly lived and ate food in the same area for most of their lives. This was a successful strategy, as we were to learn than an average of 90-94% of the adult subjects in each county still lived in the same county where they were born. When we were done we had more than 8,000 statistically significant associations between lifestyle, diet and disease variables. We had a study that was unmatched in terms of comprehensiveness, quality and uniqueness. We had what the New York Times termed "the Grand Prix of epidemiology." In short, we had created that revealing snapshot of time that we had Originally envisioned"

They revealed some significant differences in the diet of the Chinese population as compared to the diet of the U.S. population.

CHART 4.3. CHINESE AND AMERICAN DIETARY INTAKES

Nutrient	China	United States
Calories (kcal/day)[7]	2641	1989
Total fat (% of calories)	14.5	34–38
Dietary fiber (g/day)	33	12
Total protein (g/day)	64	91
Animal protein (% of calories)	0.8	10–11
Total iron (mg/day)	34	18

In North America, 15-16% of our calories come from protein and up to 80% of that protein come from animal based foods. In China, on the other hand, only 9-10% of total calories come from protein and only 10% of that protein comes from animal based sources. The major difference between most studies on nutrition done in the West is that scientist here tend to compare diets rich in animal based foods to diets very rich in animal based foods. What was so radical in this study is the comparison between animal based diets and plant based diets, and what effect each has on our health.

The media called this a "landmark study" and that this project "should shake up medical and nutrition researchers everywhere." Some said a similar study like this could never be done. It was truly a monumental task, which would, *as they hoped*, bring about major changes in the way we see nutrition.

I really like and totally agree with what Dr. Campbell states: "It doesn't take a scientist to figure out that the possibility of death has been holding pretty steady at 100% for quite some time. There's only one thing that we have to do in life, and that is to die. I have often met people who use this fact to justify their ambivalence toward health in- formation. But I take a different view. I have never pursued health hoping for immortality. Good health is about being able to fully enjoy the time we do have. It is about being as functional as possible throughout our entire lives and avoiding crippling, painful and lengthy battles with disease. There are many better ways to die, and to live."

We are supposed to be healthy and full of vitality until the day we die. The reason for any of this information is so you can enjoy every minute of every day in optimal health. So you don't have to spend time in the hospital, or spend great amounts of money on medication that will only make you sicker, so you don't have to be operated on, and so you can *enjoy* your life in *full health*.

When all the data was collected and analyzed, and all diseases were cross-listed in a way that allowed every disease rate to be compared with every other disease rate, two major groups of disease emerged; those typically found in more economically developed areas (diseases of affluence) and those typically found in rural agricultural areas (diseases of poverty).

CHART 4.4. DISEASE GROUPINGS OBSERVED IN RURAL CHINA

Diseases of Affluence (Nutritional Extravagance)	Cancer (colon, lung, breast, leukemia, childhood brain, stomach, liver), diabetes, coronary heart disease
Diseases of Poverty (Nutritional inadequacy and poor sanitation)	Pneumonia, intestinal obstruction, peptic ulcer, digestive disease, pulmonary tuberculosis, parasitic disease, rheumatic heart disease, metabolic and endocrine disease other than diabetes, diseases of pregnancy and many others

Each disease in each list tended to associate with diseases in its own list; that means people in certain geographical areas became sick with only certain diseases and not others. For example, people in "richer" areas of the country tended to get heart disease and cancer, and people in "poorer" areas of the country tended to get pneumonia, intestinal, and digestive problems. This explains that certain diseases cluster together in the same geographical area, implying that they have similar shared causes. Now the goal was to find out what those causes were.

As a developing population accumulates wealth, people change their eating habits and sanitary conditions, and as more wealth accumulates, people die more and more from the "rich" diseases of affluence than the "poor" diseases of poverty. Because the diseases of affluence are so strongly linked with eating habits they may as well be called "diseases of nutritional extravagance," which most people in the U.S. and Western countries tend to die from. This is why they are often referred to as "Western" diseases. The goal of further investigation was to figure out which dietary habits linked to each disease.

They found that the strongest predictor of Western diseases was blood cholesterol. Cholesterol levels in the U.S. are around 215 mg/dL while in China it is only 127 mg/dL. And even though some myth maybe present that low blood cholesterol is dangerous, in reality it is the opposite; lower blood cholesterol levels are linked to lower rates of heart disease, cancer, and other Western diseases, even at levels far below those considered "safe" in the West. They found that as blood cholesterol decreased from 170 mg/dL to 90 mg/dL, cancers of the liver, rectum, colon, male lung, female lung, breast, childhood leukemia, adult leukemia, childhood brain, adult brain, stomach, and esophagus (throat) decreased. We are currently aware that high cholesterol is a sign to worry about heart disease, but not many know that it is also a sign that you might need to worry about cancer as well!

Now imagine a country where the inhabitants had blood cholesterol levels far higher than the Chinese average of 170 mg/dL. It might be expected that some relatively rare diseases such as heart disease and some cancers would be much more prevalent in that country, perhaps even be leading killers! This is exactly what we see in the West. What they found was that the death rate from coronary heart disease was seventeen times higher among American men than rural Chinese men. The American death rate from breast cancer was five times higher than the rural Chinese rate. Another absolutely astonishing find was amongst the inhabitants of a southwestern Chinese provinces of Sichuan and Guizhou. During a three year observation period between 1973 and 1975, *not a single person died of coronary heart disease before the age of sixty four, among 246,000 men and 181,000 women*!

When Dr. Campbell made these cholesterol findings public, he then learned from three very prominent heart disease researchers and physicians, Drs. Bill Castelli, Bill Rogers, and Caldwell Esselstyn, Jr., that in their long careers they had never seen a heart disease fatality among their patients who had blood cholesterol levels below 150 mg/dL.

The most important question still remains, how does food affect blood cholesterol? Without any exceptions in ***all cases***, animal based foods were correlated with *increasing* blood cholesterol, and nutrients from plant based foods were associated with *decreasing* levels of blood cholesterol. Many other studies prove the same; animal protein increases blood cholesterol. In addition, animal protein increases blood cholesterol *much more* than dietary cholesterol, this means it is much more important to watch out for animal protein rather than cholesterol in your food.

CHART 4.5. FOODS ASSOCIATED WITH BLOOD CHOLESTEROL

As intakes of meat,[I] milk, eggs, fish,[I-II] fat[I] and animal protein go up…	Blood Cholesterol goes up.
As intakes of plant-based foods and nutrients (including plant protein,[I] dietary fiber,[II] cellulose,[II] hemicellulose,[I] soluble carbohydrate,[II] B-vitamins of plants (carotenes, B_2, B_3),[I] legumes, light colored vegetables, fruit, carrots, potatoes and several cereal grains) go up…	Blood Cholesterol goes down.

Also please note that ***the only significant source of cholesterol is from animal products***. Do not be fooled by the "no cholesterol" tags on bottles of olive oil or other plant based foods, those are just for better sales.

If you walk into almost any doctors office and ask which dietary factors affect blood cholesterol, the reply you are going to hear is saturated fat and dietary cholesterol. What you will never hear is animal protein, even thought an abundance of evidence clearly shows that animal protein was much more strongly correlated with blood cholesterol levels than saturated fat and dietary cholesterol.

Fat, Is It Really All That Bad?

If there was a prize given to the amount of confusion surrounding a nutrient, I think fat would be right behind protein on this one. For over forty years the questions regarding fat are still unanswered. How much fat can we have in our diets? What kind of fat? Is polyunsaturated fat better than saturated fat? Is monounsaturated fat better than either? What about those special fats like omega3, omega-6, trans fats and DHA? Should we avoid coconut fat? What about fish oil? Is there something special about flaxseed oil? What's a high-fat diet anyway? A low-fat diet?

As early as 40 years ago the fat debate started and it seems like it is still going on. Today, the percentage of recommended fat is hovering around 30% or total calories, but that was not always the case. At the beginning some were arguing for more fat, but as of recently many are advocating that less is better. Much debate spurred and even touched upon breast cancer quite heavily. The unique attention given to fat was motivated by international studies showing that the amount of dietary fat consumed was closely associated with the incidence of breast cancer, bowel cancer, and heart disease.

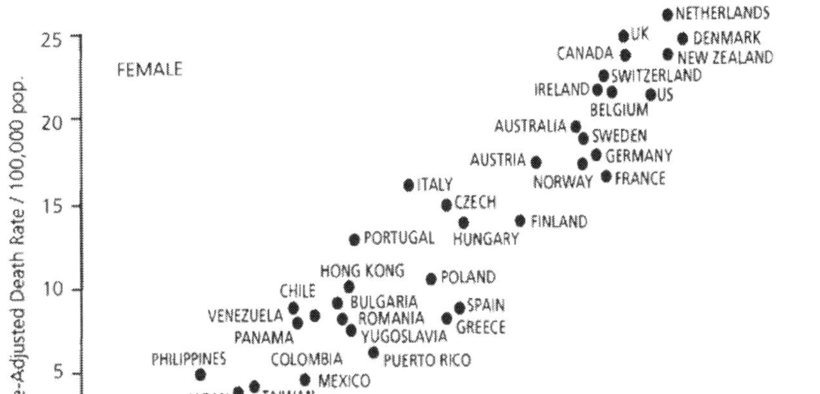

It seemed that the less fat one consumed, the less likelihood they will develop cancer implying that diet and lifestyle were the principal causes of these diseases. Adding to this, a very prominent report by Sir Richard Doll and Sir Richard Peto of the University of Oxford submitted to the U.S. Congress summarized many of these studies and concluded that only 2-3% of all cancers could be attributed to genes. The data from all those studies clearly suggests that we can definitely lower our breast cancer to almost zero if we make perfect lifestyle choices. The debate raged on, but what the most important aspect to this whole debate was ignored. Breast cancer was associated with animal fat intake but ***not with plant fat***.

CHART 4.8: ANIMAL FAT INTAKE AND BREAST CANCER

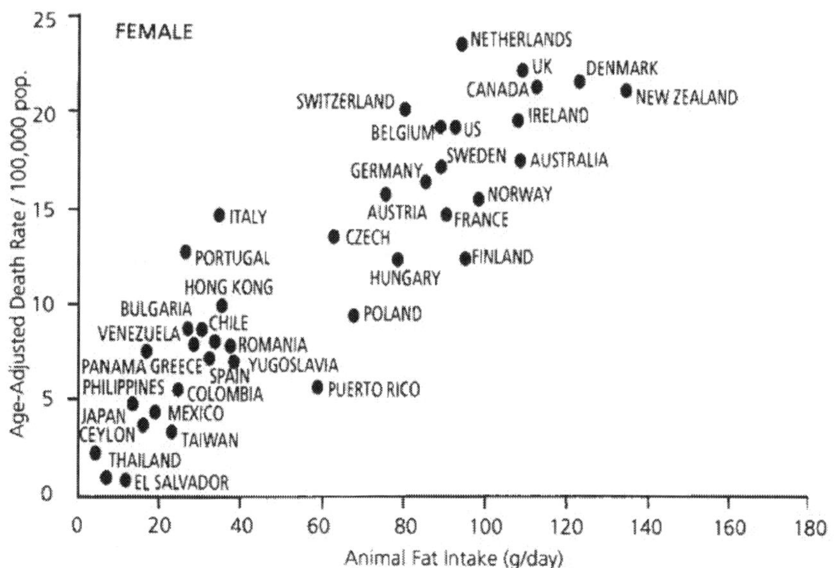

CHART 4.9: PLANT FAT INTAKE AND BREAST CANCER

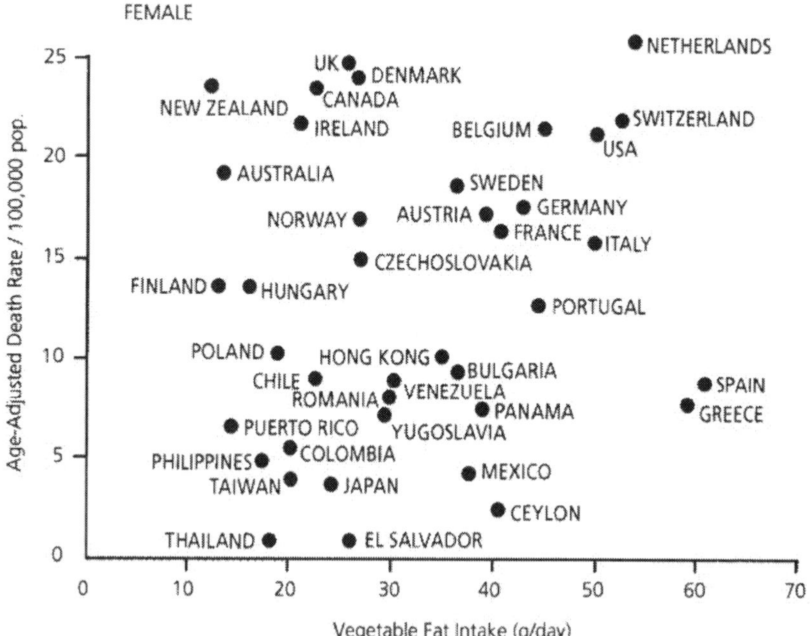

In reality, it doesn't matter how **much** fat, rather it matters ***where it comes from***! The correlation between dietary fat and animal protein seen in rural China was very high, at 70-84%, similar to the 93% seen when comparing different countries. This means the amount of fat consumed was primarily from animal sources. And the high correlation between fat and breast cancer and other types of cancer was not really because of the fat, but what that fat was attached to. Since the fat most of us eat (around 90% of it) comes from animal sources, this means we are eating a lot of animal protein. So they were studying the correlation of dietary fat on cancer, when they really were studying the effect of animal protein on cancer; the association between fat and breast cancer might really be telling us that as consumption of animal based foods goes up, so does breast cancer. No correlation between plant protein and cancer, or any other disease, has ever been found.

Findings from rural China showed that reducing dietary fat from 24% to 6% was associated with lower breast cancer risk. However, lower diatary fat in rural China meant less consumption not only of fat, but more importantly, of animal based foods!

The connection of breast cancer with dietary fat, or more accurately with animal based foods, brought into consideration other factors that also place a woman at risk for breast cancer:

- Early age of menarche (age of first menstruation)
- High blood cholesterol
- Late menopause
- High exposure to female hormones

How did the China Study augment these risk factors? It showed that higher dietary fat is associated with higher blood cholesterol, and both of these factors, along with higher female hormone levels, are associated, in turn, with more breast cancer and earlier age of menarche. The much later age of menarche in rural China is remarkable. 130 villages, with 25 women each, were surveyed and the average age of menarche was seventeen years, while the U.S. average is roughly eleven years!

Many studies have shown that early menarche leads to higher risk for breast cancer. Menarche is triggered by the growth rate of girls, the faster they grow, the earlier the menarche which also usually means there are high levels of blood hormones such as estrogen. High blood hormone levels were shown to raise the risk of breast cancer.

The strong association of a high animal protein, high fat diet with reproductive hormones and early age of menarche, both of which raise the risk of breast cancer, is an important observation. It is quite clear that we should not have our children eating a diet high in animal based foods. An interesting observation made by Ms. Magazine founder Gloria Steinem, is that eating a proper diet could reduce teen pregnancy by delaying the age or menarche.

In the China Study, animal protein intake was convincingly associated with the prevalence of cancer in families (with 99% statistical significance). What makes this conclusion especially compelling is the fact that it occurred at unusually low intakes of animal based foods.

The China Study also provided evidence that a high fibre intake was consistently associated with lower rates of cancers of the rectum and colon. A high fibre diet also was associated with lower levels of blood cholesterol. And of course, high fibre consumption reflects a high plant based diet rich in foods such as beans, leafy vegetables, and whole grains.

They also studied the iron/fiber issue very carefully in the China Study and as it turns out, fiber is not the enemy of iron absorption as so many experts claimed to be. They measured how much iron the Chinese were consuming and how much was in their bodies. The results clearly showed that increasing fiber intake did not impair iron absorption in the body. In reality, high fiber foods, like wheat and corn (not the white polished rice consumed in China) are very high in fiber, meaning the higher the consumption of fiber, the higher the consumption of iron. The view that eating a low animal food diet leads to iron deficiencies in the body, as viewed by Western scientists, is unfounded and untrue. The China Study also revealed that a high fiber, plant based diet, was consistently associated with lower rates of cancers of the rectum and colon and was associated with lower levels of blood cholesterol.

Antioxidants

In the China Study, Dr. Campbell and his team assessed antioxidant status by recording the intakes of vitamin C and beta-carotene and measuring the blood levels of vitamin C, vitamin E and carotenoids. Among these antioxidant biomarkers, vitamin C provided the most impressive evidence.

The most significant vitamin C association with cancer was its relationship with the number of cancer-prone families in each area. *When levels of vitamin C in the blood were low, those families were more likely to have a high incidence of cancer. Low vitamin C was prominently associated with higher risk for esophageal cancer, for leukemiaand cancers of the nasopharynx, breast, stomach, liver, rectum, colon and lung.* "It was esophageal cancer that first attracted NOVA television program producers to report on cancer mortality in China. It was this television program that spurred our own survey to see what was behind this story." Vitamin C primarily comes from fruit, and eating fruit was also inversely associated with esophageal cancer."

"Cancer rates were five to eight times higher for areas where fruit intake was lowest. The same vitamin C effect existing for these cancers also existed for coronary heart disease, hypertensive heart disease and stroke Vitamin C intake from fruits clearly showed a powerful protective effect against a variety of diseases. The other measures of antioxidants, blood levels of alpha and beta-carotene (a vitamin precursor) and alpha and gamma tocopherol (vitamin E) are poor indicators of the effects of antioxidants. These antioxi- dants are transported in the blood by lipoprotein, which is the carrier of "bad" cholesterol.

So anytime we measured these antioxidants, we were simultaneously measuring unhealthy biomarkers. This was an experimental compromise that diminished our ability to detect the beneficial effects of the carotenoids and the tocopherols, even when these benefits are known to exist. We did, however, find that stomach cancer was higher when the blood levels of beta-carotene were lower. Can we say that vitamin C, beta-carotene and dietary fiber are solely responsible for preventing these cancers? In other words, can a pill containing vitamin C and beta-carotene or a fiber supplement create these health effects? No. The triumph of health lies not in the individual nutrients, but in the whole foods that contain those nutrients: plant-based foods. In a bowl of spinach salad, for example, we have fiber, antioxidants and countless other nutrients that are orchestrating a wondrous symphony of health as they work in concert within our bodies (Vitamin intake is vital even with a proper plant based because of genetically modified seeds, unhealthy soil, poor farming practices, selling unripe produce, and other factors which significantly lower the vitamin and mineral content in our fruits and vegetables as compared to even 50 years ago).

The message could not be Simpler: ***eat as many whole fruits, vegetables and whole grains as you can, and you will probably derive all of the benefits noted above as well as many others.***" – Dr. Campbell, *The China Study*

The Atkins Craze

What is the one thing in nutrition that most people are afraid of these days? Carbs! The "low-carb" diet has become extremely popular with almost all diet books on store shelves promoting one theme; eat as much protein, meat, and fat as you like, but stay away from those "nasty" and fattening carbs. As you have seen already, with massive amounts of evidence and proof, eating this way is perhaps ***the single greatest threat to the health of our entire population we currently face***.

It is difficult to know where to even begin to refute the waves of misinformation and false promises commonly made by authors completely untrained in nutrition, authors who have never conducted or even bothered to look at any peer-reviewed, professionally based experimental research. These books are very popular, and this is because at first glance it *seems* that people are losing weight, at least in the short term.

It was far from being as glamorous as they made it out to be. In reality, their subjects were severely restricting their calorie intake. An average American consumes about 2250 calories per day, but their study participants were consuming and average of about 1450 calories per day. That's a 35% reduction in calories! It doesn't matter what diet you are on, if you reduce you calorie intake by 35%, you will lose weight and your cholesterol levels might even improve in the short run. It's a matter of simple math and common sense that a person cannot sustain such a diet over a period of years or decades without suffering serious health complications. Such calorie restricting diets are known to be notoriously unsuccessful over any long period of time, and that is why there has yet to be a long term study that shows success with the "low-carb" diets.

In some studies funded by the Atkins Center for Complementary Medicine they declare that over the course of six months, people on their diet lost an average of twenty pounds and their cholesterol levels decreased slightly. Good figures right? The media though so. But, nobody really bothered to look any further than the headlines, or closely examine at what really happened during their studies.

This was only the beginning of the problems. "At some point during the twenty-four weeks, twenty-eight subjects (68%) reported constipation, twenty-six (63%) reported bad breath, twenty-one (51%) reported headache, four (10%) noted hair loss, and one woman (1%) reported increased menstrual bleeding. " They also refer to other research, saying, "Adverse effects of this diet in children have included calcium oxalate and urate kidney stones ... vomiting, amenorrhea [when a girl misses her period], hypercholesterolemia [high cholesterol] and ... vitamin deficiencies (ref. cited). "47 Additionally, they found that the dieters had a stunning 53% increase in the amount of calcium they excreted in their urine, which may spell disaster for their bone health. The weight loss, some of which is simply initial fluid may come with a very high price.

A different review of low-carbohydrate diets published by researchers in Australia concludes, "Complications such as heart arrhythmias, cardiac contractile function impairment, sudden death, osteoporosis, kidney damage, increased cancer risk, impairment of physical activity and lipid abnormalities can all be linked to long-term restriction of carbohydrates in the diet." One teenage girl recently died suddenly after being on a high-protein diet. You can also lose weight by undergoing chemotherapy or starting a heroin addiction, but I would not recommend those either.

These days there are a lot of crooks who will do almost anything for money. And with the power of savvy marketing techniques they can fool a lot of people into believing whatever they want. There is plenty of evidence showing that the healthiest diet you can possibly consume is a *high carbohydrate plant based diet*. It has been shown to reverse (aka cure) heart disease, diabetes, and countless other diseases. And yes, it has been shown many times to cause significant weight loss.

*High carbohydrate does not mean the sugary, processed, refined products like pasta, chips, soda, sugary cereals, candy bars etc. Carbohydrates must be consumed in their unprocessed, unrefined, and natural state when they are in their so called "complex" form. This means they can be properly broken down in a controlled, regulated manner during digestion. Foods in their natural and unrefined, uncooked state preserve all the vitamins and minerals which would otherwise be almost totally nonexistent after processing and cooking. Fresh fruits, vegetables, and *whole* grains are the healthiest foods you can consume, and they are primarily made of carbohydrates. The junky fast food carbohydrates are the ones giving the good stuff a bad rep, devoid of all their minerals and vitamins and being pretty much no better than sugar. Don't think that pasta or bread made from refined flour, chips, or sugary cereals are what we are talking about here, absolutely not. You will gain no health benefit from such a diet. Fresh fruits, vegetables, sprouted grains and other whole grains are what the conversation is about!

These days, it is almost impossible to avoid carcinogens in our everyday lives, but whether they lead to full blow tumours, cancer, heart disease, diabetes, and other diseases depends mostly on your ***nutrition***. Our food choices every day will decide whether we will be sick or healthy; and I think it's time that you made the right choice.

These findings are more than impressive, more than just a headline, they should be on every single news hour, in every health magazine and medical journal, they should be in every textbook on diet and nutrition, and they should be known by the entire world population. The fact that none of this has happened really shows how this industry is really run. Nobody is interested in your health; they will do everything in their power to stop you from getting the truth. The largest medical studies in the world by some of the most prominent scientists in the field show such compelling evidence about cancer and nutrition, yet NOTHING is being done about it. They are continuing to cause terrible pain and suffering needlessly to millions of people worldwide. This HAS TO STOP!

"Plato, in this passage, made it perfectly clear: we shall eat animals only at our own peril. Though it is indeed remarkable that one of the greatest intellectuals in the history of the Western world condemned meat eating almost 2,500 years ago, I find it even more remarkable that few know about this history. Hardly anybody knows, for example, that the father of Western medicine, Hippocrates, advocated diet as the chief way to prevent and treat disease or that George Macilwain knew that diet was the way to prevent and treat disease or that the man instrumental in founding the American Cancer Society,

Frederick L. Hoffman, knew that diet was the way to prevent and treat disease. How did Plato predict the future so accurately? He knew that consuming animal foods would not lead to true health and prosperity. Instead, the false sense of rich luxury granted by being able to eat animals would only lead to a culture of sickness, disease, land disputes, lawyers and doctors. This is a pretty good description of some of the challenges faced by modern America!

How did Seneca, one of the great scholars 2,000 years ago, a tutor and advisor to Roman Emperor Nero, know with such certainty the trouble with consuming animals when he wrote "An Ox is satisfied with the pasture of an acre or two: one wood suffices for several Elephants. Man alone supports himself by the pillage of the whole earth and sea. What! Has Nature indeed given us so insatiable a stomach, while she has given us so insignificant bodies? ... The slaves of the belly (as says Sallust) are to be counted in the number of the lower animals, not of men. Nay, not of them, but rather of the dead .... You might inscribe on their doors, These have anticipated death."

How did George Macilwain predict the future when he said that the local theory of disease would not lead to health? Even today, we don't have any pills or procedures that effectively prevent, eliminate or even treat the causes of any chronic diseases. The most promising preventions and treatments have now been shown to be diet and lifestyle changes, a constitutional approach to health. How did we forget these lessons from the past? How did we go from knowing that the best athletes in the ancient Greek OlympicS must consume a plant-based diet to fearing that vegetarians don't get enough protein?

How did we get to a place where the healers of our society, our doctors, know little, if anything, about nutrition; where our medical institutions denigrate the subject; where using prescription drugs and going to hospitals is the third leading cause of death? How did we get to a place where advocating a plant based diet can jeopardize a professional career, where scientists spend more time mastering nature than respecting it? How did we get to a place where the companies that profit from our sickness are the ones telling us how to be healthy; where the companies that profit from our food choices are the ones telling us what to eat; where the public's hard-earned money is being spent by the government to boost the drug industry's profits; and where there is more distrust than trust of our government's policies on foods, drugs and health? How did we get to a place where Americans are so confused about what is healthy that they no longer care?

Calories, Are They The Enemy?

Calories, calories, calories, it's the one thing everyone thinks they can do without. With regards to weight loss, the China Study has some interesting conclusions based on their research. The researchers thought that China had a food problem, that it was prone to famines, and basically that there was not enough calories to go around. Although China has, during the last fifty years or so, had its fair share nutritional problems, the research team were to learn that these views on caloric intake were completely wrong.

They compared the caloric consumption in China and America. To overcome the vast difference in calorie intake and expenditure they divided the Chinese into five groups according to their levels of physical activity to match those in the U.S. They figured out the calorie intake of the least active Chinese, which would equal an office worker, and compared those to the average American. What they found was quite shocking.

Average caloric intake, per kilogram of body weight, was 30% higher amongst the least active Chinese than among average Americans. Yet, their body weight was 20% *lower*. How can they eat way more calories and be way more slimmer?

CHART 4.11: CALORIE CONSUMPTION (KCAL/KG) AND BODY WEIGHT

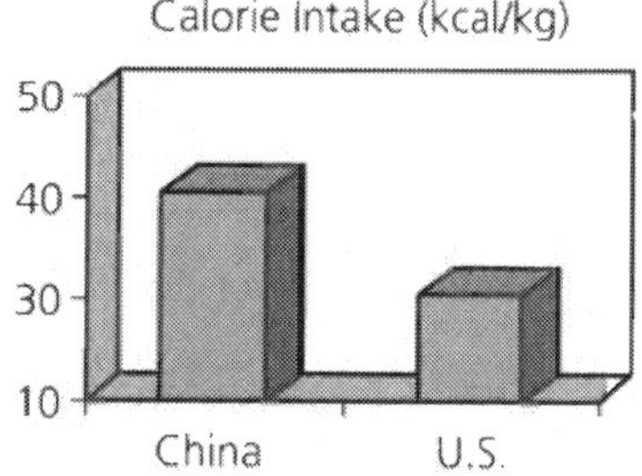

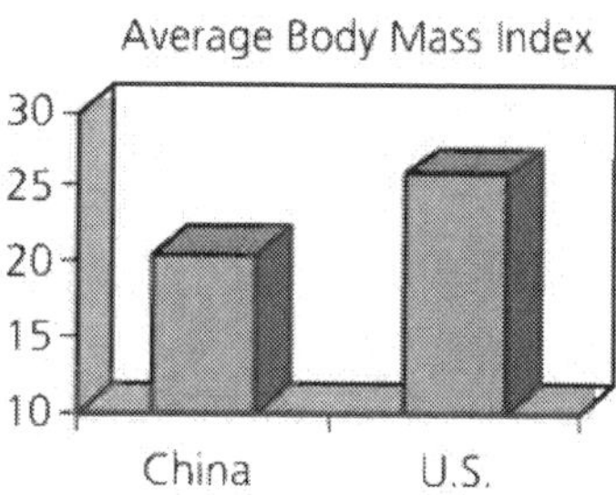

Well, there might be a few explanations. Some might say that they have a high rate of metabolism, or "it's in their genes." Such people are the ones, who seem to eat all they want and still not gain any weight, then there are most of us who have to watch what we put in our mouths or the pounds will come on quick. This is an easy interpretation. The China Study research team had a much more complex and comprehensive interpretation based on their own research and the studies of others. The reason behind it is more interesting. People who eat a high fat, high protein diet simply retain more calories than they need, storing them as body fat in all those wonderful places like our behind, midsection, and thighs.

And even though very few calories are actually needed for significant weight gain (even an extra fifty calories per day can lead to an extra ten pounds per year, and eventually fifty pounds over only five years), our attempts are calorie restrictions are imprecise and unwise, whether we do it by limiting carbohydrates or fat. Despite any short term caloric restriction regimes we may take up, our body will always decide what it wants to do with those calories through its own very fine mechanisms.

The body has immensely intricate ways in which it uses calories and distributes energy throughout the body. The only thing we can do is eat the right kind of food which will allow the body to partition the calories away properly, away from body fat, and use it for more desirable actions like keeping our body warm, running body metabolism efficiently, and supporting and encouraging physical activity. The body knows how to use the calories we give it; all we have to do is supply the proper fuel.

Here is the amazing part; calories in the form of fat or protein get stored as fat, but calories in the form of plant based foods get used and "lost" as body heat! Wouldn't you rather have your calories get used up as body heat rather than get stored as fat? The data from the China Study shows exactly this. Chinese consume more calories but because they are more physically active and due to their low fat, low protein diets, they shift their calorie metabolism from fat storage to getting burned off as body heat.

The same trend was seen in their experimental animals fed low protein diets. They routinely consumed more calories, gained less weight, burned off more calories as body heat, and even voluntarily exercised much more often, *all the while having far less cancer than animals on standard diets*! Observation shows that people who consume low fat, low protein diets composed mostly of whole plant food have far less difficulty with weight problems and are much healthier than their counterparts. How is that for a diet? Eat as much as you want, burn fat like butter on a skillet, and cure your so called "incurable" diseases.

Protein Is Muscle, Right?

So we just learned that a low protein, low fat diet is the answer for stable and healthy weight loss, but what about weight *gain*? Our culture these days is quite obsessed with the belief that animal protein is the only thing that will make the body grow and gain muscle. The desire to become bigger is pervasive in most cultures. During the colonial period in Asia and Africa, Europeans even considered smaller people to be less civilized. Body size is seen as a mark for manliness and dominance.

Most people have the idea that bigger and stronger can only be achieved by eating protein rich, animal based foods. The idea that meat protein is absolutely required for physical power and strength has saturated our culture becoming a very common notion.

As we already discussed, the problem with consuming a animal based high protein diet is that the people who do eat that way have the most heart disease, cancer, and diabetes. In the China Study, animal protein consumption was associated with more cancer and heart disease. It seems that being bigger has its very serious risks. But is that the case for all protein types? Is it possible to achieve maximal growth potential and gain muscle while minimized the risk for all major diseases?

In the study, consuming more protein was associated with greater body size for men and women. But, this effect was almost totally attributed to plant protein since it makes up almost 90% of the total Chinese protein intake. Animal protein was indeed associated with greater weight, but at the same time greater plant protein intake was closely linked to greater height and body weight. The fact is; *body growth is linked to protein in* ***general*** *and* ***both*** *animal* ***and plant proteins*** *are effective*!

What this means is that an individual can achieve their genetic potential for growth and body size by consuming a plant based diet. So why is it that we see people in developing nations, who consume little or no animal based foods, are always smaller than Western people? This is because plant based diets in poor areas of the world usually have insufficient variety, inadequate quantity and quality, and usually have poor public health conditions with prevalent childhood diseases. Under these conditions growth and development is stunted, not allowing full physical genetic potential. In the China Study low adult height and weight were strongly associated with areas having high mortality rates for pulmonary tuberculosis, parasitic diseases, pneumonia, intestinal obstruction, and digestive diseases.

This means that it is absolutely possible to achieve full growth, development, and muscular size by consuming a diet low in animal based foods and high in plant based protein while lowering the risk of cancer, diabetes, heart disease and more, to almost zero.

"Almost all of us in the United States will die of diseases of affluence. In our China Study, we saw that nutrition has a very strong effect on these diseases. Plant-based foods are linked to lower blood cholesterol; animal-based foods are linked to higher blood cholesterol. Animal-based foods are linked to higher breast cancer rates; plant-based foods are linked to lower rates. Fiber and antioxidants from plants are linked to a lower risk of cancers of the digestive tract. Plant-based diets and active lifestyles result in a healthy weight, yet permit people to become big and strong. Our study was comprehensive in design and comprehensive in its findings. From the labs of Virginia Tech and Cornell University to the far reaches of China, it seemed that science was painting a clear, consistent picture: we can minimize our risk of contracting deadly diseases just by eating the right food"

So, how about that? Eat as much as you want, lose weight, cure cancer and heart disease, gain muscle and achieve your full genetic growth potential, while becoming healthier and happier! I think everyone would want to go on such a diet.
*All charts, graphs, summaries, quotes, information and section above were taken from Dr. Campbell's book *The China Study*.

World Hunger

Did you know that there is more than enough food to feed the entire population of the world? Well, the fact is that most of the grains, corn, and soy is funnelled directly to the meat industry for cattle feed. If we speak strictly in terms of efficiency, raising cattle is the most inefficient form of food because of the huge amounts of resources needed.

Worldwide, an estimated 2 billion people live primarily on a meat-based diet, while an estimated 4 billion live primarily on a plant-based diet. The US food production system uses about 50% of the total US land area, 80% of the fresh water, and 17% of the fossil energy used in the country. Here are some interesting facts:

- Energy conservation: it takes 78 calories of fossil fuel to produce 1 calorie of beef protein; 35 calories for 1 calorie of pork; 22 calories for 1 of poultry; but just 1 calorie of fossil fuel for 1 calorie of soybeans.
- Water Conservation; it takes 3 to 15 times as much water to produce animal protein as it does plant protein.
- Soil conservation; when grains & legumes are used more efficiently, our precious topsoil is automatically made more efficient in its use. We use less agricultural resources to provide for the same number of people.
- Agricultural Chemicals: being higher on the food chain, animal foods contain far higher concentrations of agricultural chemicals than plant foods, including pesticides, herbicides, etc.
- Exposure of livestock to drugs and vaccines: There are over 20,000 different drugs, including sterols, antibiotics, growth hormones and other veterinary drugs that are given to livestock animals. These drugs are consumed when animal foods are consumed. The dangers in secondary consumption of antibiotics, are well documented.

It takes 16 pounds of grain to produce 1 pound of meat. This means that we could be producing 16 times the amount of food that we are currently producing with cattle farming, and end world hunger in one day. Just imagine, since we have figured out that plant protein is actually better for health and well being, if those 2 billion people switched to a high plant based diet we could totally eliminate world hunger, and almost completely wipe off cancer, heart disease, diabetes, and all those horrible diseases! Switching to a high plant based diet is the fist and biggest step towards health and wellbeing.

So, not only are plant eaters saving themselves, they are also saving the earth.

The Digestion Mechanism

Now let's go a little bit further. We have learned that animal based foods cause a myriad of health problems. Ok, so plant based foods are where the health "is at", as the cool kids would say, and people who eat more of it are the healthiest. But that's not all, now we have to talk more about the chemical properties of the food you eat and what happens to all that goodness when it is fried, baked, boiled, broiled, steamed, or otherwise heated to high temperatures.

Most people think our digestive system is a pipe filled with digestive juices with two holes at each end; something goes in, gets broken down by acid, something gets absorbed, then something else comes out. This perspective however is far from what scientist from many countries have shown in the 21st century. The digestion of food is not at all what we think of it.

The most important aspect of health is obviously the food we eat, yet there is something that is rarely talked about. How cooking affects even the seemingly healthy choices you make is the Achilles heel of true health and weight loss. The science behind it is simple. When you burn your finger, the skin tissue will die; the same idea applies to food. Nutrients, vitamins, minerals, proteins, carbohydrates and even fats are progressively destroyed during the heating process turning them from natural ingredients to indigestible toxic substances.

We will now examine the serious chemical changes that take place to individual nutrients as heat is applied to them. It is well understood and recognized in scientific literature that heat breaks down vitamins, amino acids, enzymes and produces undesirable cross-linkages in proteins, particularly in meat. When food is cooked above 117 degrees F (47 degrees C) for three minutes or longer, the following harmful changes begin, and progressively cause increased nutritional damage as higher temperatures are applied over prolonged periods of time.

The following section will go into a detailed analysis of what happens to the food you eat. I can't stress enough how important it is for you to know the following information. It might be a little technical but I tried to make it as simple as I could. You need to know these details so you can become a powerful, confident, and independent consumer. Knowing the following secrets will make it impossible for greedy diet and medical companies to ever use you as a cash cow. You gain your independence by knowing the facts. I didn't want to give you some washed out basic information that is littered all over the internet these days, I wanted to give you something that actually matters, the information which can help you regain your lost health.

Protein Denaturation

Protein molecules under ideal eating and digestive conditions are broken down into amino acids by gastric enzymes. Every protein molecule in your body is made from these amino acids. Protein you consume IS NOT used as protein: it is first recycled or broken down into its constituent amino acids AND THEN used to build protein molecules the body needs.

There are 23 different amino acids. They link together in different combinations in extremely long chains to create protein molecules, like individual rail cars form a train.

The amino group gives each amino acid its specific identifying characteristic that differentiates it from the others. Excessive heat breaks off or decapitates the amino group. Without this amino group, the amino acid is rendered useless and is toxic.

As you can see from the figure, a protein is a combination of amino acids which are shown as spherical structures. Cooking denatures protein. According to Encyclopedia Britannica, denaturation is a modification of the molecular structure of protein by heat or by an acid, an alkali, or ultraviolet radiation that destroys or diminishes its original properties and biological activity.

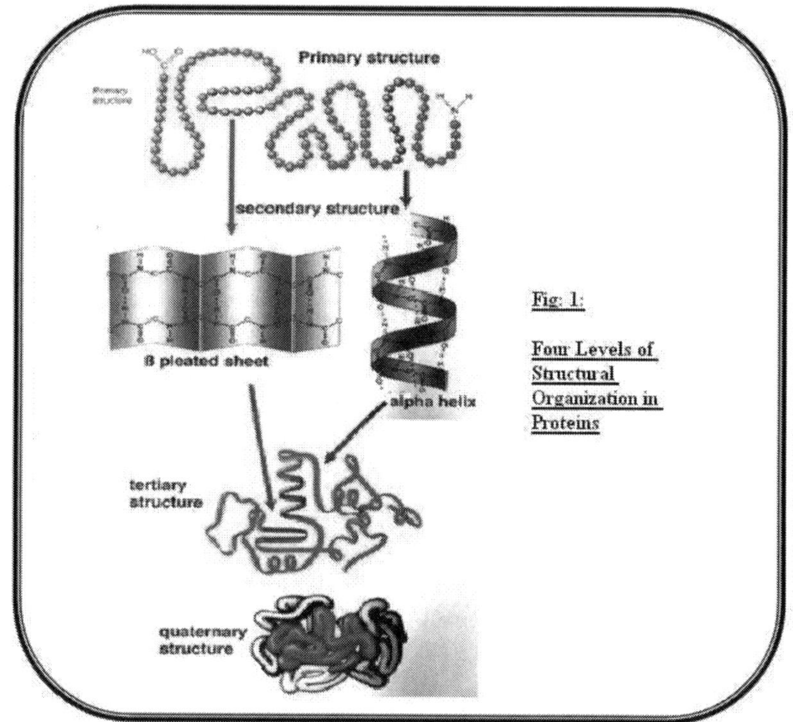

Fig: 1:

Four Levels of Structural Organization in Proteins

Denaturation alters protein and makes it **unusable or less usable**. According to Britannica, protein molecules are readily altered by heat. Unlike simple organic molecules, the physical and chemical properties of protein are markedly altered when the substance is boiled in water.

Further, all of the agents able to cause denaturation are able to break the secondary bonds that hold the chains in place. Once these weak bonds are broken, the molecule falls into a disorganized tangle **devoid of biological function**. This is because proteins are bound in a specific shape for ease of use and digestion, once cooked the protein string looses its original shape and becomes tangled and disorganized turning into unusable biological waste that is **indigestible**.

The most significant effect of protein denaturation is the loss of its biological function. For example, enzymes lose their catalytic powers (the power to jump start biological reactions, cellular metabolism, etc.) and hemoglobin loses its capacity to carry oxygen. The changes that accompany denaturation have been shown to result from destruction of the specific *pattern* in which the amino acid chains are folded in the native protein.

When proteins are subjected to high heat during cooking, enzyme resistant linkages are formed between the amino acid chains, meaning our enzymes **cannot break apart the proteins we eat**. The body cannot separate these amino acids. What the body cannot use, it must eliminate. Cooked proteins become a source of **toxicity**: dead organic waste material acted upon and elaborated by bacterial flora.

In other words; amino acids are like Lego's that combine together to form a big Lego structure, and this combination of Lego's is what a protein is. Let's say you made a car with the Lego's; each individual piece is the amino acid, and the whole car is the protein. This car you just made has a specific order and arrangement, otherwise it would be just a random thing that doesn't make sense. What cooking does is it breaks apart some of the Lego's, which turns the pretty car into a jumbled mess. Your body can't use the jumbled mess, it **can't** digest it, so it turns into a waste product rotting inside your body.

This is why the term dead food, referring to cooked food, is often used. A result of denaturation is lowered solubility. This means amino acids become all tangled up forming a clump that cannot be used, cannot be digested, and turns into a waste product even before it hits your tongue.

According to the textbook Nutritional Value of Food Processing, 3rd Edition, (by Karmas, Harris, published by Van Nostrand Reinhold) which is written for food chemists in the industrial processed food industry, changes that occur during processing either result in nutrient loss or destruction. Heat processing has a detrimental effect on nutrients since thermal degradation of nutrients can and does occur. Reduction in nutrient content depends on the severity of the thermal processing.

Protein Coagulation

You can see coagulation of protein that takes place on a macroscopic level when you fry an egg. The clear protein gel surrounding the yolk whitens, thickens, and coagulates into a glue-like consistency. Digestive enzymes in our stomachs (called peptones and proteases) cannot readily break down coagulated protein molecules once they fuse together. Not only are heated proteins unavailable to your body, worse yet: they are indigestible. The coagulated protein molecules tend to rot as bacteria in the body feed upon this dead organic matter (we will discuss this further as it is a very important point).

As bacteria feed on the rotting mess that is stuck in your digestive tract, they produce enzymatic by-products which are carcinogenic, meaning the waste the bacteria produce is cancer-causing. Coagulation occurs on a microscopic level in all cooked protein molecules whether witnessed or not. It makes the protein you eat useless.

Utilize raw fruits, vegetables, nuts, seeds, hemp protein, bee pollen, and spirulina as your source of protein. By eating more fresh, raw produce, you are assured of maximum biological value of protein and other consumed nutrients.

As you consume more fresh produce as a staple, the body progressively requires less food. As you eat more nutrient rich raw food, the body steadily becomes healthier, and its metabolic efficiency increases. So does its ability to absorb and use more nutriment. Most people get their protein from meat or fish which needs to be cooked making it useless to your body. Compared to a raw diet, you would need less than one-half the amount of protein if eaten raw from plant food (via nuts and seeds) because all that protein is usable.

Carcinogen Generation

From the book Diet, Nutrition and Cancer published by the Nutritional Research Council of the American Academy of Sciences (1982) and the FDA (Food and Drug Administration) Office of Toxicological Sciences, additional carcinogens in heated foods include: Hydroperoxide, alkoxy, endoperoxides and epoxides from heated meat, eggs, fish and pasteurized milk

Carcinogens in heated foods:

- Ally aldehyde (acrolein)
- Butyric acid
- Nitropyrene
- Nitrobenzene and nitrosamines from heated fats and oils
- Methyglyoxal and chlorogenic atractyosides in coffee
- Indole
- Skatole
- Nitropyrene
- Ptomatropine

- Ptomaines
- Leukomaines
- Ammonia
- Hydrogen sulfide
- Cadaverine
- Muscarine
- Putecine
- Nervine
- Mercaptins in cheese
- And many more

Fats Are Rendered Carcinogenic:

Simply speaking, a fat is a combination of carbon molecules combined together to form a chain. Various combinations of the carbon molecules make different types of fats. There are saturated and unsaturated fats. Saturated fats can only have a straight structure, unsaturated fats on the other hand can be have a bent shape (cis mono or polyunsaturated fats like omega 3, 6) or a straight shape (trans unsaturated fat). The reason trans fats and saturated fats are considered bad is because they are straight and can clump together and clog arteries.

Naturally occurring fatty acids generally have the *Cis* configuration which means the molecular structure of the fat is bent. When the fat is *Trans*, then it is straight in shape.

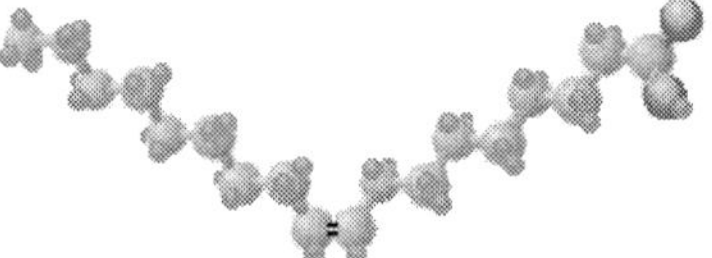

Cis-9-octadecenoic acid
(Oleic acid)

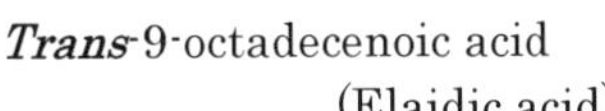

Trans-9-octadecenoic acid
(Elaidic acid)

When we fry or hydrogenate healthy unsaturated fats, making them straight, our body recognizes the chemical structure and tries to use it in the same places and for the same purposes that it uses the natural bent cis form. But the trans form (straight shape) stacks together just like saturated fats, which sabotages the flexible, porous functionality the body needs from the unsaturated. Our diet was never meant to be composed of so much trans fats like in margarines, shortenings, and fried oils which is found in most of the food on grocery shelves.

The cell wall is made up of fats, mostly from the good essential fats (essential fats are those that cannot be manufactured by the body) like omega 3 (walnuts, hemp, flaxseed), omega 6 (hemp, flax seed) which combine together to form the cellular membrane.

When the essential fatty acids are missing from the diet (essential fatty acids are very volatile and are removed from our foods to get a longer shelf life), cells have no choice but to substitute inappropriate fats (margarine, shortenings, fried fats, animal fats) into their structure, resulting in type II diabetes and perhaps cancer. These fats when used in the cell wall interfere with the absorption of nutrients and damage the mitochondria (an organelle inside our cells that produces energy needed for the cell to live), thereby interfering with production of ATP (the energy source or "food" for our cells), then this can cause significant damage to the cell because ATP is needed for important cellular processes such as membrane transport, lipogenesis and protein synthesis.

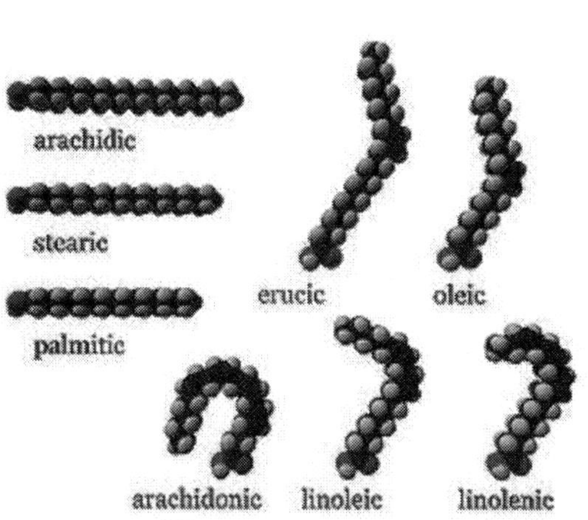

With damaged mitochondria, for its very survival the cell has no choice but to revert to the more primitive system of anaerobic respiration that is characteristic of cancer cells (more on this later). Sometimes the damage is reversible, in which case the cell can be healed. Sometimes the damage is irreversible, and a way must be found to destroy the cell.

High heat applied to oils during frying turns them into hydrocarbons that can cause cancer. Typical frying temperature is about 400 degrees F and can reach up to 600-700 degrees F. When fats / oils are heated to such temperatures the good healthy fats (CIS fatty acid) are converted to the bad TRANS fats. The unsaturated good fats then begin to behave like saturated bad fats.

When heated, they raise rather than lower serum cholesterol levels (about 50% of the cholesterol increasing effect of saturated fat) and can raise LDL cholesterol by nearly as much as saturated fat. Besides the extra fat consumed, this is another reason why fried foods contribute to hardening of the arteries.

When oil is reheated to frying temperatures (as in deep fryers), the fat is more likely to develop the cancer producing agents acrolein and benzopyrene. Very hot temperatures also destroy vitamins and alter major proteins. Temperatures up to 1000 degrees F especially when one re-uses cooking oil (as in fast-food restaurants), breaks down the polyunsaturated molecule and free radicals then form.

Simply speaking; a free radical is a free floating molecule that is unstable, and to become stable it steals electrons from other healthy cells turning those healthy cells unstable. When a healthy cell becomes unstable, it begins to age very quickly and can die. The free radicals are toxic due to their strong oxidizing (rusting) capacity, as they damage and destroy cells. Antioxidants are molecules that donate their electrons to the free radicals so they don't have to steal them from your cells; thereby preventing damage and destruction to your body.

These fats that have been changed by heat are incorporated into the cell wall where they interfere with the respiration and oxygen transport of the cell. This means they invade your cell and prevent it from working properly.

Acrolein, nitrosamines, hydrocarbons and benzopyrene are generated when fats are heated. Each are carcinogenic, cancer causing substances.

Deep-fried foods are the worse such as fried chicken, french fries, onion rings, potato chips, corn chips, cooked beef, chicken and just about all cooked meats due to their high fat content. Cancer is the number one killer of children in the United States and this is one significant reason why.

Paul Addis, professor of food science and nutrition at the University of Minnesota, says "Rancid oils are one of the factors that are important in heart disease. Oils turn rancid when the fats are broken down in cooking, and it's unarguable, these fats are toxic" Addis says.

Caramelization of Carbohydrates

While the heat of baking denatures protein, the quality of protein is adversely affected by nonenzymatic (chemical type) browning: the Maillard reaction. This is the browning seen on fried, baked, or toasted foods. They have absolutely no nutritional value for our system.

Almost all amino acids are destroyed during this process. In breads made with flour, significant losses of all essential amino acids except tryptophan occurs showing tremendous negative impact on protein quality.

If you bake some yams or sweet potatoes, you might notice the sweet sticky substance that oozes from the skin turns to ash from the heat. This is sugar molecules caramelizing, fusing together. Just like protein coagulation, caramelization also occurs on a microscopic level when foods are heated.

When sugar molecules (such as those in potatoes or bread) are carmelized or fused together after cooking, amylases (digestive enzymes) in your body cannot separate them into simple sugars for use as an energy source (our bodies need to break apart the large sugar molecule into smaller part to be used, just like a protein molecule needs to be broken down into amino acids). The cooked potato or piece of bread you just ate was nothing more than waste which your body will have to somehow dispose of.

This means the browning you see on your cookies, pastries, or any other bread product is actually indigestible and is treated as waste because it cannot be broken down.

Vitamins are Destroyed

When we treat foods with heat, we lose up to 97% of the water-soluble vitamins (Vitamins B and C) and up to 40% of the lipid soluble vitamins (Vitamins A, D, E and K).

Minerals Turn Unusable

Heat treatment also greatly affects the absorption and utilization of certain minerals primarily through splitting of complexes that makes these minerals less absorbable. In other words, the iron in your broccoli is much different than the iron in the ground. You can't just pick up a piece of iron and eat it, yet somehow it is safe in fruits and vegetables. How? Through photosynthesis (how plants use sunlight to convert carbon dioxide in the air into their food – sugar), the broccoli turns the inorganic iron in the ground that cannot be used by our bodies, into an organic iron that **can** be used by our bodies.

Cooking turns some of that usable iron back into the unusable iron that our bodies have to get rid of.

Vitamins and minerals need to be consumed in an "organic colloidal and naturally chelated molecular form" meaning "all natural" to be absorbed, and used by your cells and tissues during metabolic and digestive processes. Heat distorts the molecular arrangement of vitamins and minerals, thereby freeing its carbon. They are returned to an inorganic, ash-like form as found in soil.

All Enzymes are Destroyed

All enzymes are destroyed when heating food over 117 F (47 C). When you consider that the instructions on your frozen food items sitting in your freezer state to preheat oven to 300-400 degrees, not much will be left in those seemingly healthy vegetables.

Enzymes are specialized protein molecules that perform numerous catalytic physiological functions including breaking down food during digestion. Expose food enzymes to heat and nearly all are inactivated, unusable, destroyed. The body then must utilize energy to generate more of its own digestive enzymes instead of using the enzymes already present in the raw food. Heat of less than 117 degrees does not denature the food enzymes, however. Using food dehydrators that blow hot air on food until it cooks at low, safe temperatures allows for delicious, creative recipes such as using uncooked dehydrated garbanzo beans to make raw falafel, and dehydrated live crackers of various flavors.

This means you use your own energy to produce enzymes that were already present in the raw food but were destroyed as a result of cooking.

Other Detrimental Effects of Heating

Pesticides that are present in our food are restructured into even more toxic compounds.

Valuable oxygen is lost producing free radicals.

Cooking causes inorganic mineral elements to enter the blood and circulate through the system, which settle in the arteries and veins, causing arteries to lose their elasticity, causing blood pressure disorders, hardening of the arteries and a many other diseases.

The body prematurely ages as this inorganic matter that cannot be digested in our body is deposited in various joints or accumulates within internal organs, including the heart valves. This causes stones, arthritis, hardening of tissue and organs, and prematurely ages the body.

Natural fibers break down and cellulose (often referred to as 'dietary fiber' or 'roughage') is completely changed from its natural condition losing its ability to sweep the alimentary canal.

As temperature rises, each of these damaging events reduces the availability of individual nutrients. Alien food substances are created that the body cannot metabolize.

It is no wonder that since 1950 as processed foods increased, cancer rates in the United States have steadily climbed as well and are now at the highest point in history. We are dying from malnutrition, because the food we eat has less and less nutrients. Not only is our soil devoid of natural minerals from which grows nutrient lacking food, we load them up with pesticides, herbicides, genetically modify them, and then cook them to completely destroy whatever good was left. The result is something that looks like food, it might smell like food, it might taste like food, but nutritionally speaking it is as nutritious as a sponge.

This is the reason so many people are overweight and constantly hungry; your body needs nutrients to survive, and since the food you eat has so little nutritional value, you want to eat more and more to fulfill your body's needs. This is why people are constantly hungry, you are not hungry for food, you are hungry for nutrients which your food is not giving you. The body is then forced to draw up its decreasing supply of nutrients and remains chronically hungry, even though the stomach is full. When our nutrient reserves dwindle to nothing, then disease occurs.

It goes something like this; you have a perfectly made building (your body), and day by day it deteriorates, day by day things get used and worn. The owner of the building (you) doesn't know better and sends in lazy repair people who sit on the job and don't do nothing (nutrient lacking food) yet you keep paying them and think that the job is being done. As your building deteriorates you begin to notice some leaks, some cracks, etc. (minor ailments) and instead of fixing the piping system or the walls you send in the painters and the sealers (drugs).

So instead of fixing the problem they merely mask it by painting the walls and sealing the piping (drugs treat symptoms not the cause). As time goes by the building begins to really show signs of wear, the floors crack, major leaks begin to happen, the electrical system is malfunctioning and again you call the construction company (your doctor) who also doesn't know any better and again they put wood over the cracks, the paint over the walls with heavier paint, and they try to tape up the broken wiring (heavier drugs).

But nothing is being done on the CAUSE of all this damage and the old and broken parts are not replaced. Then all of a sudden the wall collapses or your floors fall through (a major illness like cancer, stroke, heart attack etc.) and you are in a panic. But again the foolish construction company tries to fill in the broken wall or fill in the broken floor (serious drugs like chemo or surgery etc.) without addressing the CAUSE of the damage and merely focusing on the broken parts.

This is why no diet will ever work until you begin eating nutrient rich food. It is impossible to be overweight when you eat nutrient rich, raw food. We overeat because our bodies are starving for nutrients **NOT** food! When you begin eating properly your body will automatically find a balance, it will automatically want to eat less thereby losing weight and naturally curing any disease that you might have.

The Difference Between Heat from Cooking and Digestive Chemistry

Some physiologists claim that cooking and human digestion are the same thing. They say cooking acts like a predigestion mechanism where heat hydrolyzes (breaks down) nutrients that would be similarly hydrolyzed (broken down) at body temperatures through digestion. This "predigestion" in cooked food does take place, but it is extremely *unnatural and unhealthy*.

There are two ways to denature, or break apart, proteins in order for them to get digested by our body: chemically using digestive enzymes, or through the use of heat (frying, baking, etc). Via heat, the body does not have the ability to utilize damaged broken down protein amino acids and rebuild them once again into usable protein molecules. This means that our bodies *do not have the ability to use broken down amino acids after they have been fried/cooked/baked or treated with heat*, therefore they turn into unusable waste that turns rancid, clogs our digestive system, and becomes food for the bacteria.

This is due to the enormous heat exposure during cooking, that denatures (breaks down) the protein molecule past a point of being usable, whereas body heat is too low to effect the protein molecule at all. The body does not require heat to reduce proteins into amino acids. It does a fine job of this chemically through enzymes. Chemically digested protein can be reused, whereas most of the heat destroyed protein molecules cannot.

This is the million dollar secret which nobody wants to talk about. Anything you eat that has been treated by cooking heat is then handled by your body as a toxin, because it turns into unusable waste. The trick is to include as much raw food as possible in your diet, if you don't know how delicious raw foods can be, you are missing out! But we will talk more about this later on.

So what happens when this unusable waste enters our body?

When cooked food enters our bodies, all it has to do is touch our tongue, and instantly white blood cells, or leukocytes (the soldiers of our immune system), from every corner of our body rush towards our digestive tract. This is known as *leukocytosis*. The same reaction occurs when our bodies get invaded by foreign bacteria when we are sick. **This means that our body treats cooked food like a bacterial infection and rushes to protect us from it.** What these leukocytes try to do is prevent the denatured (broken down) amino acids, fused carbohydrates, carcinogens, unusable vitamins and minerals, and all the other toxins from getting digested by your body.

Because the leukocytes left their guard posts from around your entire body, all your organs and tissues become vulnerable to invading bacteria and viruses while the white blood cells are busy preventing the cooked food from entering your system.

In the meantime, your regular body cells continue to live and produce waste products which the white blood cells would normally remove, but since they are now fighting the meal you just ate, there is nobody left to clean the fluid around your cells and they begin to swim around in their own waste.

So while the food remains in the digestive tract for 4-8 hours, the white blood cells are not able to stop invading bacteria, germs, viruses, and are unable to clean the extracellular fluid from the waste products of cellular metabolism.

The cells of your body which breathe, eat, and drink from the fluid around them, and expel excrement into it, begin to feel distress because they can no longer receive the necessary nutrients they need due to the increasing toxic environment around them. How would you like to sit and eat your own waste for hours on end?

Now imagine if you eat this dead food three times per day, you will be in leukocytosis constantly! This means that for days, months, years, for your entire life you will be lacking white blood cells and there will be nobody to rid your cells and extracellular fluid from excrement, toxins, dead cells, and invading bacteria. This leads to a severe increase in toxicity, reduced oxygen, increased acidity and reduced electrical potential between cells making them sick and diseased.

If you are also under stress you are adding to the deadly mix. Any form of stress can cause oxygen deficiency because of the chemicals produced by your body during stress. Stress due to chemical toxicity after eating cooked food leads to a reduction in oxygen as the body attempts to clean itself by oxidizing the accumulated toxins.

Emotional stress produces adrenaline and adrenaline-related hormones, requiring the body to draw down its oxygen reserves for their production and eventual removal (infection also depletes the body of oxygen which it uses to combat bacteria). Even the stress of a chronically heavy workload will deplete the body of much needed oxygen. In short, oxygen deficiency will result from any excessive stress, whatever the cause.

Some symptoms of oxygen deficiency due to a toxic environment are overall bodily weakness, muscle aches, depression, dizziness, irritability, fatigue, memory loss, irrational behavior, chronic hostility, circulation problems, poor digestion, acid reflux, lowered immunity to colds, flu and infection, bronchial problems, tumors and deposit build-ups, bacterial, viral and parasitic infections. These are all precursors to cancer, diabetes, heart disease, and other chronic diseases which will develop if the body is not detoxified.

In response to the heavy toxicity, bacteria begin to accumulate in your body. Bacteria act like garbage men that begin to eat up the excrement, dead cells, toxic materials from the food, and all the other garbage floating around. It is an emergency situation for your body, when the white blood cells are off on other duties, you must employ bacteria, which flourishes and acts as the last line of defence to help detoxify your organism.

However, if things are not fixed and the white blood cells spend all their time in the stomach rather than evenly spread inside your body, you will be in a constant state of leukocytosis. Because of this, the bacteria begin to thrive and as your normal cells die off since they can't survive in this dirty environment, they get consumed by the bacteria who now thrive.

After years of living like this, your body becomes infested with simple microorganisms like bacteria, trichomonads, fungi, microbes etc which live off the garbage that is constantly being put in. So instead of growth and development by your cells to promote a perfectly healthy body capable of living hundreds of years, bacteria and simple organisms flourish and develop, feeding on the waste, toxins, and your dead cells. At this point growth stops, teeth deteriorate, hair loss begins, and every single disease and illness begins to develop since the environment is perfect for it.

It is interesting to note that when you eat cooked food, bacteria that feast on this food flourish, but when you switch to raw foods, the reverse process begins with bacteria dying and healthy cells being restored. With regular exercise and various cleanses, the process can accelerate doubling the recovery progress.

Throughout the digestive tract down into the large intestine your white blood cells are actively defending your body from the denatured unusable amino acids, sugars, fats, vitamins, and minerals. This dead unusable food is hundreds of times larger by volume and is no match for your leukocites. As it is completely unusable by your body, it becomes food for the growing bacteria colonies which feast on the decomposing and rotting substances. The healthy cells in our bodies can only eat raw healthy foods which bacteria do not eat, this is why the digestive tracts of people on a raw food diet are nearly sterile.

As bacteria colonies increase in number, they slowly become invisible to the white blood cells which can't see them or differentiate them from the rest. This allows them to "have a say" and began to demand whatever they need from the body by secreting different chemicals. This is why we have cravings for fried or baked foods, candy, meat, coffee, tea, chocolate etc. In truth, our bodies do not need these things to survive because our healthy cells can't even use them as food! Scientists say that around 900,000 different kinds of bacteria occupy our bodies which number in the billions. At around age 50 bacteria and simple organisms can equal almost half of our body weight sitting in our fat, digestive tract, colon and many other places.

The only way to evict the invaders from our body is to detoxify our system and start eating as much raw foods as possible which will starve the bacteria allowing healthy cells to take back their place and bring your body back into balance. The lack of cooked food also allows your white blood cell count to increase tremendously allowing them to clean up your body and do what they were meant to do; help you stay young and prevent disease.

Miraculous Bacteria

In response to the heavy toxicity, bacteria begin to accumulate in your body. Bacteria in your body act like tiny garbage men that begin to eat up cell excrement, dead cells, toxic materials from the food, and all the other garbage produced by your bodily functions that is floating around. When the white blood cells are off on other duties, your body goes into a panic situation and must now employ bacteria, which flourishes because of the abundance of decomposing matter and acts as the last line of defense to help detoxify your organism.

Bacteria are a miracle of our world; they are the only living things on the planet that turn dead organic matter back into soil. Without them there would be no soil, and without soil there would not be life. A very interesting thing is that bacteria can not destroy or decompose anything that is still *alive*. They only feed on dead organic matter, on decomposing and rancid substances that have no life in order to recycle them back into nature. There is always plenty of bacteria, everywhere, ready to decompose and recycle any dead organic matter.

Think about that for a minute; every single cooked meal you eat is treated by your body as dead matter that feeds your bacteria which decompose the rotting rancid waste inside of you. As a result of the toxicity, lack of oxygen, and lack of nutrition, your own living healthy cells begin to die, bacteria begin to thrive, and your body slowly begins to decompose itself! This is called disease and aging.

Louis Pasteur

In 1857 Louis Pasteur discovered bacteria. As he looked in his microscope on healthy and sick tissue, he discovered some living things, bacteria and germs, which were all over the sick tissue, and none on the healthy tissue. He then proclaimed that germs were the cause of all disease. Have you ever noticed that there are fire trucks next to fires and flies around piles of poop? The germs cause disease statement is as silly as saying that fire trucks are the cause of fires or that flies cause piles of poop to appear on the ground. On his deathbed, Louis Pasteur **admitted that he was wrong**, he said that it is not bacteria that cause disease, but the opposite, that **disease cause bacteria**!

Today we are more afraid of germs than we are of chemicals. You should be much more afraid of chemicals than of germs because the damage they do is hundreds of times worse. Let's look at it this way; do you think something rotten smells bad? If you said yes then imagine a forest, does it smell bad? No. How come? There are millions of decomposing leaves, there are bugs and insects and animals all leaving their waste as well as dying, but it still smells nice. How come? Well, during the 1800's when oil was used to make about 100 different chemicals, things began to change in the natural cycle.

Before that time, everything that humans used was natural, organic, and biodegradable. Today, just from crude oil, we make over 83000 chemicals! All those chemicals are NOT biodegradable and cannot be recycled by bacteria to go back into the soil. When the hard working bacteria meets things like Styrofoam, plastic, glass, petrochemicals in your food, shampoos, clothing etc. it cannot decompose it, and it mutates. The good, simple, bacteria mutates into a totally different species which becomes a pathogenic bacteria, a dangerous bacteria.

All those chemicals that our society enjoys have terrible consequences. They go into nature and wreck havoc on the natural cycle of things. Recent blood samples of newborn polar bears on the North Pole revealed **62 different chemicals**!

Let's look at soap. In 1812 some French people developed rose water, the first predecessor to modern soap. It was made to smell nice, not to kill bacteria. But then some people discovered that with fear, you can make people buy a lot more stuff. They developed soap and began using the fear tactic to get people buying and buying this new substance that would rid them of this awful newly discovered "bacteria." Do you know how the linens of the Russian tsar family were washed? They were taken to the river, then in large containers filled with clay they were beaten with wooden sticks for an hour or so, then rinsed in the water and hanged out to dry in the sun. No bleach, no chemicals, no soap, no detergent, no softeners – but much better results. Did you know the sun's rays can kill more bacteria than any of these antibacterial detergents ever can?

It may make you feel better to see a hospital orderly wiping down every surface in your room with an anti-bacterial wipe. But according to a new study, that wipe isn't killing bacteria on contact, and may be simply picking up bacteria from one surface and distributing it to others.

Due to a lack of nutrients along with the 75,000 new environmental toxins that didn't exist prior to 1930's it's no wonder our bodies have absolutely no resources to deal with even the simplest illnesses. Fragrances are a major contributor to a host of diseases; things like fabric softeners, toxic washing and laundry liquids, air fresheners etc. (if your child has ADD/ADHD and you wash everything your child comes in contact with in natural detergent, only use natural washing liquids, and eliminate all toxic cleaners/air fresheners, you will notice dramatic improvements in your child, and your own health)

In an era where antibiotic-resistant "superbugs" like MRSA are a growing threat in hospitals, nurses and orderlies have understandably been wielding the wipes diligently. But when a team led by microbiologist Gareth Williams tested wipes after their use at several hospitals in Wales, they found that MRSA in particular could easily be spread by those handy little moist towelettes.

Dr Williams said: "What is remarkable is that some of these wipes actually have the words 'kills MRSA' written on the box." We found that, under the conditions we observed in actual hospitals, this wasn't the case" [*BBC News*].

So what's a nervous nurse — or kindergarten teacher, or fitness club manager — to do? Williams recommends that a wipe be used one time, to clean one surface, and then discarded. But all those institutions that have adopted the anti-bacterial wipes as a symbol of cleanliness and sanitation might be better off with a scrub brush. Commenting on the story, professor Donna Duberg of Saint Louis University said the public's over-enthusiasm for disinfecting products can have damaging results over the long term.

"We use way too many antibacterial agents," Duberg said, adding that the overuse of products like wipes, soaps and cleansers that contain these substances can lead bacteria to become resistant to our methods of extermination. "I personally believe there isn't anything that good, hot soapy water can't clean," she said [*ABC News*].

On the surface of our body we have lots of good bacteria that are standing guard ready to defend our system from any foreign invaders. When we use soap or body wash we destroy all that natural defense, and open up the doors for any foreign invader to freely come and attack. We purposefully and willingly fire all of our body guards. But how did people wash their hands before soap? With dirt, clay, sand etc, and in India, they wash with ash (which is a great dish washing substance as well). Clean in our society means lots of chemicals. Everywhere you go you see signs like "Kills 99.99% of germs" but germs are not the enemy, the chemicals are the real enemy. We are killing the fire trucks near the fire and hoping that there will be no more fires, we are killing the flies near the poop and hoping there will be no more poop. The chemicals will kill us, not the bacteria. If your body's immune system is in top shape, it can kill most of the germs it comes into contact with. How in the world did we live 20 years ago before the advent of all these anti-bacterial products? These companies are just cashing in on our fears.

A natural shampoo and shaving cream can be simply made with some flax seeds soaked in water overnight, then blended. A good soap substitute is simple baking soda or hydrogen-peroxide, you may wash dishes as well as all fruits and vegetables in them safely without using any harsh and dangerous chemicals.

Hunters will tell you that wild animals **have no parasites** in them. If we look at animals who come in contact with city food, they all have parasites (in the intestines, brain, lungs, heart, liver etc). Parasites, just like bacteria, are scavengers, they feed on dead organic matter, on the toxins that our healthy cells cannot use. They are helping us get rid of all that rotting stuff. Think about a mushroom, it can only grow on something that is decaying.

How does cooked food lead to diseases of the digestive tract?

Your body has a much harder time digesting and removing cooked food, not to mention it is a lot denser than raw foods. Before any food can pass into the small intestine, it must first become alkaline, for which the pancreas is responsible for. Due to the high acidity and density of cooked foods, pancreatic juices are unable to pass into the small intestine in necessary amounts leading to the pancreatic ducts being congested. This leads to inflammation; pancreatitis. The same thing happens to liver and gallbladder ducts leading to gallbladder inflammation; cholecystitis.

It is well known that the amount of digestive juices that will be released into the digestive tract equals the amount of food that touches the taste receptors in the mouth. If there is inadequate chewing and very quick swallowing, the amount of juices that will be releases from the pancreas and the liver will not be enough for the complete breakdown of the food. It is unable to digest and the sphincter leading further into the small intestine does not open, while more and more food keeps entering the stomach. Only under the increasing pressure does the sphincter open and the undigested food enters the small intestine. However, due to the fact that the intestinal ferments and enzymes only work in non-acidic, alkaline environments, they are unable to digest the still acidic food.

Yet again the undigested food in its own acidic environment is treated as waste by your body, eliminated undigested, and leaves your cells hungry for nutrients.

Leukocytosis also leads to a dramatic decrease in the peristalsis (wave-like contractions of muscles which move the food along the digestive tract) of the intestines. After intake of cooked food, the peristaltic movements occur at a rate of about 4-6 per minute which allows all of the food to pass through the digestive tract in about 24 hours. During the intake of raw foods however, peristalsis is 4-8 times faster leading to a 3-6 hour trip through the digestive tract. If you have normal peristaltic movements, then you should be going to the bathroom as many times as you eat, the more the better. A few hours after intake of food your intestines should be empty.

Congestion in the liver and the pancreas shuts down their ability to filter blood. Since the blood leaving the intestines must pass through the portal vein into the liver, which is congested, it must go through secondary veins, and enters the body uncleaned. The kidneys are left as the last filtering defence and as a result of the high stress placed upon them, they quickly clog up leaving no other blood filtering capabilities. This leads to high blood pressure, heart pains, headaches, warts etc. which are all indications that the blood is not being cleaned as a result of eating cooked food. If you happen to have low blood pressure this means that the heart muscle has become congested and weak.

Throughout our life we accumulate these toxins, pollutants, stagnant bile, other fluids, parasites, bacteria, and other nasty things. This, in addition to the lack of nutrients, is the reasons we get all the various diseases which plague our society today. This is why detoxing and cleansing your system is absolutely vital to health and longevity.

After switching to raw foods, people who are overweight can expect to lose 10-20 lbs without dieting and feeling absolutely fantastic. A proper colon cleansing program removes the toxins as well as the mucoid plaque from the colon which builds up during the intake of cooked food. Even a thin layer of mucoid plaque weakens the body. Nature intended mucoid plaque to be removed. But due to stress and diet, most Americans have many hardened layers of mucoid plaque. The healthy colon weighs about 4 pounds. One autopsy revealed a colon choked with 40 pounds of impacted mucoid plaque! A proper colon cleanse, detoxification program, and raw food prepares your body for optimal health.

This is the magic of raw foods; your body will automatically adjust, lose weight, cure itself of disease, and make you feel and look younger, without any foolish calorie counting, without watching every bite of what you eat, without taking any expensive supplements, and without the headache. Im not going to expect everyone who reads this to switch to raw foods (those who do I applaud you because you are true heroes of your health), yet I do stress eating as much raw foods as possible with every meal (un-cooked fruits and vegetables).

In 1834, Sylvester Graham, inventor of the cracker that still bears his name, switched to raw foods during the cholera epidemic in America. He, as well as his followers, were not affected by the disease at all. Raw foods help alcoholics and smokers forever kick their habits. Women who stick to the raw food diet notice that during menstruation they no longer have blood flow, no more PMS, no more cramps, and while they enjoy *every* day of the month, the ovulation process strengthens in the mean time bringing about benefits to childbirth and healthy offspring.

In recent years it was shown that a raw food diet helps people restore weak organs, teeth, hair, improve sexual vitality, and increases our ability to withstand radiation up to three times as much as regular eaters. It is interesting to note that when one is on a cooked food diet, every year 1% of healthy tissue is replaced by bacteria, but when you switch to a raw diet the process in the other direction is almost twice as fast replacing bacteria with healthy cells by 1.5-2% per year. This number can increase with fasting and various cleanses, and if you regularly exercise you can double the regenerative process.

Everyone who switches to raw foods becomes younger from the inside and the outside. That's because your white blood cells are now able to do what they were meant to do; remove waste from the extracellular fluid, eliminate dead cells and bacteria. This leaves no more food for the billions of microbes and parasites which die or turn into cysts that are also removed by your white blood cells. There are numerous cases of people who, after switching to a raw food diet, physically become younger and after being tested by medical doctors appear have the biological age decades and decades younger. Your body's biological age will actually get younger!

When all your body reaches 100% healthy cells, you might start looking decades younger, you might notice that all your diseases are cured (if you had any), you might notice that you are stronger than ever, you might notice that your sex drive has reached levels not seen before, and you might notice your life has changed.

Food Absorption

Cooked food promotes the production of mucous in the digestive tract which prevents the absorption of the food. This acts like a protection barrier preventing the cooked food waste from entering your body. This is why people who eat cooked food are always hungry. Not only is the food we eat devoid of almost all the nutrients, vitamins, and minerals, not only is the remaining nutrients destroyed by heat, not only is cooked food unusable by our bodies as discussed earlier, but the body adds a further protection barrier in the form of mucous to further prevent absorption of the toxins.

Here is a table showing the percentage of absorption of cooked and raw foods and their interaction.

% Raw Food	% Cooked Food	% Absorbability Into Body
5	95	0.03
10	90	0.06
25	75	0.1
50	50	0.3
75	25	1
99	1	3
100	0	30

Even a fully raw diet does not provide 100% absorption. Can you imagine how hard our bodies have to work under "normal" conditions of fast food and junk food? Can you imagine what our bodies go through in presence of this chronic malnutrition? This is why our bodies are full of diseases! Healthy people today are a rarity because under these conditions our body physically **cannot** be healthy!

The Food Diversion

The cells in our bodies are constantly dividing, and throughout many years do not show any degeneration or aging, which was proved by German biologist August Weismann who was ranked by many as the second most notable evolutionary theorist of the 19th century, after Charles Darwin. He showed that with proper nutrition and oxygenation, unicellular organisms like our cells are immortal. In a massive organism like our bodies, when the extracellular fluid is polluted, when there is no proper nutrition and oxygenation, the cell ages and dies. The situation changes when you switch to a raw living diet, in which case the extracellular fluid becomes clean, there is plenty of nutrition and oxygenation, and the body becomes virtually ageless. This means you can live to 100 years of age and even much longer, and there are many cases of people who are this old, you just don't hear about them.

How is it that in many religious and ancient texts we hear of people living to 600, 800, even 1000 years of age and suddenly in our day most of us die before we get to 80? The ancient Egyptian Coptic texts write that as soon as people lost "knowledge", they became weak and died young. What is this knowledge that we have lost?

The presence of leukocytosis is evidence that cooked food began to be used only very recently. We would have developed some sort of adaptive reaction over time which would enable the body to easily deal with cooked foods, but we do not have such ability. Cooked food is an attack on the immune system which weakens the body to any foreign invaders, creating a life of sickness and disease. We are meant to be healthy throughout our entire life, being vibrant and energetic every day, being sick is **not normal**.

Those who profit from the population living in a constant state of disease is pushing and promoting this unnatural, chemically lased, genetically modified junk while knowing full well what it can do. And the interesting thing is that we buy it, and pay good money for it! We have seen an almost total elimination of more than 10 different kinds of edible grains which have been replaced by hard sorts that require cooking. Such grains like sorgo or emmer wheat and many others that are very close to the human nutritional requirements were taken out of our rations and replaced with hard sorts like rice, wheat, oats, etc. which must be eaten cooked.

The table of a raw food eater is actually very diverse and delicious. Raw vegetables and fruits, nuts, greens, berries, honey, some types of raw mushrooms, dried fruits, seeds, and a variety of grains. With a dehydrator you can create raw bread, crackers, chips, sweets, cakes etc. For a gourmet eater this opens a world of possibilities never thought possible. And the most important thing is that from all this you never get fat and old, but young and healthy!

A Life Story

When we ate cooked food for the first time as we were children, our bodies produced the first mucous. Part of this mucous is left on the walls of the digestive tract, and the other part is collected by the lungs. Mucous however cannot stay in the lungs for too long because the lungs are not meant to be mucous collectors, and similar to the peristalsis of our intestines, it is moved up from the lungs into the throat and nose, and you notice your child has a runny or stuffed nose. If we feed our child mucous producing foods (all cooked foods, sugary foods, sodas), they will always have runny and stuffed up noses because the body is readily removing the mucous in the most normal, and quickest way possible; the mucous is removed through the nose and the lungs remain clean.

What is the typical parental reaction in this case? "I have to help my child and take him to the doctor." The doctor will write out a prescription for some medication or nose drops, and we feel better because we did everything we think we could for our child. However, the medication or nose drops were not needed. Your child has no need for them because they are extremely toxic. They are so toxic that the normal mucous removing reaction is stopped so that the body can focus on removing the poisonous medication from the body! The detoxification process is stopped, the nose stops running, and the mucous goes right back into the lungs. We look at our child and say "This medication worked, my child is healthy."

What we don't understand is that the nose stopped running because the body has concentrated all of its energy on removing the toxic medication. A red runny nose is not as serious as lungs full of mucous and a body weakened by the toxic medication. The mucous layer in the lungs and intestines becomes thicker, which makes it much harder for the body to cleanse itself. When the toxic medication is removed and our body regained its strength once more, it starts the detox process again by removing the mucous through the nose. After a few months we notice our child has a runny nose yet again, and we do the same thing as before; go to the doctor and get more medication. We take our child to our physician who says we need stronger drugs since the mucous has become more concentrated, there is now more of it, and as a result the glands have become swollen and inflamed. In addition, since the mucous rises along the trachea and leaves residue on the vocal chords, the voice weakens and becomes hoarse.

The new stronger medication is so toxic that the body stops its detox process dead in its tracks, and again focuses its energy on the removal of the new toxic drug. This process will take a few months until the body has regained its strengths once more to begin the mucous removal.

Think about this for a moment. When you do you usually get sick? Is it not a coincidence that every time you are either on vacation, or a weekend, or on some relaxing down time that you usually get sick? As soon as you get some extra energy your body quickly tries to use that extra boost to detoxify itself before you spend it on something else. This is why we get sick when we have time for rest.

When your body is severely polluted it must revert to serious measures; we get sick with a fever. In order to speed up the process of detoxification and increase the enzyme activity, the body raises its temperature, which in itself is a very complicated process requiring a large amount of time and energy. The body has to work very hard to raise its temperature; the heartbeat increases by 20-30 beats per minutes, all the hormonal glands work twice as hard, and other processes increase their capabilities which is why fatigue sets it.

To preserve its energy which would usually be used to digest food, your body creates a situation when you do not want to eat. Your tongue becomes covered with a heavy coat of mucous to block the taste sensation, your nose is stuffed to block the smell sensation, and your glands have swollen to make swallowing more difficult.

When you get a fever your body begins to sweat to allow the toxins to leave the body with the sweat through the pores. This sweat is somewhat slimy due to the increased mucous leaving the body.

What do we do when our body spent so much time and effort producing the fever to help us detox? We take temperature lowering drugs, Aspirin (made from coal tar which is very toxic) Tylenol, etc.

Our bodies do not expect such evil and despicable action on our part. These medications are so toxic that our bodies simply do not have enough energy to continue the healing process which simply stops dead in its tracks. Your body works so hard and becomes so weak trying to remove the poisons of newly ingested drugs that it cannot sustain the fever which falls below normal. We become weak from the medication and not from the fever itself.

Have you heard of complications during a fever? This is not due to the fever, but due to the food or medication we take! Then the doctors say "fever is so dangerous, you have to lower it or you might die!" The only thing you might die from is the toxic drugs that you stuff inside your hard working body, in other words you can die from not cooperating with your body and doing something unnatural. When you get a fever you might be going through hot and cold spells, listen to your body and take off the covers when you get too hot, and when you get too cold put the covers back on. There were cases of seizures during fevers, it happens because the body is too hot, put yourself (or your child) under lukewarm water and the seizures will stop. If you get a fever the best remedy is to listen to your body, you can help it by fasting for a few days, doing enemas, and taking plenty of vitamin C. For goodness sake do not take any toxic medications!

It takes a lot of energy and resources by the body to rid itself from the medication, and we might not get sick for a long time after that because the body has no energy for detoxification. This is why most adults do not experience such high fevers as children, because adult bodies are weak and barely have enough energy for any healing process.

As we continue to sabotage our body's natural detoxification process, we continue to collect mucous which turns from colourless clear to green, orange, yellow, or brown. To rid itself from such a huge amount of mucous our body turns on another backup mechanism; pneumonia. Our bodies put forth heroic strength, much more than with a fever, to clean up the mucous which makes us even more fatigued and tired. If you develop pneumonia that means your body is urgently trying to clean itself up, its an emergency call for action, but yet again we sabotage the process with drugs which makes our bodies weaker than ever.

Our bodies have to be very strong to raise our temperature and we must be glad this even happens! It means that your body is actively detoxifying and cleaning up making you healthier. When you are sick, help your body and fast for a few days, take hot and cold alternating showers, go to a sauna, do cold water dousing, and drink 3 litres of water per day. Most importantly listen to your body, if it feels like lying down with no covers, then lie down with no covers, if it feels like taking a bath rather than a shower, then take a bath.

After regular prescription drug abuse your body will give up trying to detoxify for many years, apart from some light bouts of the flu. Your lungs will continue to collect mucous until they are about two thirds full! Then when the lungs are full to capacity, the mucous begins depositing in the nasal and vocal cavities, and then under the skin making it rough, bumpy, and porous. If we then take a short walk, we begin to sweat which allows for this acidic mucous to escape through the pores of the skin. The mucous irritates the skin, and we call this skin allergies.

Allergies occur because our bodies are severely intoxicated by the large amounts of mucous. Sometimes we have so much mucous in our bodies and lungs that breathing becomes difficult; we develop asthma and other breathing problems.

To test whether you are polluted with mucous, you should take a short run, if your nose starts running then you have lots of mucous. If your nose does not run and you can breathe freely then your lungs are not full of mucous, but it does not mean they are completely clean though.

Have you ever noticed professional athletes or runners? They are always spitting, blowing their nose, and clearing themselves from mucous. Even if they are vegetarian they still eat high caloric, cooked, mucous producing foods. *Raw food* athletes don't have this problem.

When you begin a raw food diet, you must be prepared for the detox process that your body will go through. About two to three weeks after the switch you might start feeling the effects of detox, or healing crisis as it is called. This may mean fatigue, weakness, blood pressure changes, various forms of skin irritation, headaches, diarrhea, fevers, past illnesses coming back, pains in various body parts, vomiting, and many other detoxification symptoms which you should welcome with open arms because you are finally becoming healthier! Your body finally has enough energy to start cleaning itself out.

Sadly, most people mistake this as something that is wrong, start blaming the new raw diet for their poor health and go right back to their old sick selves. Many people who have tried going vegetarian with the same results often go back to meat and then think that meat is the one keeping them "healthy" since their body is so weak it can't even clean itself out.

The severe symptoms of detox will stop in a few weeks, but will continue until your whole body is free from bacteria and all the microorganisms that feed on cooked or dead food. The process occurs because these microorganisms are dying in very large quantities activating the immune system fighters, the white blood cells, and putting pressure on the filtering organs like the kidneys, liver, and lungs, which are unable to clean them in time, leading to all the symptoms listed. A 24-36 hour water or juice fast will accelerate the detox process. Think about it, your body has to get rid of tens of pounds of dead microbes, germs, microorganisms and toxins. It tries to do this as fast as possible and through every pore.

Cravings for cooked and dead food will still occur for a few months after you begin, but it is better to withhold for these short months rather than give in and suffer much longer.

"*I believe the strain on our enzyme "bank account," caused by diets of cooked food, is one of the paramount causes of premature aging and early death. I also believe it is the underlying cause of almost all degenerative diseases.*" - **Dr. Edward Howell,** The Status of Food Enzymes in Digestion and Metabolism, 1946.

The only thing stopping you is knowledge, which will in turn change you behaviors. We need to change our perspective, our ideas, and our understandings. We need to move closer to nature, not add pills or supplements. Only nature and you body can cure itself.

How to Help Your Body During Detox

There are basically two paths your cleansing process can take, the detox route or the crisis route. The detox route is when your body has enough energy and is able to deal with all the toxins that are coming out from "hiding" from various parts of your body. During a crisis, your body is unable to deal or doesn't have enough energy to deal with the toxins and intoxication occurs.

During a crisis your body does not have enough calcium, other minerals and antioxidants, which could easily be replaced by eating fresh greens or taking quality supplements. If your memory becomes worse that means you do not have enough omega 3 and omega 6 fats in your diet. The crisis is further stimulated by stress, fatigue, not enough sleep, and not enough sunlight.

To help your body to detoxify it is recommended you partake in physical exercise which will help to literally squeeze the toxins out of your tissues and cells through sweat. The best "medicine" to detoxify your body is fasting, dry fasting (no food or water) or water/fresh juice fasting for 3 days or more. This will give your body extra strength to deal with the waste that is leaving the body and provide an accelerated cleansing reaction. Fasting by itself is the strongest and quickest way to detoxify your body.

For those who think they are ready there is a very quick, yet challenging way to completely clean up your body, that is to totally and fully get rid of all toxins, of all parasites, and of all bacteria. That is a 21 or 30 day dry fast, meaning no food or water for 21 days. If you think that is impossible, think again, there are thousands of people across the world that can vouch for fasting this long without any harmful side effects. To get ready for this fast you must complete a 3 day dry fast, a 7 day dry fast, and a 14 day dry fast to get your body ready.

At certain times fasting can actually save your life or save one of your organs. I know of a young man who was suffering from severe kidney failure and was one day away from an operation to get rid of one of the kidneys. He went on a 7 day dry fast, and was completely cured. The man didn't know the magical benefits of fasting, and being one day away from having only one kidney, he was absolutely furious when he went back to the doctor who was going to slice him up.

Mainstream medicine does not want to cure you, it does not want you to be healthy, and it will do anything it can do keep it this way. They are more satisfied when they can stuff you full of toxic medication or put you on the operation table; this makes them money and keeps you coming back. The reason some things may seem farfetched, or some cure unbelievable is because the medical mafia for decades has been brainwashing the people into believing their lies. If you know how disease starts, then it will become clear how it can be cured.

If you are not yet ready to go on a 100% raw food diet but want to detox and clean up your body then you must do at least a 3 day dry fast. If you are overweight or very unhealthy then you can start with a 3 day water or freshly squeezed juice fast (water is better). If you are ready to take this step forward in your life and choose a 100% raw food lifestyle then you can also start with a 3 day dry or water fast to speed up the results. It is not necessary to go 100% raw right away, you may choose to go 70-30 or 50-50 at first, the most important thing is start eating as much fresh natural foods as possible. We will get into the details a little later on.

What Happens During Digestion?

Most people think that the digestive system is a tube that is filled with digestive juices and acid, and the process of digestion is the breaking down of food with the acid. They think that they can throw in anything and the acid will break it all down. This is far from being true as proven by many scientists in the 20th century.

As we have already learned, eating cooked food requires a lot of our own strength to manufacture the necessary enzymes, nutrients, and other elements for the proper digestion, or shall we say removal, of the food we have eaten. Raw food on the other hand goes through a completely different process in our digestive system; autolysis. Autolysis can be explained by a simple experiment. The experiment involved filling two containers with the stomach acid of a carnivore, and then placement of an uncooked frog in one container, and a cooked frog in the other container, both filled with the exact same digestive juice. The results were much unexpected.

The raw frog completely dissolves, with all the bones, within a short time, while the cooked frog merely changed color. If our digestive acid truly did break down food, then the results should have been the same in both containers, which was not the case. In the presence of digestive juice, the raw frog turned on the process of complete self dissolvement and digestion through its **own** enzymes!

Autolysis is a very simple process. After raw food is masticated (chewed) and swallowed, it enters our stomach, which is already full of digestive acid. Stomach acid is basically hydrochloric acid which contains lots of free hydrogen ions. Free hydrogen has immense penetrating and destroying abilities making it a perfect digestive force. In every living cell there are special vesicles called lysosomes which are cube shaped organelles that contain enzymes. When the raw living food enters the stomach, the hydrogen atoms quickly penetrate the cells and destroy the lysosome, allowing all the natural enzymes to escape and begin to self digest the food from the inside as well as from the outside. Cooked food on the other hand does not have any remaining natural enzymes. With raw food your body does not need to do anything else except absorb all the nutrients (instead of using up its own enzymes and nutrients to try and break down cooked food), talk about energy savings!

What should have taken only 20-30 minutes (how long it takes on average for most raw fruits and vegetables to fully digest), now takes a "normal" 6-24 hours for cooked food.

Raw food is stock full of enzymes ready for its self digestion! Nature has provided every single raw food with a specific balanced set of enzymes, minerals, and vitamins for the most complete and easy digestion and absorption process. Cooking food completely ruins that balance. This means our digestive system is fully ready and built only for raw foods; it can however run on cooked food, but only in emergency situations and will bring disease with it. Just like a car that is meant to run on supreme gasoline, you can fill it up with 92, but the engine will become dirty and will not run properly.

According to Dr. Zalmanov from his book "Sacred Wisdom of Human Body" when we eat three cooked meals a day, our bodies produce 2 gallons of digestive juices per day! When we eat raw foods, we only produce about two cups. Can you imagine how much energy it takes to produce 2 gallons of digestive juices? This takes up to 80% of our entire body energy reserves.

Our body is fully prepared to face times of hunger and emergency situations and has built in safety mechanisms to accept cooked, canned, or otherwise dead food. In the animal kingdom carnivores sometimes feed on grass or leaves, and herbivores sometimes even feed on meat. The result of this diet is disease; our bodies are not meant to **live** on such a diet!

The Overeating Safety Mechanism

Nature has provided our body with a very simple, yet very effective, safety mechanism against overeating, and absorbing things from our digestive tract that we don't need. Nobel Prize laureate Pavlov discovered that the relationship between the amount of hydrochloric acid in our digestive juices and our body's need for nutrients is directly correlated. In other words, if our body needs nutrients, we will have more hydrochloric acid in our stomachs for digestion, and if our bodies do not need any nutrients, there will be no hydrochloric acid for digestion, simple. So in the case that our body does not need any nutrients, if we do ingest some food, it simply will not digest and come out the same way it came in.

So how come people are still overweight and obese? Did the mechanism stop working? The mechanism is fine; it all has to do with the type of food we eat. Nutritionists, doctors, and chemists tell us that cooked food is much better absorbed because during the heating process, it breaks down, meaning complex structures are broken down into simple structures. This bypasses what your saliva and your stomach acid are supposed to do. So when we eat cooked food it comes as somewhat pre-digested, but here lies the ultimate evil. If raw food enters our digestive system and is not needed, it is simply not broken down and exits in the same shape that it came in. But cooked food, since it is already broken down, **bypasses** this safety mechanism and is absorbed no matter what, whether it is needed or not!

Our body is completely defenceless against cooked food!

As an example let's look at raw protein and simplify what happens during digestion. As a raw form of protein enters your body, it is usually in a very tight roll that is quite large. If your body has no need for protein, no hydrochloric acid is produced, it is not digested, and it leaves your body the same way it came in. And since it is still raw, it does not become food for your bacteria and does not become a toxin.

On the other hand, if a denatured and dead protein enters your body, it will bypass the lack of hydrochloric acid safety mechanism, and some of it will bypass the mucous membrane (another safety mechanism as discussed previously) and get absorbed straight into the blood. These denatured, dead particles are treated as an invader by your body and will be attacked by the white blood cells (remember leukocytosis?). Some other particles will stick together forming plaques that will attach themselves to various capillaries, and day by day this amino acid garbage will pile up inside your body and clog up your arteries, kidneys, liver etc. Add to this the denatured, dead particles of carbohydrates, fats, inactive vitamins, inorganic minerals, all the additives like pesticides, preservatives, flavour enhancers, and other toxic substances, and you will have a poisonous concoction floating around your body.

Some biochemists and doctors will tell you that our body is able to remove all those toxins, and if it not able then we must resort to various organ cleanses. This is a lie. Our body does not, and cannot, remove such massive amount of toxins; it was not built for this. Toxins get deposited throughout the whole body, in all of our organs, in fat, in blood vessels, and under our skin. Our hard working body does not have the time, energy, or resources to deal with such an onslaught 3-4 times per day, every day.

It turns out our toxin elimination system was **only** built for the removal of **our own** bodily toxins and products of natural metabolism! Since raw food does not need any defence mechanism or removal process, our body is only supposed to deal with its own by-products of normal life (eg. cellular waste). But we add to this process massive amounts of foreign toxins, and things our body have never even seen before and does not know how to remove like pesticides and herbicides, preservatives, colorants, taste enhancers etc.

In most cases, due to our weakened immune system, when foreign matter enters our system, it can't even be properly taken care of. In this case it is simply encapsulated in a membrane and left floating around our body. The immune systems "knows" about these incapacitated invaders and "remembers" their structure creating antibodies for all similar matter. This is when allergies are at full swing. Even if you take away a product that you might be allergic to, as doctors say, you will get an allergy to something else because your body reacts to all similar things.

If the foreign matter is not encapsulated, your immune system creates antibodies for it, leaving this matter incapacitated, this is called an immune complex, and it is left floating around your circulatory system, or it gets stuck to your blood vessel, or it gets stored in your organs. Since this immune complex is not removed from your body, your immune system will react to everything similar that enters your system – creating an allergic reaction.

Doctors do not know the reason why these immune complexes are not properly removed from your body. But it is evident; your body simply does not have enough energy to remove such enormous quantities of these immune complexes as well as all other foreign matter. In nature there is never such a high quantity of denatured and destroyed proteins, fats, and carbohydrates, apart from maybe a forest fire or a volcanic eruption, "cooking" does not occur in nature. Doctors are now beginning to find atherosclerotic plaques on blood vessels and immune complex deposits in the liver and spleen, in young children! This is frequently called dietary allergies, which many regard as a fundamental cause of chronic diseases.

Antibiotics do not recognize encapsulated matter or immune complexes and are useless against them, all they do is completely destroy the natural balance in your digestive system. A fast, or a raw food diet, is the only way to allow your body to remove all the atherosclerotic plagues, deposits, immune complexes, and all the other toxins from your system. On a raw food diet your body no longer has to put up such strong defences and protection against the food, and begins to do what it does best; live a healthy life. All the so called "incurable" disease are easily removed, painlessly, and side-effect free.

Why Do You Feel Warm After Eating Cooked Food?

This is one of the most frequently asked questions about eating raw. People commonly believe that without a bowl of cooked food on a chilly winter day they would not be able to stay warm. I know many people who quit the raw food lifestyle because they were afraid that they would become too cold during the winter.

A hot meal, a cup of coffee, or an ice-cold shot of vodka all warm our body in a similar manner. When any impure substances get into our blood through the walls of the intestines, they irritate our adrenals, the endocrine glands located above the kidneys. The adrenals immediately begin to produce epinephrine, norepinephrine and a variety of steroid hormones. These hormones stimulate our sympathetic nervous system, which is why we feel awake at first. They also force our heart to beat faster and to pump larger amounts of blood through our body, which makes us feel warm. This feeling doesn't last long and we pay a high price for it. After 10-15 minutes our body gets exhausted from performing extra work, the heart requires rest, the nervous system becomes inhibited, and we feel tired, sleepy and even colder than before.

However we remember only the feeling of getting warmer after eating cooked food and repeat such stimulation again and again. This harmful practice wears the body out and by the end of the winter many people feel exhausted and depleted.

Winter after winter of eating quantities of cooked food doesn't help the human body to withstand cold weather better. On the contrary, weakened adrenals eventually won't be able to work properly even at warm temperatures. For example, older people feel cold even in the middle of the summer.

Another reason why it is hard for many of us to tolerate cold temperatures is because eating a cooked food diet severely impairs our capillary circulation. According to Dr. Alexander Zalmanoff, author of "Sacred Wisdom of Human Body" (Paris, 1961) 80% of all the blood in any human body is located in the capillaries (small blood vessels), and only 20% in arteries and veins. Tiny capillaries get clogged easily by unnaturally large particles of cooked food, immune complexes, plaques, which results in poor circulation, poor blood flow, and such symptoms as cold hands and feet.

If you truly want to feel warm during the cold season, a raw food lifestyle is inevitable choice for you. During your first "raw" winter you may experience some cold due to the weakened adrenals, so put on an extra sweater, take a hot bath, or do some pushups. If you will continue staying raw, your adrenals will rest and recover, your capillary circulation will improve, and your nervous system and your heart will naturally strengthen without any artificial stimulation.

Natural Evidence

Have you ever seen Cola running through a mountain stream? How about a double cheeseburger hanging from a tree? Ramen noodles with chicken strips sprouting up from the soil? Maybe in your dreams, but not in reality. It is as simple as asking this question, if nature truly did want us to eat such a variety of cooked and processed food, it would have made it available in nature. Nature has created a world where we can survive with minimal effort and minimal resources, pretty much anywhere on the planet. In our malnutrition society with food that barely even has a fraction of the nutrition is used to have, yes we do need to supplement, but to say that we **need** the countless different foods, vitamin pills, and supplementation in nature, is simply not true.

A koala feeds exclusively on eucalyptus leaves, and it is completely healthy, it has magnificent fur, teeth, and claws. It is able to make perfect soft tissue, bones and muscles. Look at squirrels who feed only on nuts and seeds. What about carnivores who are able to feed sometimes on only one type of animal. Elephants, giraffes, antelopes, zebras etc. feed only on leaves and grass yet are completely healthy and have huge amounts of muscle. Humans are no different. Our bodies are designed in such a way that we can easily live off of a simple raw diet, and we will be much healthier as a result.

Liver – Our Synthesising Sensation

Research in the 20th century showed that our body is able to synthesize proteins when only carbohydrates are the source of food. Our liver is the place where the magic happens, where the necessary proteins are synthesized for use. When we eat cooked food, including meat, the foreign protein is seen as an invader that needs to be removed. This meat protein is digested in the liver into uric acid and is then directed through the kidneys for removal. This is completely useless work placed upon your organs, which requires great amounts of digestive enzymes and ferments provided and made by your system. Your body goes through a lot of work to remove what you constantly put in.

Parallel to this, your liver has to deal with all the waste and toxins from the food, as well as your body's own products of metabolism, and while this is happening, it has to synthesize the needed amino acids, haemoglobin for your blood, glycogen, vitamins, and enzymes. How long do you think your liver will last under these extreme working conditions? You guessed it, not long at all.

As a result your liver becomes exhausted and overworked leading to inflammation and a reduced ability to function. This allows toxins to freely enter your blood and circulate around your system. Many people who switch to raw foods, after years on unhealthy diets, report pain in the liver which is a sign that this vital organ is going through major detoxification. The liver in carnivorous animals is able to synthesize all the necessary elements only from the amino acids in raw meat, so there is no need for carbohydrates. There is no need to feed your dog or cat any cooked food, raw meat or fish is what they were born to eat.

The only difference is that adults are free to choose whether they want to continue poisoning their body, but children are forced to eat what surrounds them. It is imperative that they eat a large variety of fruits and vegetables, and even if they are used to eating junk food, after a very short while they will get so used to eating raw, that cooked food will bring as much disgust as broccoli once did.

The Beginning of Malnutrition

A few hundred years ago when canned food was invented, it quickly became not only a status symbol but was touted as more healthy and beneficial for the body than raw food because it was thought to be "pre digested" and thus more beneficial. After the American people foolishly switched their diet from fresh raw produce to more and more canned goods, in good faith that it was actually more healthy, there was a very quick rise in ailments such as beriberi (deficiency in vitamin B1), pellagra (deficiency in vitamin B3, in 1915 in the United States 10,000 people died from this disease in one month), scurvy (deficiency in vitamin C), and other simple ailments all due to malnutrition.

People are getting sick and dying due to malnutrition. A few decades from now we might look back at heart disease, diabetes, and cancer just the same as we look at scurvy now, which was a major ailment at its time and treated with ridiculous methods such as bloodletting, mercury creams, and sulphur drinks (they said at that time these methods were quite successful). Will current therapies such as thermotherapy which has a 2% cure rate, or major medication or surgery be seen as ridiculous a few decades from now? They seem quite ridiculous now days.

Max Gerson writes in his book that 180 years ago cancer was so rare that to find one case to show young medical students took weeks upon weeks of searching the country! Today they say that every third person develops cancer.

A Balanced Diet – Fact or Fiction

It seems nowadays that diet and nutrition is some cosmic, extraordinary process that is only understandable by astronauts and Ivy League university graduates. At first glance it does seem so. This is because medicine has unveiled graphs and tables measuring every gram of calories, every unit of vitamins and minerals, every amino acid, so many different enzymes to make your head spin, so many beneficial nutrients to fill magazines and books until no end, so many new discoveries in health to make any sane information seeking individual to raise their hands up in the air and say “I give up!”

It started in the late 18th, early 19th century when the method of measuring calories was discovered. A special commission in Germany gave orders to scientist to find out the minimal amount of calories that a factory worker needed to work 15 hours per day. The method is simple, just burn the food and measure how much heat it produces. To get the amount of calories in a food, they just calculated the amount of energy it takes to raise one gram of water by one degree Celsius.

1 gram of Protein = 4 Calories
1 gram of Carbohydrate = 4 Calories
1 gram of Fat = 9 Calories
1 gram of Alcohol = 7 Calories

Food labs today rely on conversion factors first assembled more than 100 years ago by the agricultural chemist Wilbur O. Atwater, who literally *did* burn things like beef and corn in a device called the "bomb calorimeter." While today's calorimeters look a lot more sophisticated, Atwater's was more or less a fireproof container enclosed in water and hooked up to a thermometer. He used it, along with a larger device capable of measuring the heat output of an active person, to figure out how much usable energy different foods possess.

The major issue with the nutritional value number seen on all the cooked food packages is that most of those proteins, carbohydrates, fats, vitamins and minerals are unusable by your body and treated as toxins. So it doesn't matter how much vitamin C or calcium you see on your packaged cereal, box of frozen vegetables, or loaf of bread, it is treated as toxins by your body.

This archaic method is very good for business and is still used today to find out the calorie content of most foods. It enable the pharmacological and diet industry bombard us with useless numbers, figures, graphs, and then stuff us full of pills and diet "secrets." We are not supposed to live with a calculator at hand mindlessly adding and subtracting numbers and constantly thinking what vitamin to take when and what mineral we are supposedly lacking. Adequate and proper nutrition is the key to the golden door of health, it is the "secret," it is the answer, and it is the "miraculous" diet that so many of us are looking for.

Nutrition Masquerade

Nature has built into us some very amazing skills and abilities so we can function properly in the world, and find the best food that we need for survival. What abilities did Mother Nature provide us with? Our five senses; but most importantly sight, smell, and taste. By looking, smelling, and tasting the food, we are able to gauge whether we need something or not, and determine the nutritional value of the food.

Food chemists have brilliantly been able to create countless different man made flavour, sight, and smell enhancers to fool our natural senses and masquerade absolutely useless food into being seen by our body as nutrition.

After years on cooked food, our natural abilities are suppressed and we are not able to correctly judge whether or not a particular food is actually beneficial for us. When we begin to eat raw food, our natural mechanism will begin working allowing us to choose only the food that we need, and protect us from the foods that we do not need. You might have noticed sometimes that you crave a certain food one day, but can't stand it the next. This is your natural mechanism at work, telling you what your body needs naturally, without the need for any calculators or nutrition manuals.

Have you ever wondered why animals in the wild are so strong and healthy? How come wild animals don't get any diseases and illnesses that plague us humans, compared to even our house pets that suffer the same terrible sicknesses as we do? The reason is that they eat a monoculture (meaning one thing) diet. They eat what nature has created and perfected over thousands of years, we eat what man has created a few decades ago.

Today, food is treated as something that gets rid of our hunger, it is treated as an act of pleasure, a tradition, or a process to spend time with someone, it is treated as a mindless and quick activity to throw something down the tube. It has long lost its main principle of filling our body with vital nutrients and providing adequate energy for optimal functioning.

Experiments showed that if a neuron which is attached to the pleasure center in the brain of a mouse, and if that neuron is drawn outside the brain allowing the mouse to stimulate it with the push of a pedal, the mouse will not move, eat, or drink; it will pleasure itself until it dies. We are just like that mouse, stimulating our taste sensation with various foods and absolutely no regard for any consequences.

Culinary art has transformed to create the most delicious foods, a cocktail of tastes to pleasure the people. Our food has "evolved" to stimulate as many taste receptors as possible. Most people are not aware that they are in a dangerous game of taste addiction that is cultivated from our youngest years. Taste, as a natural means of sorting what food we need and what food we don't need, has been evolutionary hardwires inside our brains. What tastes good we eat, what doesn't taste good we don't eat, a very efficient mechanism. When we are surrounded by chemicals, we cannot make the right decision, we will always be fooled.

When we go back to the natural way of eating, our body will automatically readjust. We will no longer even want any cooked or dead food, we will crave different fruits, vegetables, nuts, seeds, grains, just like some of us crave chocolate, hamburgers, sweets, and other cooked and dead food. Our body's built in mechanism will begin to work perfectly, it will detoxify, cleanse, and become a well oiled organism that is free from disease, ailment, fatigue, and lack of energy. You will be able to live well into you 100s, you will have more free time and energy, your will begin to experience and feel things you have never felt before, see things you have never saw before. You will have a brand new body, and a brand new life!

Back to Nature

Going raw does not mean you need to take on a certain "wild" lifestyle as some think, or go and sell your house, live in the forest, and grow your own food. You don't need to say no to phones, computers, showers, or toilets. Not at all.

We are only talking about your body, which is capable of making you healthy no matter where you are or what you do. A body that will be able to defend itself from the onslaught of pollutants that every one of us inhales and eats on a daily basis. A body that forgets the word disease and illness. Don't you want to receive compliments on a daily basis of how much weight you lost and how great you look? That's what happens to everyone who switches, people notice.

The many positive effects of a raw vegetarian diet include: lightness, happiness, constant good mood, peace, more tolerance to hot and cold temperatures, less sweating, no bodily smells, inability to get a cold or flu, disappearance of all diseases and ailments, no fatigue (especially after meals), unbelievable physical stamina and psychological well being, improved concentration, increased focus, perfect hormonal balance, increased sexual performance, increased sex drive, improved sleep, improved look of skin, physical age decreased by decades, and some very nice benefits like no more need to cook and a lot of free time. The positive effects go on and on, but they are only positive because we are used to being sick, everything listed is how a person should always feel, look, and function.

A very important skill you need to learn is to listen to your body, eat what you like when you like, do not go with what you "should" eat, or what someone tells you to eat, eat what your body craves, it will naturally direct you to the most proper food at the most proper time, that is of course if it **raw** food, not a double cheeseburger or a chocolate fudge cake! Those things are food for the bacteria, they cannot be taken seriously. When you switch to raw foods you will begin to crave a variety of different things that your body needs. You must learn to listen to your body, something that we have completely forgotten to do. Sometimes those cravings will be for things that you don't even know, for something that you can't identify. This is a natural way for your body to get what it needs, like a vitamin pill, but since we have never eaten such a variety of natural fruits and vegetables, sometimes we don't even know what we want! Kids do this all the time; they stand in front of the open fridge searching for something, not even knowing what they want.

Instead of introducing ourselves and our children to over 12 different kinds of seeds, more than 18 kinds of nuts, more than 200 kinds of vegetables, and over 300 varieties of fruits, we introduce ourselves to over 18 kinds of cereals, 200 varieties of candy, and 300 varieties of pizza.

When a baby reaches 3 or 4 years old and is ready to chew hard foods, we should be priming their body to receive information from all those varieties of raw foods. The brain, like a computer, will digest and absorb the foods and record all the information about each individual item scanning for all the vitamins, minerals, enzymes, and nutrients so when the body needs something, it sends a craving, and you know exactly what you want because you have all the information about those foods. It's a very clever system. No matter where on earth you are, you will alsways intuitively know what to eat.

But if you don't have the necessary information about each food, then you won't know what you want. A very interesting thing you might find is that when start eating what you crave (raw foods of course), you will eat a **lot less**.

You are going to become what you should have been; a perfectly healthy and happy human being!

Are You Ready?

Victoria Boutenko, author of "12 Step to Raw Food" discusses an easy way to switch to raw food. First you must consciously make the decision to take this easy step in your life. You must think about it and fully agree to dedicate yourself to it. Then it is recommended write down three reasons why you want to take this step, and to make it easier to accomplish your goal, it helps to find another person to take on this challenge with; a family member, a friend, or even someone across the country, and every time you feel like eating cooked food, call your friend who will dissuade you from the craving, who will remind you about the benefits of eating raw, and most importantly remind you of the reasons why you switched. Your brain can betray you, but your friend will never do.

When you make the decision, you can read and familiarize yourself with books, articles, and testimonials from raw fooders. You can go on forums or actually talk and see the people who live the lifestyle. When you are satisfied you can go to a grocery store, and head straight for the vegetable/fruit section. Here you can start using your natural mechanisms of smell and sight, and fill your cart with everything that looks and smells good for you. Forget about what you "think" is good, or what someone told you is beneficial, or what you read in a magazine, or calories, or fats, or carbohydrates, choose whatever you feel is good for **you**. Your body will begin telling you what you need, trust your senses and eat what you crave. Remember, when eating fruits and veggies there is no such thing as gaining weight or watching your cholesterol, carbs, calories, sugar, fat, or any other things made up by today's society - mother nature has thought of all of that for us and she'll never let us get out of shape. You can never become sick or overweight by eating too many fruits and veggies.

Another aspect with raw foodism/vegetarianism is dealing with your friends and family members who will try to dissuade you, or tell you that you are wrong and you need meat or cooked food for health. You do not have to argue with them or try and make them eat the same food. You can just tell others that you are on a diet, a healthy diet to detoxify. And if you are in a situation where others are eating cooked food, like a barbeque or a get together, you can just ask your friends for help “help me stay on this diet guys, remind me that I can only eat raw foods, or I might give in!” They will gladly help you, but if you argue, things might not go as well. Just refrain from using the words “I switched to raw foods,” or “Im going raw,” best to just say you are on a healthy diet otherwise people might not understand.

After a year on this diet, people will look at you and notice how you got younger, lost a lot of weight, increased your energy levels, your vibrancy, and soon enough everyone will accept your lifestyle and you will easily be able to spend time with anyone in any situation. Let everyone else judge your lifestyle by what you will become later on, after they see the new you, many other people will want to switch. It is very important however that you leave everyone else’s choices to themselves, even if your family or friends are not ready yet, let them choose for themselves. The best way you can influence others is by **your own actions**, not by arguments or forcing your will. They will eventually see how you changed, and will want to be like you!

Raw food IS delicious if you just know a few simple recipes. In general, raw food is very easy to make, it is very nutritious, and many times even more delicious than cooked food. Just like many people now can't fathom how someone can eat veggies all day, after a short while on the raw diet you won't be able to believe how people can eat so much processed and unhealthy food either. A raw food lifestyle is the cure to ALL diseases and of ALL ailments.

Recently in Switzerland some facts were publicized that revealed bodies of people buried within the last few decades do not decompose. After many months, bodies look like they have been buried a few weeks ago. The reason is the massive amounts of preservatives and chemicals that we ingest with our food and put on our bodies in the form of creams or makeup. If you eat a so called “normal” diet your body probably will not decompose for decades. The purpose of preservatives is to destroy or prevent bacteria from acting upon the matter. If bacteria cannot act upon the dead organic matter, it does not decompose.

Raw foodism is not a diet, it is a normal, and healthy lifestyle from the perspective of regular bodily functions.

When one switches to a raw food diet, all their bad habits disappear, like smoking, drinking or drugs. People who have these habits are not aware that they just stop smoking, drinking, or doing drugs, it happens automatically, some don't even notice that they stopped! One man remembers after he switched to raw foods, that as he woke up and went about his day, at one point he stopped and realized that he completely forgot to smoke!

Vegetarianism - the First Path to Total Health

The word " Vegetarian " was coined by the Vegetarian Society of the United Kingdom in about 1847. The word does not come from vegetable as is generally assumed; it is a derivation of the Latin word ' vegetari ' which means to **enliven**. The practice of vegetarianism, however, goes far back in history. Many noted philosophers and religious teachers urged their followers to avoid a flesh diet. Brahminism, Jainism, Zoraostrianism and Buddhism acknowledged the sacredness of life and the need to live without causing suffering ; so did many of the early Christians.

There are various types of vegetarians. " Vegans "are the strictest vegetarians who eat only plant foods and exclude all animal by-products such as eggs, milk, cheese, curd, butter, ghee (clarified butter) and even honey. There are "lacto vegetarians " who eat plant foods as well as dairy products and " lacto-avo vegetarians " who eat eggs besides plant foods and dairy products. Vegetarians are those who choose not to eat animals (fish and seafood, and warm blooded animals as well) on personal or religious reasons.

As you have already read, eating an animal based diet leads to all the major diseases and has shown absolutely no benefit over a plant based diet. Every time you eat meat you are feeding the disease in your body.

Meat seems to have assumed an exaggerated importance nutritionally. It is generally mistakenly believed that nutritional deficiencies, especially of proteins and vitamin B12 and poor health may result if animal foods are eliminated. Studies however, have indicated no health problems or deficiency diseases for those on a vegetarian diet.

Of the 22 amino acids - the essential components of proteins - needed by the body for its normal functioning, only nine need be supplied by the diet as the body synthesizes the remaining 13.

On a quality rating scale of 1 to 100 (the higher the value, the more protein something has), egg protein is 95, milk is 82, fish 80, meat and poultry are 67, grains are between 50 to 70, and legumes, nuts and seeds are between 40 and 60. The so-called protein deficiency in a vegetarian diet is in fact more imaginary than real as the contribution of the protein value of the green vegetables has been ignored and the true protein requirement is less than that assumed. **Green vegetable protein is as high in quality as milk protein** and thus makes a very valuable contribution to the vegetarian's protein nutrition. The high quality of protein balances the lower quality of other vegetarian proteins such as nuts and beans. As discussed earlier every single raw food item that is full of enzymes means it is full of protein since an enzyme is made up of amino acids, the building blocks of ALL proteins.

The recommended daily allowance of 70 value proteins is 44 grams per day for women and 56 for men. Researchers have now discovered that the actual protein requirement is much less, being 15 grams per day of 100 value protein or 21.5 grams of 70 value protein or 30 grams of 50 value protein. A wholesome vegetarian diet can, therefore, easily meet the body's protein needs. Moreover, it is possible to combine two low-value plant proteins to get a protein of higher quality.

As regards the adequacy of B12 nutrition, laco-avo vegetarians and lacto-vegetarians should not feel concerned on this score, as the B12 needs can be easily supplied by dairy products. A quarter litre of milk per day will supply the recommended daily allowance. B12 is stored in the liver.

Reliable scientific studies have found **no evidence** of B12 deficiency diseases. It is therefore, presumed that this vitamin can be **synthesised in the body**.

Auto-Intoxication

As we have discussed earlier, most diseases of the human body are caused by auto-intoxication or self-poisoning, the toxicity of the cellular environment caused by dead food. Meat is the worst toxin that we can ever put inside our bodies and it is the most acidic food after alcohol.

The flesh of animals increases the burden of the organs of elimination and overloads the system with animal waste matter and poisons. Chemical analysis has proved that uric acid and other uremic poisons contained in the animal body are almost identical to caffeine, and nicotine, the poisonous stimulating principles of coffee, tea and tobacco. This explains why meat stimulates the animal passions and creates a craving for liquor, tobacco and other stronger stimulants.

Excessive uric acid resulting from meat-eating also causes diseases such as rheumatism, Bright's disease, kidney stones, gout and gall stones. Most of the meat is already a decomposing matter unfit for consumption which then gets cooked, and when it enters our digestive system its almost wholly unusable, rotting, putrid substance that feeds all our bacteria and germs.

Meat proteins cause putrefaction twice as rapidly as do cooked vegetable proteins. The morbid matter of the dead animal body is foreign and incompatible to our excretory organs. Our body goes through great difficulties to eliminate animal tissue from our system. Moreover, the formation of ptomains or corpse poisons begins immediately after the death of the animal and meat and poultry are usually kept in cold storage for many days and even months before they reach the kitchen. A very interesting fact; in 1902 a French scientist discovered that appendicitis occurs **only** in those who eat meat.

Another powerful influence tends to poison the flesh of slaughtered animals. As is well known, emotions of worry, fear and anger actually poison blood and tissues releasing chemicals such as adrenaline, corsisol, growth hormone, norepinephrine, ect. If you think animals are kept in spacious conditions, given good quality meals, and slaughtered in a loving manner then you really don't know how this business works.

This is how it goes; as the animal is born it is neutered without painkillers, calf are taken from their mothers resulting in terrible fear and stress, they are kept in cages just big enough for their bodies, they are fed corn which fattens them up and makes their meat much different than its supposed to, and then they are injected hormones and vaccines. When slaughter time comes, imagine the animals' stress after many days of travel to the slaughterhouse, closely packed in shaking vehicles - hungry, thirsty, scared enroute to their deaths. Many die even before the end of their journey. Others are driven half dead with fear and exhaustion to the slaughter pans, their instinctive fear of death augmented by the sight and odour of the blood shambles.

Flesh is often a carrier of disease germs. Diseases of many kinds are on the increase in the animals, making flesh foods more and more unsafe. People are continually eating flesh that may contain tuberculosis and cancerous germs. Often animals are taken to the market and sold for food when they are so diseased that their owners do not wish to keep them alive any longer. And some of the processes of fattening them to increase their weight and consequently their market value produce disease. Shut away from light and pure air, breathing the atmosphere of filthy stables, perhaps fattening on decaying foods, the entire body now becomes contaminated with foul matter. Is this what you want to put inside you?

There were even cases of tumour tissue (cancer tissue) that was found in meat products!

Benefits of Vegetarianism

A vegetarian diet can have many nutritional benefits, if it is rich in fruits and vegetables, and contains moderate amounts of seeds, nuts, whole grains and legumes. One of the main benefits of a proper vegetarian diet is its high content of vitamins, enzymes, amino acids, and minerals allowing your body to eat less while receiving more. The other benefit is its low caloric content in relation to the bulk supplied, which helps maintain ideal weight.

Another benefit of the vegetarian diet is the much lower intake of fat, if dairy products, seeds and nuts are eaten sparingly. This accounts for lower serium cholesterol levels found in vegetarians, which considerably reduces the risk of developing heart diseases , breast and colon cancer.

Another nutritional advantage of the vegetarian diet is its high fibre content. Fibre, being indigestible, increases the bulk of the faces, keeps them soft and makes them easy to expel.

One study has indicated that lacto-avo vegetarians consume twice as much and vagans four times as much fibre as non-vegetarians. High fibre intake has been associated with decreased risks of diseases of the colon, appendicits, cancer of the colon and rectum, hiatus hernia, piles and varicose veins.

McCarrison, one of the greatest aurhoties on food, has outlined a perfect diet. According to him, "a perfectly constituted diet is one in which the principal ingredients are milk, milk products, any whole cereal grain or mixture of cereal grains, green leafy vegetables and fruits. These are the protective foods. They make good the defects of other constituents of the diet, protect the body against infection and disease of various kinds, and their use in sufficient quantity ensures physical efficiency. " Remember if you do drink milk, make sure you drink it at the right time, between 6pm and 6am, otherwise it will not digest properly.

Vegetarianism is thus a system based on scientific principles and has proved adequate for the best nutrition free from the poisons and bacteria of diseased animals. It is the best diet for man's optimum, physical, mental and spiritual development.

You might be saying to yourself that there are so many rules and so many laws regarding food and lifestyle, why can't I just live the way I live! Life should be simple and easy, this is too much! When I hear these things from people I can't help but feel pity for the amount of ignorance that has clouded our views and perspectives. If your car break down and you go and open up the hood, you don't say "oh man there are so many hoses and metal parts, and why does the oil have to go here and this fluid have to go there, it's just so complicated I just want to drive forever and never take it to a mechanic!"

When you go for your driver's licence you don't say to the issuing officer "you know what, I just want to live my life simply, so I'll just go ahead and forget the rules and laws and drive the way I want." You don't go and pick and apple when its unripe and you don't come out at night and demand that the sun come up at once; there are rules and laws that govern the whole universe. We take such great care of our cars and clothes, yet when it comes to our own bodies, one of the most complex mechanisms on the planet, we are so careless and so ignorant sometimes.

Your body is much more complex than your vehicle, yet we always change the oil on time, put in proper gasoline, and keep it clean and never do we say "it's too much work changing the oil and putting proper gasoline in, ill just do it the way I want." Yet that is what most people say when it comes to their own bodies, they don't even know the basics of how it works yet they think they can eat and drink whatever they want and think it is a good choice. It is a miracle that we even live to the age of 70 (most people won't even live this long).

There are human laws and there are universal laws. You can break a human law and speed a few miles over the limit and it might be fine, but when you break a universal law, no matter how much you hide it, no matter what you hide it in, no matter if anyone sees you or not, the law will act upon you whether you like it or not. If you eat meat, you **will** get serious chronic diseases, if you eat cooked food, you **will** die at a much younger age than what you can live to, if you smoke or drink alcohol you **will** ruin your health, etc.

The rules are very simple, but due to ignorance or lack of knowledge we don't even know these laws exist, yet continue to live the way we live and expect to be healthy and happy.

Mass media has done a great job in making us more worried about what brand of clothing we are going to wear or what music player we have in our pockets than how healthy we are. It has done a great job in making us forget about the truly important things and focus our attention on things that do not matter.

They have purposefully constructed a society that is running to disease and illness, that is voluntarily **paying** for disease and illness. When you purchase a soda or a fast food meal, you have given up some of your time and effort to make the money to buy these products, so you are giving up your time and your strengths for something that is killing you. We are basically working for our own deaths, and loving it!

Then when we get sick we spend more of our time and strength to buy the toxic poisons called medication, or get expensive operations which only do you more harm.

We forgot what it is like to live a happy, healthy, and prosperous life. We are under the belief that being sick and diseased is ok and that is how it should be. We are under the impression that drugs and medication are the only way to health. I wrote this book and compiled all this evidence to show you a totally different perspective on health and wellness, an natural view on how you can look at your body and your wellbeing.

Scientific Research Proves Raw Food Protects Against Cancer and Heart Disease

Scientific evidence shows that raw vegan diets decrease toxic products in the colon (From: J Nutr 1992 Apr;122(4):924-30). Shifting from a conventional diet to an uncooked vegan diet reversibly alters fecal hydrolytic activities in humans, according to researchers, Ling WH, and Hanninen O, of the Department of Physiology, University of Kuopio, Finland. Results suggest a raw food uncooked extreme vegan diet causes a decrease in bacterial enzymes and certain toxic products that have been implicated in colon cancer risk.

Researchers have also found that a diet rich in raw vegetables lowers your risk of breast cancer, and eating lots of fruit reduces your risk for colon cancer, according to a study published in the May 1998 issue of the journal Epidemiology. Including fresh fruit as part of your daily diet has been associated with fewer deaths from heart attacks and related problems, by as much as 24%, according to a study published in the September 1996 issue of the British Medical Journal.

Increasing your fruit and vegetable intake to at least 50% of all your meals is the fastest, most direct, healthiest way to start cleansing your system and regaining your body's health. It is also many times more beneficial than beginning poisonous medical treatment. For cancer it is 12 times more beneficial than chemotherapy; and your side effects instead of more disease and ailments will be increased energy, a healthy body, healthier skin, improved love life, weight loss, and about a hundred more benefits.

In "The China Study", the largest health study ever undertaken, professors from the United States teamed up with scientists from China to look at how our nutrition affects our lives. They studied 6500 people over many years and here are some of their startling results:

"The China Study included a comparison of the prevalence of Western diseases (coronary heart disease, diabetes, leukemia, and cancers of the colon, lung, breast, brain, stomach and liver) in each county. It was based on diet and lifestyle variables, and found that one of the **strongest predictors of Western diseases was blood cholesterol.** The study linked lower blood cholesterol levels to lower rates of heart disease and cancer. As blood cholesterol levels decreased from 170 mg/dl to 90 mg/dl, cancers of the liver, rectum, colon, lung, breast, leukemia, brain, stomach and esophagus (throat) greatly decreased."

"The authors write that "several studies have now shown, in both experimental animals and in humans, that **consuming animal-based protein increases blood cholesterol levels.** Saturated fat and dietary cholesterol also raise blood cholesterol, although these nutrients are not as effective at doing this as is animal protein. In contrast, plant-based foods contain no cholesterol and, in various other ways, help to decrease the amount of cholesterol made by the body." They write that "these disease associations with blood cholesterol were remarkable, because blood cholesterol and animal-based food consumption both were so low by American standards. In rural China, animal protein intake (for the same individual) averages only 7.1 grams per day whereas Americans average 70 grams per day." [source]

To put it simply: eating meat causes heart disease, diabetes, leukemia, and countless cancers. This is not a "maybe"; this has been proven 100% in scientific studies in animals and humans.

The scientists discovered that cancer doesn't just randomly appear, these cancerous cells get into our bodies as a result of all the carcinogens we put into it - carcinogens can be found in processed foods, cooked foods, in chemicals added to our food as flavour enhancers or preservatives, in our laundry detergents, shampoos, the air we breathe, nearly everywhere! These lingering cancer cells are only triggered when our food intake comprises of more than 10% animal protein. And while animal protein raises the risk of cancers and other diseases, vegetable protein does the reverse and lowers the risk them.

Another recent British study comparing meat-eaters to vegetarians found that "...vegetarians appeared to have much lower risk of getting cancers of the lymph and blood. When these were grouped, vegetarians had about 50 per cent lower risk than meat eaters. And in one rare cancer in particular, multiple myeloma, a cancer of the bone marrow, vegetarians were 75 per cent less likely to develop the disease compared to meat eaters." [source]

If you think vegans are all skinny and weak, here are some athletes disproving the notion:

*Triathlete Dr. Ruth Heidrich ('terminal' cancer cured via vegan diet)
*B.J. Armstrong (Chicago Bulls, former all-star guard)
*Andreas Cahling (Bodybuilding Champion)
*Nicky Cole (1st woman to walk to N. Pole)
*Cory Everson (6 time Ms. Olympia)
*Desmond Howard (Jacksonville Jaguars, NFL)
*Carl Lewis (Olympic Sprinter)
*Bill Manetti (Power-Lift Champion)
*and many, many more

So there you have it; the less meat you eat and the more fruits and veggies you ingest, the lower your risk of all the diseases plaguing the western world.

Why Are We Sick?

Have you ever wondered why we are sick? Why do people keep dying from disease and illnesses? Why is being sick considered normal? Was human kind always sick? Why did nature create such weak humans who are unable to withstand disease? It is all quite simple, we are sick because of what we eat, remember the saying "you are what your eat."

Large food manufacturers keeps feeding you this stuff because it is profitable to keep you sick and unhappy. Companies don't use the best ingredients, they don't use natural things, if they can cut corners and make more money by putting chemical additives, or preservatives or flavour enchancers, they will. They do not care about your health, only their bottom line. A sick and unhappy individual is a lot profitable than a healthy and happy one. A sick person will always need some sort of medication, treatment, or procedure, for their entire lives. And an unhappy person is a great customer; you offer him some new gadget, some new attraction, some new experience and they will be glad to fork out the cash. A sick and unhappy individual is a walking money machine for the giant corporations.

A healthy individual does not need medications, they don't need the pills, they don't need the diets and "magic" weight loss "secrets" that litter every magazine and television program. A healthy person does not need the whole "health" industry, **IT NEEDS YOU**! This is why they keep feeding you these toxins under the name of "food" and keep you in the dark as to the real reason of your diseases and ailments. If you are healthy then you are most likely happy, and a happy person is not afraid. As you know, fear is a key tactic to keep you buying and buying. Without fear you are no longer under their influence and you can think for yourself. The only reason these companies are still in business is because people keep buying their products!

The whole food and drug industry is like the big bad wizard of OZ. When you strip away the curtain from your eyes, you see that it was nothing more than smoke and mirrors, diversion tactics, and lots of huff and puff. The real reasons were hidden from view, clouded by numbers and figures, useless calorie counting, countless diet "tips" and techniques, so called health "discoveries," health "gurus" coming out with their "new" secrets, and a so much mumbo jumbo that I'm amazed that people haven't gone crazy yet.

True health is **very simple**, if you just know the foundation of how our body works, and how food works; then it all makes sense.

Fat Nation

We all weigh on average 25 pounds more today than we did 25 years ago. The fact is we are all getting fatter. There is even an epidemic of obese 6 month olds! (Kim et al, 2006)

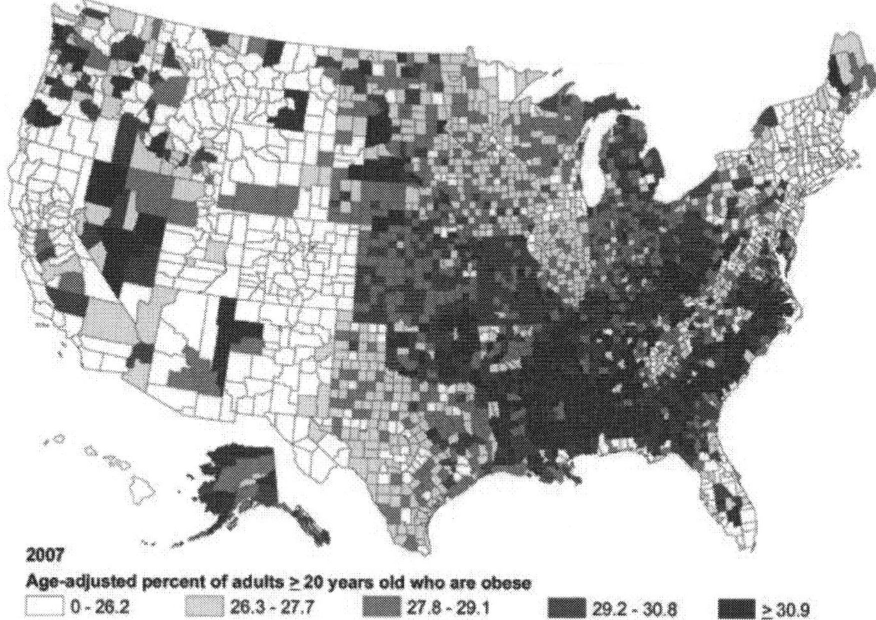

In 1900 life expectancy in the United States was less than 50 years. During the past 100 years life expectancy has increased by 60% due mostly to lower infant mortality, plus better diet and improved hygiene which together resulted in reduced infectious diseases. If we can increase the present day lifespan of 80 years by 60%, the result is nearly 130 years of life. A 60% increase was achieved during this past century as an unexpected side benefit from other changes in society. Can we do it again by putting conscious attention on it?

Seems farfetched? A hundred years ago people dying in their 40's and 50's thought that you couldn't live any longer that than either.

The typical species in its natural untouched environment lives seven times past its age of maturity. This means animals in their normal habitat, as a normal process of life, live seven times past their age of maturity. Humans normally mature in their late teens to early twenties. Our average potential life span in robust wellness is actually in the range of 120-140 years! This means we are doing something wrong. Take a look at the Hunzas or the Okinawas, their lifespan is pretty much in that exact range.

Several studies of healthy people over age 50 indicate that the death rate from all causes (including cancer and heart disease) can be reduced by about 50% and longevity increased an average of **eleven years** by taking nutritional supplements. The higher intake of vitamin C is most important, and also valuable are two of the B vitamins (B6 and niacin), vitamin E, vitamin A, calcium and other minerals.

In fruit flies and rats, a 30% reduction in calories eaten results in a **30% extension of life span**, and the rats experienced a **one third reduction in cancerous tumors**. The physiological changes in the rats on the reduced calorie diet are also seen in an ongoing study (since 1987) of monkeys on a reduced calorie diet, suggesting that systematic under eating ("under nutrition without malnutrition" aka “health fasting”) may be a useful part of an overall plan for human life extension.

People tend to over eat when the food they are consuming does not contain sufficient **nutrients** to satisfy the requirements of the body ("empty calorie foods"). Overeating depletes digestive **enzymes** and reduces the efficiency of the digestive system. What is needed is a **nutrient-dense diet** that provides abundant nutrients with fewer calories. Attaining such a diet for individuals and our whole society is the purpose of the nutritional supplements and superfoods, freshly squeezed juices and foods loaded with natural enzymes, vitamins, and minerals.

GMO (genetically modified organism) foods, cooked foods, processed foods all have significantly less nutritional value than raw foods. The nutritional value of “fast food” is so low that there is no point even talking about it. There is something important to understand here; our bodies need enzymes, vitamins, and minerals.

Did you know that an enzyme is a combination of amino acids? Did you know that proteins are combinations of amino acids? That means that every single fruit and vegetable is stock full of protein! So why have you heard that fruits and vegetables have absolutely no protein? Because the machines that test food can only test cooked food, and we all know that cooking something over 118 degrees Fahrenheit (47 Celsius) for more than one minute destroys most of the nutritional value of the food including all the enzymes, vital minerals and vitamins. If someone comes up with a machine to test the nutritional value of food that has not been cooked, **they will find that every single leaf and apple is full of protein**!

Next time you are eating that juicy fresh piece of fruit, know that you are also eating a natural protein shake!

"You don't have to walk around hungry. If you change the quality of what you eat, you can be satisfied with lower calories. There have been experiments in both people and rats that if you give them the so-called "cafeteria diet" - a junky American diet - and let them eat as much as they want, they will eat about 3,000 calories. If you take the same people and give them a high-quality diet, and let them eat as much as they want, they'll settle for about 2,500 calories. So right off, you can knock off 500-600 calories just by eating better food." - Dr. Roy Walford.

No special diets, no special supplements, just by eating nutrient rich food your body will need less of it.

Animals and humans eating unhealthy fats "eat six times as much fat and six times as much food. A lot of money is saved by buying the right kind of fat." - Budwig pages 22, 33.

Healthy fats include clarified butter (ghee), regular butter, coconut oil, olive oil, and flax oil. Unhealthy fats include all hydrogenated oils, all oils heated to high temperature, rancid oils, and most of the modern vegetable oils (due to genetic modification, pesticide use, herbicide use, poor soil, and the lack of "good" fats like omega 3 and 6 in most vegetable oils).

According to the "USDA's Continuing Survey of Food Intakes by Individuals", a major amount of people do not consume enough essential vitamins and minerals in their diets compared to the Recommended Dietary Allowances (RDAs). Below are some statistics from the survey which list the percentage of people (age 20 and over) who do not meet the RDAs for:

- **Vitamin A:**

Males: 60.9%
Females: 59.6%

- **Vitamin E:**

Males: 64.4%
Females: 73.0%

- **Vitamin B6:**

Males: 52.6%
Females: 64.2%

- **Calcium:**

Males: 55.4%
Females: 78.0%

- **Magnesium:**

Males: 65.7%
Females: 75.7%

- **Zinc:**

Males: 67.6%
Females: 82.6%

Just to stress the importance of these facts; the intake amounts stated by the RDA prevent us from falling seriously ill, that is how low their recommended intake amounts are, **and more than half the population barely even get the bare minimum**. And people wonder why there is so much disease and illness.

Eating all your vegetables was a lot better for you in the '50s. Store-bought veggies weren't as pretty back then, but according to USDA data, they were packed with a lot more nutrients than their modern counterparts. The likely reason for the nutritional drop is that hybrid crops are often bred for size and color, not nutrients.

"Changes in USDA Food Composition Data for 43 Garden Crops, 1950 to 1999,"
http://www.jacn.org/cgi/content/full/23/6/669

Balancing Acid/Alkaline Foods

A surprising number and variety of physical problems and diseases can be caused by foods that produce acid after digestion. Today the vast majority of the populace in industrialized nations suffers from problems caused by the stress of acidosis, because both modern lifestyle and diet promote acidification of the body's internal environment.

The current typical Western diet is largely composed of acid-forming foods (proteins, cereals, sugars). Alkaline-producing foods such as vegetables are eaten in much smaller quantities. Stimulants like tobacco, coffee, tea, and alcohol are also extremely acidifying. Stress, and physical activity (either excessive or insufficient amounts) also cause acidification.

Many foods are alkaline-producing by nature, but manufactured processed foods are mostly acid-producing. It is important to consume at least 80% alkaline-producing foods in our diet, in order to maintain health. We need plenty of fresh fruits and particularly dark green vegetables (alkaline-producing) to balance our unnecessarily high protein intake (acid-producing). And we need to avoid processed, sugary or simple-carbohydrate foods, not only because they are acid-producing but also because they raise blood sugar level too quickly (high glycemic index therefore fattening); plus they tend to be nutrient-lacking and may be toxic too.

What is the body's pH?

Water is the most abundant compound in the human body, comprising 70% of the body. The body therefore contains a wide range of solutions, which may be more or less acid. pH (potential of Hydrogen) is a measure of the acidity or alkalinity of a solution - the ratio between positively charged ions (acid-forming) and negatively charged ions (alkaline-forming.) The pH of any solution is the measure of its hydrogen-ion concentration. The higher the pH reading, the more alkaline and oxygen rich the fluid is. The lower the pH reading, the more acidic and oxygen deprived the fluid is. The pH range is from 0 to 14, with 7.0 being neutral. Anything above 7.0 is alkaline, anything below 7.0 is considered acidic.

Human blood pH should be slightly alkaline (7.35 - 7.45). Below or above this range means symptoms and disease. If blood pH moves below 6.8 or above 7.8, cells stop functioning and the body starts to die. The body therefore continually strives to balance pH. When this balance is compromised many problems can occur.

An imbalanced diet high in acidic-producing foods such as animal protein, sugar, caffeine, and processed foods puts pressure on the body's regulating systems to maintain pH neutrality. The extra buffering required can deplete the body of alkaline minerals such as sodium, potassium, magnesium, and calcium, making the person prone to chronic and degenerative disease. Minerals are borrowed from vital organs and bones to buffer (neutralize) the acid and safely remove it from the body. Because of this strain, the body can suffer severe and prolonged damage--a condition that may go undetected for years.

"...bile contains alkaline salts that are often absorbed to help maintain the proper pH of the blood (which is slightly alkaline at 7.4). Since the Standard American Diet emphasizes more meats and refined foods at the expense of raw unrefined vegetables (resulting in acidic blood), the absorption of alkaline salts from the gallbladder is required to help bring the pH back into balance. When salts are removed from the bile, it becomes thicker. In turn, thicker bile makes the removal of cholesterol from the gallbladder more difficult - leading to the formation of **gallstones**." - Dr. David Williams, *Alternatives* newsletter, June 2006.

Health problems caused by acidosis

Research shows that unless the body's pH level is slightly alkaline, the body cannot heal itself. So no matter what means you choose to take care of your health, it won't be effective until the pH level is balanced. If your body's pH is not balanced, for example, you cannot effectively digest and absorb vitamins, minerals and food supplements. Your body pH affects everything.

Acidosis will decrease the body's ability to absorb minerals and other nutrients, decrease the energy production in the cells, decrease its ability to repair damaged cells, decrease its ability to detoxify heavy metals, make tumor cells thrive, and make it more susceptible to fatigue and illness.

An acidic pH can occur from an acid-forming diet (meat, alcohol, sugar, coffee, all cooked food), emotional stress, toxic overload, and/or immune reactions or any process that deprives the cells of oxygen and other nutrients. The body will try to compensate for acidic pH by using alkaline minerals. If the diet does not contain enough minerals to compensate, a buildup of acids in the cells will occur. Acidosis can cause such problems as:

Cardiovascular damage.
Weight gain, obesity and diabetes.
Bladder conditions.
Kidney stones.
Immune deficiency.
Acceleration of free radical damage.
Hormonal problems.
Premature aging.
Osteoporosis and joint pain.
Aching muscles and lactic acid buildup.
Low energy and chronic fatigue.

Slow digestion and elimination.
Yeast/fungal overgrowth.
Lack of energy and fatigue.
Lower body temperature.
Tendency to get infections.
Loss of drive, joy, and enthusiasm.
Depressive tendencies.
Easily stressed.
Pale complexion.
Headaches.
Inflammation of the corneas and eyelids.
Cancer.

Loose and painful teeth.
Inflamed, sensitive gums.
Mouth and stomach ulcers.
Cracks at the corners of the lips.
Excess stomach acid.
Gastritis.
Nails are thin and split easily.
Hair looks dull, has split ends, and falls out.
Dry skin.
Skin easily irritated.
Leg cramps and spasms.

Test Your Body's Acidity or Alkalinity with pH Strips

It is recommended that you test your pH levels to determine if your body's pH needs immediate attention. By using pH test strips (Litmus Paper), you can determine your pH factor quickly and easily in the privacy of your own home. The best time to test your pH is about one hour before a meal and two hours after a meal.

Saliva pH Test: Simply wet a piece of Litmus Paper with your saliva. While generally more acidic than blood, salivary pH mirrors the blood and tells us what the body retains. It is a fair indicator of the health of the extracellular fluids and their alkaline mineral reserves. The optimal pH for saliva is 6.4 to 6.8. A reading lower than 6.4 is indicative of insufficient alkaline reserves. After eating, the saliva pH should rise to 7.5 or more. To deviate from an ideal salivary pH for an extended time invites illness. If your saliva stays between 6.5 and 7.5 all day, your body is functioning within a healthy range.

Acidosis, an extended time in the acidic pH state, can result in rheumatoid arthritis, diabetes, lupus, tuberculosis, osteoporosis, high blood pressure, most cancers and many more. If salivary pH stays too low, the diet should focus on fruit, vegetables, vitamins, minerals, as well as remove strong acidifiers such as meat, alcohol, sodas, coffee, fluoridated water, artificial sweeteners etc.

"Clinical research by Dr M T Morter (Arkansas, USA) has shown that if the anabolic urinary and **salivary pH** (measured immediately upon awakening) is below 6.8, we can be relatively certain that digestive support must be provided. Controlled clinical studies by Dr Paul Yanick (Pasadena, USA) have confirmed

Dr Morter's findings and recorded that intracellular assimilation of nutrients is significantly decreased when the anabolic pH is below 6.8. However as both these researchers have shown, **supplementing the diet with appropriate alkalizing agents was highly beneficial** in elevating the systemic pH by replenishing the alkaline mineral and enzyme reserves." - Dr. Peter Bartlett, Using pH as a Measure of Digestive Physiology. Available on the Internet at http://www.positivehealth.com/permit/Articles/Colon%20Health/ph.htm

Urine pH Test

The pH of the urine indicates how the body is working to maintain the proper pH of the blood. The urine reveals the alkaline (building - anabolic) and acid (tearing down - catabolic) metabolic cycles. The pH of urine indicates the efforts of the body via the kidneys, adrenals, lungs and gonads to regulate pH through the buffer salts and hormones. Urine can provide a fairly accurate picture of body chemistry, because the kidneys filter out the buffer salts of pH regulation and provide values based on what the body is eliminating. Urine pH can vary from around 4.5 to 9.0 in extremes, but the ideal range is 6.0 to 7.0. If your urinary pH fluctuates between 6.0 to 6.5 first thing in the morning and between 6.5 and 7.0 in the evening before dinner, your body is functioning within a healthy range.

Urine testing may indicate how well your body is excreting acids and assimilating minerals, especially calcium, magnesium, sodium and potassium. These minerals function as "buffers." Buffers are substances that help maintain and balance the body against the introduction of too much acidity or too much alkalinity. Even with the proper amounts of buffers, acid or alkaline levels can become stressful to the body's regulatory systems. When the body produces too many of these acids or alkalis, it must excrete the excess. The urine is the method the body uses to remove any excess acids or alkaline substances that cannot be buffered. If the body's buffering system is overwhelmed, a state of "autointoxication" is created, and attention should be given to reducing this stress.

Another very important aspect to understand is that our body cannot live in an acidic environment, and "buffers" the acids we put into it by releasing calcium from bones/hair/teeth/nails (which leads to osteoporosis, muscle weakness, fatigue, heart problems, brittle bones etc.) and releases other alkalizing minerals from its reserves.

Foods: are they Acid or Alkaline-forming?

Note that a foods acid or alkaline-forming tendency in the body has nothing to do with the actual pH of the food itself. For example, lemons are very acidic; however, the end-products they produce after digestion and assimilation are alkaline, so lemons are alkaline-forming in the body after digestion. Likewise, meat will test alkaline before digestion but it leaves acidic residue in the body so, like nearly all animal products, meat is classified as highly acid-forming.

To maintain health, the diet should consist of **at least** 60% alkaline forming foods and at most 40% acid forming foods. To restore health, the diet should consist of 80% alkaline forming foods and 20% acid forming foods.

FOOD CATEGORY	High Alkaline	Alkaline	Low Alkaline	Low Acid	Acid	High Acid
BEANS, VEGETABLES, LEGUMES	Vegetable Juices, Parsley, Raw Spinach, Broccoli, Celery, Garlic, Barley	Carrots, Green Beans, Lima Beans, Beets, Lettuce, Zucchini, Carob	Squash, Asparagus, Rhubarb, Fresh Corn, Mushrooms, Onions, Cabbage, Peas, Cauliflow	Sweet Potato, Cooked Spinach, Kidney Beans	Pinto Beans, Navy Beans	Pickled Vegetables

	Grass		er, Turnip, Beetroot, Potato, Olives, Soybeans, Tofu			
FRUIT	Dried Figs, Raisins	Dates, Blackcurrant, Grapes, Papaya, Kiwi, Berries, Apples, Pears	Coconut, Sour Cherries, Tomatos, Oranges, Cherries, Pineapple, Peaches, Avocados, Grapefruit, Mangoes, Strawberries, Papayas, Lemons, Watermelon, Limes	Blueberries, Cranberries, Bananas, Plums, Processed Fruit Juices	Canned Fruit	
GRAINS, CEREALS			Amaranth, Lentils, Sweetcorn, Wild Rice, Quinoa, Millet, Buckwheat	Rye Bread, Whole Grain Bread, Oats, Brown Rice	White Rice, White Bread, Pastries, Biscuits, Pasta	
MEAT				Liver, Oysters, Organ Meat	Fish, Turkey, Chicken, Lamb	Beef, Pork, Veal, Shellfish, Canned

						Tuna & Sardines
EGGS & DAIRY		Breast Milk	Soy Cheese, Soy Milk, Goat Milk, Goat Cheese, Buttermilk, Whey	Whole Milk, Butter, Yogurt, Cottage Cheese, Cream, Ice Cream	Eggs, Camembert, Hard Cheese	Parmasan, Processed Cheese
NUTS & SEEDS		Hazelnuts, Almonds	Chestnuts, Brazils, Coconut	Pumpkin, Sesame, Sunflower Seeds	Pecans, Cashews, Pistachios	Peanuts, Walnuts
OILS			Flax Seed Oil, Olive Oil, Canola Oil	Corn Oil, Sunflower Oil, Margarine, Lard		
BEVERAGES	Herb Teas, Lemon Water	Green Tea	Ginger Tea	Cocoa	Wine, Soda/Pop	Tea (black), Coffee, Beer, Liquor
SWEETENERS, CONDIMENTS	Stevia	Maple Syrup, Rice Syrup	Raw Honey, Raw Sugar	White Sugar, Processed Honey	Milk Chocolate, Brown Sugar, Molasses, Jam, Ketchup, Mayonnaise, Mustard, Vinegar	Artificial Sweeteners

* Note: The chart above represents a close approximate guide.

What difference does it make to have acidic blood?

In order for the body to remain healthy and alive, your body keeps a delicate and precise balance of blood pH at 7.365, which is slightly alkaline. The body does whatever it has to in order to maintain this balance. The problem is that most people have incredibly acid lifestyles. Acid is produced in your body whenever you have stress, upset emotions and when the food you eat is acid-forming.

The typical diet is significantly acidic. So what happens to your body when you're over-acid? Your body will store excess acid in your fat cells (which is why so many people have such trouble losing weight). Over time, your body will leach calcium and alkaline stores from your bones in a desperate attempt to retain the pH balance in your body (which is why some people "shrink" as they get older).

Your blood plays a very important role in your healthy and energy: it carries oxygen to all your cells! This gives you energy, and it's what keeps you alive. It also plays a key role in how energizing your sleep is. Here's a picture of healthy red blood cells:

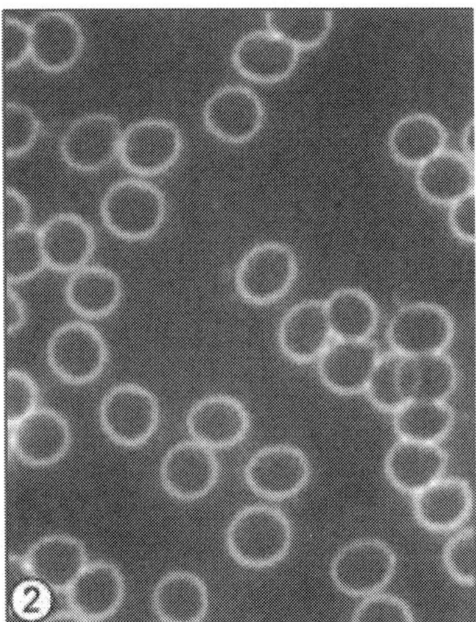

Do you see how far apart the blood cells are from each other? As a result, your blood can move freely throughout your entire body, it is able to receive proper nutrition, waste removal is easily accomplished, and it can get into all your small capillaries, so you feel like your whole body is getting energy. During deep sleep, proper blood flow and hydration is important. When your blood looks like this, your sleep is also really energizing and you need less of it!

Blood cells have a negative charge on the outside and a positive charge inside; this is what keeps them healthy and far apart from each other, this is otherwise called the zeta-potential or z-potential. However, when your body is over-acidic, the acid strips your blood of its negative charge. Your blood cells no longer have the same repelling force and clump together like this:

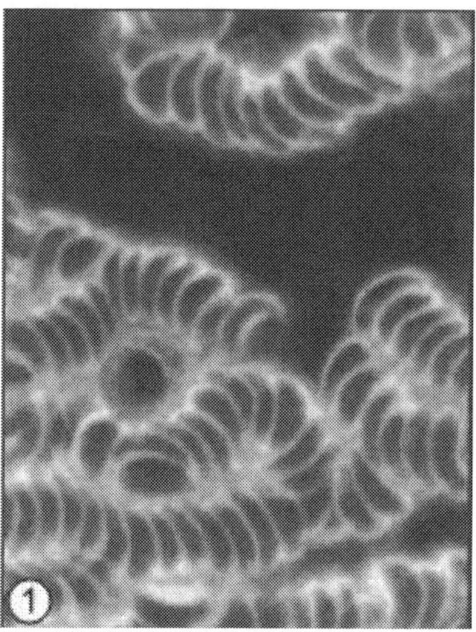

When your blood is clumped together, it no longer can get to all the little capillaries in your body to give you the life giving oxygen you need. It no longer can give every cell in your body the energizing and rejuvenating effects and proper nutrients. This is the major reason why some people feel horrible when they wake up, and why they need to sleep longer. It's also why you tend to wake up feeling de-hydrated.

Most of us, from the time we're children, have a fear installed into us by our parents that "Disease is out to get you, and viruses are flying around all over the place looking for their next victim!" It comes with sayings like: "Put on your sweater or you'll 'catch' a cold!" However, the truth is most of us create toxic and acidic environments inside of our body, the perfect breeding ground for disease and illness. It doesn't **happen** to you; instead, you **make** it happen to yourself. Remember the fire-truck analogy?

Here's a good example: Pretend you had a goldfish in a bowl, and one day you saw the goldfish was beginning to look very unhealthy. You also notice that the water is a little dirty. What makes more sense? To take the fish out and try to fix it? Or change its water? Chances are it's the water that's making the fish unhealthy, not the fish itself. When you change the water, the fish will get healthier. The fact that the goldfish (our cells) is unhealthy is actually a SYMPTOM of the **unhealthy environment <u>around</u> our cells**.

Do you know why we feel better outdoors? A forest, trees, a body of water, fresh clean air, any place far away from civilization is full of negatively charged ions which revive and rejuvenate the body. Any electrical appliance radiates positively charged ions (since any electric current produces an electromagnetic field, just like your blood cells which have a negative charge on the outside and a positive charge inside) leading to a variety of negative symptoms.

Can Vitamin/Mineral Supplements Replace a Bad Diet?

They better.

In spite of decades of intense and well-funded mass education, "70 percent of all adults and children in the U.S. do not eat the recommended five to nine servings of fruits and vegetables a day for good health," according to an April 25, 2002 press release by the National Cancer Institute. And when a "serving" of fruit may be a 6-ounce glass of juice and a "serving" of a vegetable is a mere half-cup of beans, it really makes you think. Not only are the recommended servings insignificantly small, most of us don't even get **that**.

At least half of all Americans take vitamin supplements daily, answering the question that supplements can replace a bad diet. Today, the public finally has the support of orthodox medicine. After years of disparaging supplements, the Journal of the American Medical Association has recently published the recommendation that every person take a multivitamin daily, saying that "(S)uboptimal intake of some vitamins, above levels causing classic vitamin deficiency, is a risk factor for chronic diseases and common in the general population, especially the elderly." Therefore, JAMA's intent goes beyond routine nutritional insurance for widespread bad-to-borderline diets. The goal is stated in the article's title: Vitamins for chronic disease prevention in adults. It seems to be a novel idea that should have come a long time ago.

Supplementation's harshest critics have traditionally railed against vitamins (especially in large doses) as being outright "dangerous" and at the very least "a waste of money." Even as late as this year, the New York Times expanded the attack to question folic acid supplementation and even the practice of taking a daily multivitamin, saying, "vitamin supplements cannot correct for a poor diet (and that) multivitamins have not been shown to prevent any disease."

The NY Times may have neglected to emphasize the real story: people eat terribly.

Even though they are eating less fat, westerners are more obese than ever before, and in the United States, an astounding 80% of persons over the age of 25 are overweight. Nearly two-thirds of all Americans (more than 120 million people) are overweight or obese, according to the 1999-2000 National Health and Nutrition Examination. Protein and sugar intake is still astronomically high and fruit and vegetable consumption is still ridiculously low.

While vitamin supplements themselves do not produce weight loss, persons trying to lose weight or cure a particular illness, face nutritional deficiency problems of their own. Approximately 50 million Americans admit to being "on a diet" at any given time. Virtually all popular unsupplemented weight loss plans are nutrient deficient meaning even more struggles for your nutritionally deficient body. Taking supplements can be seen as especially important for everyone, especially those on a mainstream "diet."

Dieticians have set themselves the heroic but probably unattainable goal of getting every person to eat well every day. In a real-life situation it is close to impossible to receive the necessary amounts of nutrients from our completely deficient foods. Tens of millions of women are at an even greater risk. Oral contraceptives lower serum levels of B-vitamins, especially B-6, plus niacin (B-3), thiamin (B-1), riboflavin (B-2), folic acid, vitamin C and B-12. Ladies, when is the last time your physician instructed you to be sure to take supplemental vitamin C and B-complex vitamins as long as you are on the Pill? (Did you know that taking any oral contraceptive for a period of time wrecks havoc on your hormonal balance leading to irreversible changes within your system, even leading to being unable to conceive?)

Furthermore, government vitamin recommendations are so low as to resemble a test so easy, a standard so minimal, that you would think no one can possibly fail. For example, the US Reference Daily Intake (RDI) for vitamin E is 30 International Units. It is widely appreciated that at least 400 IU of vitamin E (and probably 800 IU or more) daily is required to prevent a great deal of cardiovascular and other disease. Yet it is literally impossible to obtain even 100 IU of vitamin E from even the most perfectly planned diet.

To demonstrate this, I, as well as other nutritionists tried to create a few days of "balanced" meals, using the food composition tables in any nutrition textbook, to achieve 100 IU of vitamin E per day. We could try to attempt our mission with any combination of foods and any reasonable number of portions of each food. The only limitation was that we had to design meals that a person would actually be willing to eat. As this ruled out prescribing whole grains by the pound and vegetable oils by the cup, we could not do it. Nor can the general public. Most people do not even get 30 IU of vitamin E a day. In fact, most get only 17 IU.

"Supplements" by definition are designed to fill nutritional gaps in a bad diet. They fill in what may be surprisingly large gaps in a good diet as well. In the case of vitamin E, doing so is likely to save millions of lives. The New England Journal of Medicine had two articles in the May 20, 1993 issue showing that persons taking vitamin E supplements had an approximately 40% reduction in cardiovascular disease. Nearly 40,000 men and 87,000 women took part in the studies. The more vitamin E they took, and the longer they took it, the less cardiovascular disease they experienced.

A 1996 double-blind, placebo-controlled study of 2,002 patients with clogged arteries demonstrated a 77% decreased risk of heart attack in those taking 400 to 800 IU of vitamin E. Again, such effective quantities of vitamin E positively cannot be obtained from diet alone. 800 IU is 2,667% of the US RDI for vitamin E. Is this a lot, or is the government recommendation too low? (Vitamin E will be discussed more in detail later on.)

Even a modest quantity of vitamin C (ascorbic acid) prevents disease and saves lives. Just 500 mg daily results in a 42 percent lower risk of death from heart disease and a 35 percent lower risk of death from any other cause. Since two-thirds of the population is not eating sufficient fruits and vegetables, the only way to close the gap is with vitamin supplements.

To illustrate how extraordinarily important supplements are to persons with a questionable diet, consider this: Children who eat hot dogs once a week double their risk of a brain tumor. Kids eating more than twelve hot dogs a month (that's barely three hot dogs a week) have nearly ten times the risk of leukemia as children who ate none. However, hot-dog eating children taking supplemental vitamins were shown to have a reduced risk of cancer. It is curious that, while theorizing many "potential" dangers of vitamins, the media often choose to ignore the very real cancer preventative and health benefits of supplementation.

Critics also fail to point out how economical supplements are. For low-income households, taking a two-cent vitamin C tablet and a three-cent multivitamin, readily obtainable from any Wal-Mart or discount store, is vastly cheaper than getting those vitamins by eating right. The uncomfortable truth is that it is often less expensive to supplement than to buy nutritious food, especially out-of-season fresh produce. And those who wish to follow Linus Pauling's vitamin C recommendation to take daily 3-5 gram doses of vitamin C can do so easily and cheaply, while only a few people can afford to eat several dozen oranges a day (Ester-C brand vitamin C is better absorbed by our bodies than regular vitamin C).

Since ancient Egypt, through the time of Hippocrates, and right up to the present, poor diet has been described and criticized by physicians. Little has changed for the better, and much has changed for the worse. We eat not only for our self-indulgent pleasure but also because we are hungry, and we are hungry for nutrients! Supplementation is an easy and inexpensive way you can begin the process of a healthier diet. However, and this is a big however, you cannot continue your terrible eating habits and think that supplementing with vitamins and minerals is going to be your cure-all. Supplementation is meant to be just that, a **supplement** to your diet, not the diet itself. It is meant to help you deal with the nutritionally deficient fruits and vegetables on your grocery store shelves. Nonetheless, if you could be so lucky as to eat organic, home grown, non GMO fruits, vegetables, and grains, then you would not have to supplement as much or worry about diets or cures; your body would naturally lose weight and cure itself from disease. But since most people do not have a chance to eat so well, they must supplement.

Even though we seem to know so much about nutrition, and our diet and medical industry is so advanced, obesity, and all other diseases are still on the rise. Cardiovascular disease is still the number one killer of men and women. "Health is the fastest growing failing business in western civilization," writes Emanuel Cheraskin, M.D., in Human Health and Homeostasis. "We can say with reasonable certainty that only about six percent of the adult population can qualify as 'clinically' healthy." We can try to sort out each of the many negative behaviour variables (such as smoking) which certainly must be factored in. When we have done so, we are left with the completely unavoidable conclusion that our dinner tables are killing us.

The good diet vs. supplement controversy may be reduced to four clear and logical choices:

a) Eating right AND taking supplements
b) Eating right but taking no supplements, and being vitamin and mineral deficient for our entire lifespan, and greatly increasing our risk of sickness and death at any age.
c) Eating wrong and taking no supplements and being even more unhealthy and full of disease.
d) Eating wrong, but taking daily supplements and being a little less sick than if taking no supplements at all.

While each of these four options shows a popular choice, there is one best health-promoting conclusion: Supplements make any dietary lifestyle, whether good or bad, significantly better. Supplements are an easy, practical entry-level better-nutrition solution for the public. In the end, malnutrition is the elephant in the room which only a few seem to notice.

In 1998, the American Association of Poison Control Centers' Toxic Exposure Surveillance

System reported the following deaths from vitamin supplements:

Adult multiple vitamins: 0

Pediatric multiple vitamins: 0

(And, incidentally, ***there were no deaths from vitamin C, vitamin E, folic acid, nor from any other vitamin whatsoever.***)

On the other hand, according to David DeRose, M.D., M.P.H., "300,000 Americans die annually from poor nutrition choices" and hundreds of thousands die every year from prescription medication. I think the choice on nutritional supplements is clear.

As it has been for thousands of years of human history, so the malnutrition problem remains with us today. Only in the last century have supplements even been available. Their continued use represents a true public health breakthrough on a par with clean drinking water and sanitary sewers, and can be expected to save as many lives. A very worrying fact in the United States is that USDA Food Stamps may be used to buy a box of doughnuts, but are not allowed by law to be used to buy multivitamins, which raises many questions on how well the government really looks after its people. Vitamin supplements, like air bags, can save lives. We should advocate **good quality** supplements at **all costs**.

Vitamin supplementation is definitely better than no vitamin supplementation. But, if you have the chance and resources to buy fresh fruits and vegetables, raw milk, bee pollen, and find a good green superfood powder, these would be much better choices than synthetic vitamins.

Importance of Vitamins

Vitamin C

"Amazingly, vitamin C has actually already been documented in the medical literature to have readily and consistently cured both acute polio and acute hepatitis, two viral diseases still considered by modern medicine to be incurable."

Thomas E. Levy, MD, JD

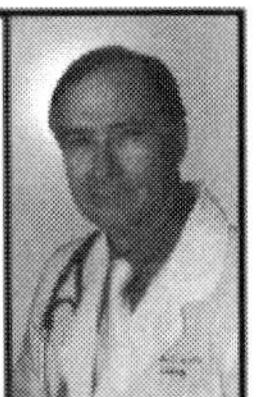

"Many viral infectious diseases have been cured and can continue to be cured by the proper administration of Vitamin C. Yes, the vaccinations for these treatable infectious diseases are completely unnecessary when one has the access to proper treatment with vitamin C. And, yes, all the side effects of vaccinations...are also completely unnecessary since the vaccinations do not have to be given in the first place with the availability of properly dosed vitamin C."

Thomas E. Levy, MD, JD

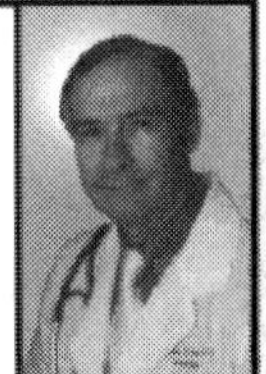

Two-time Nobel Prize winner Dr. Linus Pauling estimated that the rate of heart disease would be reduced by 80 per cent if adults in the US supplemented with 2,000 to 3,000 milligrams (mg) of vitamin C each day. As stated by Dr. Pauling, "Since vitamin C deficiency is the common cause of human heart disease, vitamin C supplementation is the universal treatment for this disease." In the US, heart disease is the number one killer. Dr. Pauling said that for those with existing heart disease the blockage of heart arteries could actually be reversed by supplementing with 6,000 mg of vitamin C and 6,000 mg of lysine (a common amino acid) taken in divided doses throughout the day. Vitamin C supplementation both lowers serum cholesterol levels and repairs lesions of arterial walls.

1998 Nobel Prize winner Dr. Louis J. Ignarro proved that supplementing with vitamin C and vitamin E significantly reduces the risk of developing arteriosclerosis.

One study looked at Vitamin E and Vitamin C supplementation in relation to mortality risk in 11,178 people aged 67-105 who participated in the

Established Populations for Epidemiologic Studies of the Elderly over a nine year period. The use of vitamins E and C simultaneously was associated with a lower risk of total mortality and coronary mortality.

In a massive study following over 85,000 nurses over a long 16-year period with a combined total of 1,240,000 person-years revealed that vitamin C supplementation significantly reduced the risk of heart disease. They found that the intake of vitamin C from food alone was insufficient to significantly affect the rate of heart disease. It was essential to supplement with high quantities of the vitamin itself to notice the protective effects. The study adjusted for age, smoking, and a variety of other coronary risk factors.

Pooled data from nine international prospective studies with 293,000 people, that included information on intakes of vitamin E, carotenoids, and vitamin C, with a 10-year follow-up to check for major incidents of coronary heart disease. Intake of antioxidants in the diet was only weakly related to reduced coronary heart disease risk. On the other hand, **subjects who took as little as 700 mg of vitamin C daily reduced their risk of heart disease events by 25 per cent** compared to those who took no supplements.

Researchers in Finland measured serum vitamin C levels in 2,419 middle-aged male participants of the ongoing Kuopio Ischemic Heart Disease Risk Factor Study. Men with a history of stroke were excluded from this analysis. Participants were followed for up to 10 years; the outcome of interest was development of stroke. During the follow-up period 120 participants suffered a stroke. After controlling for potential confounders - including age, BMI, smoking, blood pressure, and serum cholesterol - the researchers found that **men with a low vitamin C level in their blood were more than twice more likely to experience a stroke** than men with higher vitamin C blood levels..

Strokes commonly occur when a blot clot or thrombus block the flow of blood to certain parts of the brain. A thrombus or clot may form in an artery affected by arteriosclerosis. A recent study has shown how low plasma vitamin C was associated with increased risk of stroke, especially among hypertensive and overweight men.

Vitamin C strengthens the artery walls and tissue of the heart. Research indicates a reduced incidence of major coronary heart disease events at high supplemental vitamin C intakes. Recent studies have shown that vitamin C appears to reduce levels of C-reactive protein (CRP), a marker of inflammation. This is important to note because there is a growing body of evidence that chronic inflammation is linked to an increased risk of heart disease.

Conclusion: By just supplementing your diet with high levels of vitamin C, you can lower your risk of heart disease by 25-50%. This is just supplementing with a vitamin, imagine if you also started eating healthier foods and exercising more.

"I became interested in vitamin C and cancer in 1971 and began working with Ewan Cameron, M.B., Ch.B., chief surgeon at Vale of Leven Hospital in Scotland. Cameron gave 10 grams of vitamin C a day to patients with untreatable, terminal cancer. These patients were then compared by Cameron and me to patients with the same kind of cancer at the same terminal stage who were being treated in the same hospital but by other doctors--doctors who didn't give vitamin C, but instead just gave conventional treatments. Cameron's terminal cancer patients lived far longer compared to the ones who didn't get 10 grams a day of vitamin C. The other patients lived an average of six months after they were pronounced terminal, while Cameron's patients lived an average of about six years. "--Linus Pauling Interview by Peter Chowka 1996

"Vitamin C extends the lives of cancer patients, confirmed by Drs Murata & Fukumi Morishige in 1981. In their study, patients who received 5-30 grams daily as their only therapy lived an average of 6.2 times as long as those on 4 gms or less. Those suffering from cancer of the uterus who took vitamin C lived an average of 15.4 times as long than those receiving little or no vitamin C supplementation."---Passwater.

"In one case where complete remission was achieved in myelogenous leukemia...the patient took 24-42 gms vitamin c per day...it is inconcievable that no-one appears to have followed this up....without the scurvy, leukemia may be a relatively benign, non fatal condition. I wrote a paper..in an attempt to have the therapy clinically tested..I sent it to 3 cancer journals and 3 blood journals..it was refused by all....Two without even reading it."---Irwin Stone, Ph.D.

Recall how hydrogen peroxide is poured on wounds to kill germs. Well now researchers clearly show high-dose vitamin C, when administered intravenously, can increase hydrogen peroxide (H2O2) levels within cancer cells and kills them. Intravenous vitamin C was also demonstrated to kill germs and may be an effective therapy for infectious disease.

With a growing body of evidence mounting, National Institutes of Health (NIH) researchers conceded today that intravenous vitamin C may be an **effective treatment for cancer**. Last year the same researchers reported a similar study but the news media failed to publish it.

Here is the vitamin C study: http://www.ncbi.nlm.nih.gov/pubmed/16567755

The latest study, published in the Proceedings of the National Academy of Sciences, confirms the work of Nobel-Prize winner Dr. Linus Pauling who conducted cancer research in the 1970s with vitamin C. Dr. Pauling's studies were discredited at the time by poorly conducted research studies at the Mayo Clinic.

Unlike cancer drugs, intravenous (I.V.) vitamin C selectively killed cancer cells, but not healthy cells, and showed no toxicity. The ability of intravenous vitamin C to kill lymphoma cells was remarkable almost 100% at easily achievable blood vitamin C concentrations.

For inexplicable reasons, NIH researchers continue to maintain high-dose oral vitamin C can produce a limited increase in serum vitamin C concentrations, meaning high oral doses do not raise vitamin C levels in the blood. However, their earlier study published in 2004 clearly showed oral-dose vitamin C can achieve three times greater blood concentration than previously thought possible, a fact which negates the current Recommended Dietary Allowance for vitamin C. [Annals Internal Medicine 140:5337, 2004] NIH researchers refuse to issue a retraction of their earlier flawed research which mistakenly claimed humans cannot benefit from high-dose oral vitamin C supplements.

The NIH also offered no explanation why it has taken 35 years to confirm the work of Dr. Linus Pauling. If they could, they would have never confirmed his work, but the evidence is so strong, and the treatment so effective, that they couldn't look the other way any longer. Billions of dollars are at stake.

Intravenous vitamin C also does more than just kill cancer cells. It boosts immunity. It can stimulate collagen formation to help the body wall off the tumor. It inhibits hyaluronidase, an enzyme that tumors use to metastasize and invade other organs throughout the body. It induces apoptosis to help program cancer cells into dying early. It corrects the almost universal scurvy in cancer patients. Cancer patients are tired, listless, bruise easily, and have a poor appetite. They don't sleep well and have a low threshold for pain. This adds up to a very classic picture of scurvy that generally goes unrecognized by their conventional physicians.

To summarize, most organisms and animals make their own vitamin C, except humans. When they are under stress, either by illness or injury, Mother Nature has provided them with a means to facilitate healing: they produce more ascorbic acid. As a result, they are in less pain, they remain active, they can sleep, and they have a better appetite: all functions which promote healing. This is why oral vitamin C intake is so important for all people to maintain health and well being, minimum 2-3 grams per day if you are healthy.

Dr. Riordan, having his own clinic, once said that here at The Center, we don't treat cancer... we treat people who happen to have cancer. IVC (intravenous vitamin C) is a tool that allows our Center physicians to harness a healing mechanism that our human ancestors lost long ago: the ability to dramatically increase tissue levels of vitamin C. Research shows that the astonishingly high levels achievable only by IVC not only help fight the risk of infection and the pain of metastases, they actually aid in the defeat of the cancer cells themselves, through a very elegant mechanism that does no harm to healthy cells. It's a discovery that the medical world is only beginning to recognize.

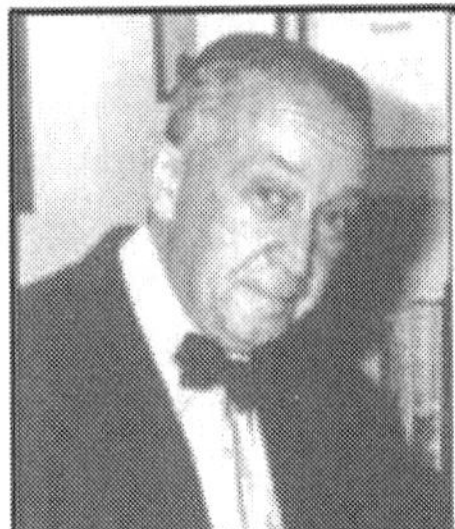

"In one case where complete remission was achieved in myelogenous leukemia...the patient took 24-42 gms vitamin c per day...it is inconcievable that no-one appears to have followed this up....without the scurvy, leukemia may be a relatively benign, non fatal condition. I wrote a paper.....in an attempt to have the therapy clinically tested..I sent it to 3 cancer journals and 3 blood journals..it was refused by all....Two without even reading it."

Irwin Stone, Ph.D.

"74% of Americans are below daily RDA requirements for magnesium, 55% for iron, 68% calcium, 40% vitamin C, 33% B12, 80% B6, 33% B3, 35% B2, 45% B1, 50% vitamin A. From 25-50% of hospital patients suffer from protein calorie malnutrition. Pure malnutrition (cachexia) is responsible for at least 22% and up to 67% of all cancer deaths. Up to 80% of all cancer patients have reduced levels of serum albumin, which is a leading indicator of protein and calorie malnutrition. At least 20% of Americans are clinically malnourished, with 70% being sub-clinically malnourished, and the remaining "chosen few" 10% in good optimal health."—Patrick Quillin, Ph.D.

Think about this; 70% of americans are malnourished, and 63% are obese or overweight. This means that your malnutritioned body is not only lacking almost every single recommended vitamin and mineral, it is becoming obese trying to extract as much of those elements as it can from the poor quality food you eat. We cannot expect ourselves be healthy when we do everything to be sick; it's like hitting your head against a wall and expecting an outcome other than a headache.

"Mr X has a lack of vitamin C and contracts a cold. The cold leads to pneumonia. Mr X dies and his body is taken to the mortuary...not with the diagnosis "lack of vitamin C", but with the diagnosis "pneumonia". This does not matter for him anymore, but matters for the rest of mankind, which is mislead in its thinking and judgement about vitamins."---Dr Albert Szent-Gyorgyi, Nobel Prize winner for discovering Ascorbate (Vitamin C).

"I have been consulted by many researchers who proposed bold studies of the effects of massive doses of ascorbate. Every time the university center, the ethics committee, the pharmacy committee, etc. deny permission for the use of massive doses of ascorbate and render the study almost useless. Seasoned researchers depending upon government grants do not even try to study adequate doses. All of this results in a massive accumulation of knowledge about very little which gives the impression that there is no more of real importance to be learned. This accumulation of minutia hides the great effects of ascorbate already known by some. The following sites reflect this problem. As you read these learned papers, you will realize that they seem to be completely unaware of the uses of massive doses of ascorbate. One of the most amusing aspects of this research are the speculations and research into the toxicity and other adverse reactions of tiny doses of ascorbate when many have used for years 20 to 100 times the amounts being discussed."--Dr Cathcart

Frederick R. Klenner, M.D. of North Carolina has seen cures of diphtheria, staph and strep infections, herpes, mumps, spinal meningitis, mononucleosis, shock, viral hepatitis, arthritis and polio using high doses of vitamin C (*Journal of Preventive Medicine*, Spring, 1974). http://www.seanet.com/~alexs/ascorbate/197x/klenner-fr-j_int_assn_prev_med-1974-v1-n1-p45.htm

Insofar as a cancer therapy, the following website lists 60 references to published studies: www.doctoryourself.com/biblio_cameron.html

What is a Recommended Dose of Vitamin C?

The current recommended daily intake of Vitamin C, as well as most other nutrients, as given by medical guidelines is what is required by your body to stay alive. There has been virtually no instruction on how much to take to stay healthy and prevent a multitude of diseases. As we now know, nobody wants you to stay healthy and prevent diseases so they will never tell you those amounts. But I am in favor of your health and I don't want you to keep giving your money away to the pharmaceutical drug mafia. As Linus Pauling states, every adult should take about 3 grams of Vitamin C per day, smaller amounts for children. If you are at risk or suffer from heart disease you must take about 5-6 grams of Vitamin C per day as well as 2-3 grams of Lysine (an essential amino acid that can be found in any health food store) per day.

Animals of different species make ascorbate at a rate of about 2-20 grams per day averaging at about 10 grams. That is about 40 – 400 times the regular RDA amount for humans. The recommended amount of Vitamin C in monkey food is about 70 times the RDA for an adult human.

We humans do not have the ability to make ascorbate in our system and that is why it is essential to have a proper intake of Vitamin C. You know you don't have enough Vitamin C if you still get colds and flu's. But as discussed earlier, if you still get sick then your body is full of toxins and mucous, and is actively trying to detoxify itself.

Another interesting thing is that collagen is formed in our bodies with the help of this miracle vitamin. Those expensive creams with collagen that supposedly reduce the aging of skin can be substituted with an increased dose of Vitamin C for a fraction of the cost, yet many times more beneficial.

To sum up, as we look back to the fact that cancer is a metabolic disease that requires an oxygen poor, acidic environment to survive (any bacteria, fungus, virus, or germ requires such an environment); anything that will increase the oxygen supply to the organism will allow your cells to turn back into being healthy. Vitamin C and E do just that, they increase the oxygen capacity in the blood thus allowing healthy cells to thrive and cancerous, disease ridden cells to die.

Large Study Shows that Those with Highest Blood Levels of Vitamin C Live Twice as Long as Those with Lowest Levels

High blood levels of Vitamin C may lower the risk of mortality due to all causes by as much as 50%. This is the conclusion from a published study conducted by Dr. Key-Tee Khaw at the University of Cambridge School of Clinical Medicine.

The researchers collected and analyzed data for 19,496 men and women 45 to 79 years of age. The subjects, who were participants in the Norfolk arm of the European Prospective Investigation into Cancer and Nutrition (EPIC) study, were followed for 4 years. Overall, those with blood levels of Vitamin C ranging in the top 20% were 50% less likely to die, from all causes, than those in the lowest 20%.

Vitamin D – The Sunshine Vitamin

Biochemist Proposes Worldwide Policy Change to Step Up Daily Vitamin D Intake

ScienceDaily (Aug. 9, 2010) — Anthony Norman, a leading international expert in vitamin D, proposes worldwide policy changes regarding people's vitamin D daily intake amount in order to maximize the vitamin's contribution to reducing the frequency of many diseases, including childhood rickets, adult osteomalacia, cancer, autoimmune type-1 diabetes, hypertension, cardiovascular disease, obesity and muscle weakness.

Vitamin D is the sunshine vitamin that is one of the oldest hormones on the planet and has been traced back 750 millions years, being made by some of the oldest bacteria on earth. Vitamin D is made from something which many people are so keen on reducing; cholesterol! You skin absorbs ultraviolet radiation and with the help of cholesterol turns into vitamin D. Your body can never make too much vitamin D from the sun because a clever system is present which works to destroy any excess vitamin D that may be made.

In 2006, CNN ran a headline news story that stated a massive study proves that vitamin D terminates 50% of all cancers. Since most of the funding for TV comes from pharmaceutical companies, the story was quickly buried. I'm guessing you have never heard of this study, so here it is:

http://edition.cnn.com/2005/HEALTH/12/28/vitamin.cancer.study/

Lets imagine that there was a drug that eliminated 50% of all cancers; it would be worth billions of dollars, it would be on television, radio, newspapers, and magazines all over the world. So here we had CNN with the hottest story of the 21st century, and because of the revenues from pharmaceutical companies the story was buried. Again and again you see how much they really care about you.

75% of breast and colon cancer deaths can be prevented with vitamin D3 and calcium - Moores Cancer Center and Department of Family and Preventive Medicine, UC San Diego

They say vitamin D needs to be between 40-60 nanograms per ml in blood plasma to be healthy. If you or anyone you know has cancer, multiple sclerosis, or heart disease, have them take a vitamin D3 test to see just how low their blood plasma levels really are.

Other doctors, such as Trump, Holick, Haney, Garland, and research centers across the world are beginning to notice the correlation between vitamin D deficiency and cancer.

Donald Trump M.D, conducted studies at Roswell Park Cancer Institute to measure vitamin D levels in cancer patients. They found that most of their patients with cancer had low vitamin D levels; below 32 ng/mL while a healthy person should have between 40 and 60 ng/mL.

Michael Holick, M.D has been talking about the importance of vitamin D for over 30 years and data proves that vitamin D deficiency and rickets is only the tip of the iceberg, and stretches into diabetes, multiple sclerosis, arthritis, infections, heart disease, and most of all cancer.

The question is, is rickets still a problem today? (In 1889 in Boston, 80% of infants had rickets) YES! There are still about a dozen cases per year of rickets which is a severe lack of vitamin D, it's like having severe malnutrition. This means people are STILL suffering from a lack of vitamin D. Doctors say that breast milk contains all the necessary nutrients, and that is a misconception. Mothers' breast milk these days only contains about 25 IU/L which is not enough to say the least. If the mother is barely receiving her required daily dose of vitamins, she cannot expect her breast milk to be fully nutritious.

Holick did another study on pregnant mothers who took multivitamins and drinking more than two glasses of milk per day and they were taking about 600IU per day which is lower than the recommended amount even with vitamins and milk!! He found 76% of mothers and 81% of newborns were vitamin D deficient! The study also found that preeclampsia (abnormal state of pregnancy characterized by hypertension and fluid retention and albuminuria) was strongly associated with vitamin D deficiency.

He also found that there was a huge correlation with vitamin D deficiency and C-section birth. This means that if you have proper amounts of vitamin D you are more likely to have a normal birth without needing a C-section. There is no question about it, infants need vitamin D at birth at a minimum of 400IU per day as requested by the Academy of Pediatrics.

Do you know why we used to take cod liver oil? Because there is not enough vitamin D in foods except oily fish like salmon which has about 500-1000 IU per 3.5oz serving. So you would have to eat it every day and even then you would still barely get enough. But wait, is there a difference between wild and farmed salmon? You bet. Wild salmon get plenty of vitamin D from their ocean environment and food chain, but farmed salmon (the stuff in all the restaurants, fast food joints, frozen dinners, cans etc) doesn't get practically any with about 100-250 IU per 3.5oz serving. If your doctor says "don't worry about sunlight, just eat more fish," you should get another doctor.

The fact is, only about 0.1% of UVB and 4.9% of UVA rays ever reach the surface of earth at the equator, this is during June, at noon time. So that 0.1% is responsible for our vitamin D production. What do you think happens during winter when the sun is weaker and you wear more clothes? Holick did another study and found that from November through February we get pretty much no vitamin D (unless you live closer to the equator).

But what about the evil sun, doesn't it cause cancer? We constantly hear that the sun causes cancer. Too much breathing can make you pass out; too much water can kill you etc. Too much of anything is not good for you, and those that do develop skin cancers are people who are already at risk and who are unhealthy. Have you ever asked the question how come countries where people are constantly out in the sun don't get cancer? Could it be something other than the sun? If you wear even an SPF 15 sunscreen you block between 95-99% of vitamin D producing capacity, and that is because SPF 15 sunscreen is supposed to block between 95-99% of UVB rays. People barely get any vitamin D from their diet, but when summer rolls around and is the best time to fill up on this vitamin, people cover their bodies in sunscreen and block it all out.

So how do you get your vitamin D? Studies found that 24 hours after 1 minimum erythemal dose (A measure of ultraviolet radiation, where 1 MED is sufficient to cause detectable sunburn) the vitamin D you would get equals about 20000 IU if you would have taken it orally. Now you can see the magnitude differences between what we get from a glass of milk (100 IU), a multivitamin (400 IU), and what we are supposed to be getting naturally from the sun.

No matter where you are, studies show that we have most concentrations of vitamin D in our blood in the summer and lowest in the winter. Most of our vitamin D should be coming from sun exposure!

The best sun exposure is just below 1 minimum erythemal dose, meaning just below that which would give you sunburn. Everyone is different, so about 15-20 minutes (could be more or less) in the sun during the hours between 10 am to 3 pm when the sun's rays are strong. The darker your skin the more time you need to spend in the sun because melanin (substance that gives skin its dark color) is a natural sunscreen which blocks UVA and UVB rays. If your skin is black then you will need about 5-10 times more sun exposure to get the same benefit as light skin individuals. This is why 30-50% of African Americans are vitamin D deficient throughout the year.

What about age? If you are 70 years old, you have about a 75% reduced ability to make vitamin D, so the older you are the more important it is that you get adequate sun exposure. Another study showed that even 15-30 minutes of sun exposure a few times per week for older adults was enough to raise their vitamin D levels.

Obese individuals need even more vitamin D to maintain the proper amount in their bodies. This is because vitamin D is fat soluble meaning it is stored in fat tissue and obese individuals have more storage places for the vitamin. Meaning about 2-3 times more or 50000 IU per week.

If you would like to know your vitamin D levels, request from your doctor a 25(OH)D Assay hydroxy test, NOT the active form of vitamin D 1,25(OH)2D which is always normal or elevated in vitamin deficiency. You are deficient if you have about 10 ng/mL, and if you are under 30 years of age then you definitely need to supplement with vitamins or be out in the sun more. If you tested people who work out in the sun (or yourself after a sunny vacation on the islands) they are going to be over 100 nm/mL and up to 200 and more, and that is absolutely fine.

Vitamin D deficiency is an unrecognized epidemic with 42% of African American women aged 15-49 who were vitamin D deficient as reported by the Centers for Disease Control. In Boston, 84% of healthy African American adults, 42% of Hispanic adults, and 30% of Caucasian adults over 50 years of age were vitamin D deficient at the end of the summer (less than 20 ng/mL). Study after study shows our population is vitamin D deficient, even after the summer because we don't practice safe sun exposure. We are made to believe that the sun is totally evil and we must soak ourselves with sunscreen and wear a parka to the beach.

Lets look at a very common disease these days; osteomalacia (softening of the bones due to defective bone mineralization). The symptoms are generalized bone pain, isolated bone pain, and muscle aches and pains. The typical diagnosis is FIBROMYALGIA or chronic fatigue syndrome. When vitamin D levels are corrected, within a few months the symptoms are almost gone. If you have bone or muscle aches and pains, if you are tired and fatigued and depressed, get a vitamin D test done and begin supplementing immediately.

People routinely show up in hospitals with aching bones, denervation, muscle atrophy, muscle weakness etc. and get an improper diagnoses. If the doctor is competent, they will test for vitamin D levels, which in most cases is the culprit, but they never do. Now there is even evidence that Parkinson's disease and dementia can also be caused by a vitamin D deficiency.

A study led by Paul Knekt and colleagues at the National Institute for Health and Welfare, Finland, examined levels of vitamin D in the blood of 3,173 Finnish men and women aged 50 to 79 determined to be free of Parkinson's disease at the start of the study. The researchers then examined the incidence of Parkinson's disease in these participants over a 29-year follow-up period. They found that participants with the highest levels of vitamin D (more than 50 nmol/L) had a 65 percent lower risk of developing Parkinson's disease than those with the lowest vitamin D levels (less than 25 nmol/L).

The higher your 25 hydroxy vitamin D levels, the higher you bone density, these are the facts, end of story. Not only is Vitamin D good for bones, it also increases muscle strength, balance, and lower extremity function. Listen up you bodybuilders and all those wanting to be a little stronger!

Dr. Holick gives his vitamin D deficient patients 50000 IU of vitamin D2 once every two weeks, forever. Toxicity? Not one bit. Over 6 years his patients taking 50000 IU were in the good 30-60 ng/mL range, and it could have been better. Holick's study on D2 vs D3 efficacy proved no difference in the effectiveness of either vitamin D2 or D3. Another study showed that even taking 10000 IU per day does not cause vitamin D toxicity. If you really want vitamin D toxicity you will have to be taking ridiculously huge amounts deliberately, every day. Otherwise you are absolutely safe. How much is too much?

One day Dr. Holick received a call from a lawyer who was going to sue him because of his recommendations. He said that 10 years ago there were no vitamin D supplements in stores so he ordered some online. The bottle was labeled as 1000 IU per teaspoon so he was taking 2 teaspoons every day for a few years and during the time of the call he was taken to the hospital with severe vitamin D toxicity. Dr. Holick asked for a sample to analyze the product he bought, and it turned out that the company did not dilute the powder. He was taking 1 000 000 IU per day! His blood vitamin D levels were 520 ng/mL; now this is toxicity.

Another interesting fact is that every cell in our bodies has a vitamin D receptor. Not only is it a vital part of our metabolism and calcium regulator, it is also very important in cancer. In 1979 Suda et al took leukemia cancer cell and incubated them with active vitamin D and showed that they became normal. This led to the vitamin D and cancer connection we read about. The connection is that active vitamin D inhibits cancer growth. Evidence shows that up to 2000 genes are regulated by active vitamin D which also has effects on the immune system explaining its positive effects on tuberculosis.

"Vitamin D plays a critical role in the human body's response to tuberculosis, according to new research ... The research also suggests a new way to fight one of the world's deadliest diseases: with a simple dietary supplement. Tuberculosis, usually caused when a person inhales tuberculosis bacteria, killed an estimated 1.7 million people in 2003 and is the leading cause of death for people afflicted with AIDS, according to the World Health Organization (WHO)." – Alvin Powell, Harvard News Office

Aloya et al in 2007 showed that women taking 2000 IU vitamin D per day reduced the risk of developing upper respiratory tract infections by 90%. Do you think the flu season only hits winter because of a lack of vitamin D which is due to a lack of sunshine? Science says so.

Do you or someone you know have psoriasis? You are in luck. Dr. Holick also conducted a study on the topical application of the active vitamin D 1,25(OH)2D and had a 92% improvement rate and a 65% complete cure rate in his subjects! The topical cream needs to have 15 micrograms per gram of base, not 3 like currently used in most psoriasis creams, to have such quick and safe effects. In the end Dr. Holick has the most psoriasis patients than any dermatology establishment in the United States. Topical vitamin D treatment needs to be the first line treatment for psoriasis.

Another huge study showed that the more sun exposure you get throughout your life the less likely you are to prematurely die (W. Grant, 2002). Knight et al, published a study showing that girls exposed to the most sunlight during their teenage years reduced their risk of developing breast cancer by more than 50%. Studies showed that taking 1100IU of vitamin D per day reduced the risk of ALL cancers by 60-70% (Lapey, Heaney).

Vitamin D deficiency is a disease of neglect. It has been linked to cause cancer, increased mortality, autoimmune diseases, type 1 and 2 diabetes, hypertension, osteoporosis, M.S, fibromyalgia etc.

A few studies showing that sun exposure actually reduced your risk of developing melanoma.

Sun Exposure and Mortality From Melanoma – Berwick et al J National Cancer Institute 2005
"Sun exposure is associated with increased survival from melanoma"

UV Radiation Exposure and Risk of Malignang Lymphomas – Smedby et al J National Cancer Institute 2005
"High frequency of sun bathing by age 20 reduced risk of non-Hodgkin lymphoma by 30-40%"

Currently, the recommended daily intake of vitamin D in the United States is 200 international units (IU) for people up to 50 years old; 400 IU for people 51 to 70 years old; and 600 IU for people over 70 years old. Today there is a wide consensus among scientists that the relative daily intake of vitamin D should be increased to 2,000 to 4,000 IU for most adults.

"Low cancer areas were far more frequent in the sun belt. What was the significance of sunlight with regard to cancer rates? Sunlight reacts with cholesterol inside and on the surface of the skin to create vitamin-D. Vitamin-

D helps the body absorb calcium and plays a major role in the body's ability to use the calcium that is available," The Calcium Connection, Dr. Cedric Garland and Dr. Frank Garland, 1989, Forside, Simon and Shuster Inc.

Discover and Time magazines have hailed vitamin D as one of the most important breakthroughs of our time. Have you heard about it? Now you have.

Now go outside and get some free medicine!

Coral Calcium

Scientists say that calcium inhibits, prevents, and even cures cancer. The best is marine grade coral calcium which has the perfect biological ratio of magnesium to calcium 2:1

"After nine months, women on magnesium supplements increased bone density by about 11%." - Journal of Nutritional Medicine

Most calcium supplements in stores are calcium carbonate which is only about 1% absorbable by your body. Calcium citrate on the other hand is a bit more absorbable but a lot more expensive. Even a mother's milk is only about 17% absorbable but coral calcium is 76% absorbable!

When the Japanese government was conducting studies on the longevity of their population, they sent teams of scientists to the Okinawa province to find out why they lived so much longer than the rest of the country and have practically no diseases(the Okinawas are amongst the world's longest lived people). The three massive studies concluded it was the coral calcium in their water. Yet when scientists and researchers tried to tell the American people of its benefits, they were threatened with jail. When some tried to sell this miracle mineral they were fined and faced terrible consequences.

When scientists studied such cultures as the Hunzas (who live to **between 120 and 140 years of age**, and are HEALTHY their entire lives), Azerbaijanis, Titikaki's in Peru, the Okinawas, they tried to figure out how come they live so long and have virtually no diseases. They found that they all consume massive amount of calcium (up to 100 times the tiny recommendation of 1000mg) AND spend hours upon hours in the sun every day.

In 1972 scientists in John Hopkins University discovered that DNA will only replicate when smothered with calcium. DNA replication is responsible for growth, development, building and maintenance of body parts, staying young etc. How much highly absorbable calcium did you get today? If you don't take some form of calcium then you are growing older 5 times faster than normal.

Recently it was reported that calcium supplements increase your risk of heart attacks. This is not news, for years it was warned about the risks of cheap, ineffective supplements. Much of the calcium used by companies today is just ground up sea shells. The body cannot identify or digest this calcium molecule and thus stores it in the soft tissue of the body including the heart. This increases your risk of heart disease and heart attacks. Only choose marine grade Okinawa coral calcium to ensure good health.

Calcium and vitamin D also cures lupus, multiple sclerosis, cardiovascular diseases, autoimmune diseases, infection etc because these diseases are also due in part to oxygen deficiencies in the cells.

"Vitamin D in Systemic Lupus Erythematosus: Clinical Studies of Vitamin D and Systemic Lupus Erythematosus" - **Diane Kamen** and **Cynthia Aranow**, Medical University of South Carolina, USA

- High prevalence of vitamin D deficiency and its association with left ventricular dilation: An echocardiography study in elderly patients with chronic heart failure. Nutr Metab Cardiovasc Dis. 2010 Apr 14.
- Vitamin D deficiency and myocardial diseases. Mol Nutr Food Res. 2010 Mar 29.
- Vitamin D deficiency and cardiovascular disease: Is there a role for vitamin D therapy in heart failure? Curr Opin Investig Drugs. 2010 Mar;11(3):309–14.
- Vitamin D receptor: a new risk marker for clinical restenosis after percutaneous coronary intervention. Expert Opin Ther Targets. 2010 Mar;14(3):243–51.
- Vitamin D and cardiovascular risk. Int Urol Nephrol. 2010 Mar;42(1):165–71.
- Extraskeletal effects of vitamin D in older adults: cardiovascular disease, mortality, mood, and cognition. Am J Geriatr Pharmacother. 2010 Feb;8(1):4–33.

- Maternal vitamin D deficiency leads to cardiac hypertrophy in rat offspring. Reprod Sci. 2010 Feb;17(2):168–76.
- Vitamin D, race, and cardiovascular mortality: findings from a national US sample. Ann Fam Med. 2010 Jan–Feb;8(1):11–8.

More studies on vitamin D and heart disease here: http://www.vitamindcouncil.org/researchHeartDisease.shtml

There is an intestinal disorder known as celiac disease that disrupts the ability to absorb calcium and vitamin D as well as other nutrients. Many people with osteoporosis actually have celiac disease. Celiac disease is the result of intolerance to the gluten in wheat, barley, oats and rye. Following a gluten-free diet may improve both digestion and bone density. If you are having difficulty increasing your alkalinity, you might try a gluten-free diet for a few weeks or months to see if it helps. Gluten-free grains include brown rice, wild rice, amaranth, quinoa, and buckwheat. Or, if you have a gluten intolerance you can always switch to sprouted grains.

Vitamin B17 - Nitrilosides (Laetrile, Amygdalin)

Over 20 years ago vitamin B17 was the subject of great controversy when many of the world's top scientists claimed that when it was consumed, the components of certain raw fruit seeds make it **100% impossible to develop cancer and will kill existing cancer in most cases.**

Immediately the pharmaceutical companies sprung on this claim and demanded that the FDA, run by the same people, look into it. Because god forbid something free will take away their billions of dollars of profit from cancer. The results of these studies are found in a book called "World Without Cancer", by G. Edward Griffin.

Vitamin B17, also know as Laetrile and Amygdalin is found in most fruit seeds, namely apricot seeds. The apricot seed was claimed as the **cure for all cancers over 50 years ago**.

It was claimed that eating 7 apricot seeds per day will make you immune to cancer, just like one can never get scurvy if they eat citrus fruit (because of vitamin C), or pellagra if they take vitamin B every day.

The pharmaceuticals companies together with the medical establishment pushed the FDA into making it illegal to sell "raw" apricot seeds or vitamin B17 with information about its effects on cancer. Even to this day, **you can't get raw apricot seeds in your health food store**, only the sun dried ones which have all the important enzymes killed off.
How does it work?

Dr Krebs and other researchers like Otto Warburg maintain that cancer is a chronic metabolic disease. A chronic disease is one which usually does not pass away on its own accord.

"The great advantage of knowing the prime cause of a disease is that it can then be attacked logically and over a broad front. This is particularly important in the case of **cancer**, with its numerous secondary and remote causes, and because it is often stated that in man alone there are over one hundred well-known and quite different kinds of **cancer**, usually with the implication that therefore we will have to find one or several hundred bases for prevention and treatment, and usually without any realization that this need not necessarily be the case now that we know that **all cancers studied have a characteristic metabolism in common, a prime cause**." - Dr. Otto Warburg, two time Nobel prize winner.

All of us probably have cancer many times in our lives. If our defence mechanisms are functioning normally, the body kills off the cancer cells, and we're never aware that anything even happened. If, however, there is a breakdown in that defence mechanism when the cancer cells appear, there is nothing to prevent the growth of those cancer cells and soon there is a tumour.

A doctor from the U.S. FDA once said that Laetrile contains "free" hydrogen cyanide and, thus, is toxic. I would like to correct that misconception:

There is no "free" hydrogen cyanide in Laetrile. When Laetrile comes in contact with the enzyme beta-glucosidase, the Laetrile is broken down to form two molecules of glucose, one molecule of benzaldehyde and one molecule of hydrogen cyanide (HCN). Within the body, the cancer cell-and only the cancer cell-contains that enzyme. The key word here is that the HCN must be FORMED. It is not floating around freely in the Laetrile and then released. It must be manufactured. The enzyme beta glucosidase, and only that enzyme, is capable of manufacturing the HCN from Laetrile. If there are no cancer cells in the body, there is no beta-glucosidase. If there is no beta-glucosidase, no

HCN will be formed from the Laetrile .

An interesting thing to note is that the enzyme beta glucosidase is used to break down sugar for energy in the cell. In our bodies only cancer cells have this enzyme. This, yet again, leads back to the basis of all cancers and most diseases, back to Otto Warburg and anaerobism; that all cancer cells live in an oxygen poor environment and unlike healthy cells they feed on sugar to survive. If you understand the basis of disease everything will become a lot simpler.

Laetrile does contain the cyanide radical (CN). This same cyanide radical is contained in Vitamin B12, and in berries such as blackberries, blueberries and strawberries. You never hear of anyone getting cyanide poisoning from any of the above-mentioned berries, because it's simply not possible. The cyanide radical (CW) and hydrogen cyanide (HCN) are two completely different compounds, just like pure sodium (Na+) - one of the most toxic substances known to mankind - and sodium chloride (NaCl), when combined together make table salt, but separated are two completely different compounds.

If the above is true, how did the smear campaign ever get started claiming that Laetrile contains "free" hydrogen cyanide? It was the Food and Drug Administration.

In a newspaper back in the late 1960's or early 1970's there was a news release from the FDA. This release stated that there were some proponents of a substance known as "Laetrile" who were saying that this substance was capable of forming hydrogen cyanide in the presence of the cancer cell. The release continued by saying that, if this were actually true, we had, indeed, found a substance, which was target-specific, and would be of great value to the cancer patient. But, the news release went on to say, the FDA had done extensive testing of this substance, "Laetrile," and found no evidence that it contained hydrogen cyanide or that any hydrogen cyanide was released in the presence of the cancer cell. Thus, they said, Laetrile was of no value.

When it was clearly established some time later that Laetrile did, indeed, release hydrogen cyanide in the presence of the cancer cell, how do you suppose the FDA reacted? Did they admit that they were wrong? Did they admit that they had done a very inadequate job in running their tests? No! They now proclaimed that Laetrile contained hydrogen cyanide and thus was toxic!

Importance of Vitamin E

"Now I've got to the point where I think we can get almost complete control of cardiovascular disease, heart attacks and strokes. [The proper therapy] can prevent cardiovascular disease and even cure it.". --Linus Pauling. Heart disease is caused by vitamin deficiencies!

Linus Pauling was hailed as "The greatest living scientist this century." He is the only scientist to ever win two unshared Nobel prizes and he has 48 honorary doctorates.

Natural Vitamin E Dramatically Reduces Heart Disease

"Supplements" by definition are designed to fill nutritional gaps in a bad diet. They fill in what may be surprisingly large gaps in a good diet as well. In the case of vitamin E, doing so is likely to save millions of lives. The New England Journal of Medicine had two articles in the May 20, 1993 issue (8,9) showing that persons taking vitamin E supplements had an approximately 40% reduction in cardiovascular disease. Nearly 40,000 men and 87,000 women took part in the studies. The more vitamin E they took, and the longer they took it, the less cardiovascular disease they experienced.

A 1996 double-blind, placebo-controlled study of 2,002 patients with clogged arteries demonstrated a 77% decreased risk of heart attack in those taking 400 to 800 IU of vitamin E. (10) Again, such effective quantities of vitamin E positively cannot be obtained from diet alone. 800 IU is 2,667% of the US RDA for vitamin E. Is that a lot, or is the government recommendation too low?

Vitamin E has been viciously and fraudulently attacked by powerful vested interests, especially researchers funded primarily by Big Pharma. This has nothing to do with real science, and everything to do with a media-backed Big Pharma PR machine trying to convince Americans to take toxic and health-deteriorating drugs instead of safe and effective vitamins. http://www.newswithviews.com/Richards/byron39.htm

"In the 1950s the Schute brothers in Ontario did some amazing work with vitamin E. Their claims were simple. They said vitamin E worked against heart disease and cerebrovascular disease. They were greeted with laughter. A couple of years ago, the Harvard School of Public Health published a huge study on vitamin E and showed that just 100 units of vitamin E per day decreased the death rate by 40 percent. Suppose they had done that in 1960? How many Americans would have been saved in the intervening 35 years had Harvard taken a responsible position and said, "We are skeptical of these claims but let's look at them"? But they wouldn't do that--it didn't fit their paradigm. So vitamin E was totally destroyed by the establishment. Think of the cost of those decisions."--Linus Pauling Interview by Peter Chowka 1996

Furthermore, according to Dr. Rath, significant documentation attests that:

"Vitamins belong to the most powerful agents in the fight against heart disease. This fact has been established by studies of thousands of people over many years. Here are some important results of recent clinical studies:

Vitamin C cuts heart disease rate almost in half (documented in 11,000 Americans over ten years) Vitamin E cuts heart disease rate by more than one third (documented in 36,000 Americans over six years.) Beta Carotene (provitamin A) cuts heart disease rate almost in half (documented in 36,000 Americans).

No prescription drug has ever been shown to help prevent heart disease similar [to vitamins A, C and E]. These results and those of countless other studies are so clear that anybody questioning the value of vitamins in the prevention of heart disease may safely be considered as uninformed." Interview of Dr Rath by Family Health News Dr Rath site http://www.rath.nl/GB/frame1.htm

A natural anti-oxidant and oxygen conservator such as Vitamin E affords the body many advantages. First, when richly supplied with Vitamin E, the cells of the body are able to perform more efficiently - not demanding as much oxygen for metabolic processes, thereby freeing more oxygen for those cells and organs needing it most. An ailing heart is also supplied with more oxygen and thus does not have to pump as hard to convey blood to the cells. Its work is considerably lessened, consequently easing the strain - which is an extremely important factor in heart ailments. Also, the heart muscle itself is more richly nourished with oxygen through its main source of blood supply, the coronary arteries. These two factors - less work and more oxygen - partially explain why the vitamin has a direct, beneficial, seemingly miraculous, effect on ailing hearts and on normal hearts as well. Researchers have stated that Vitamin E therapy is equivalent to being placed in an oxygen tent - without the inconvenience, of course.

Vitamin E is also a vasodilator: it opens arteries (particularly those all-important smallest ones, the arterioles) so that more blood can flow through the circulatory system. This is of particular significance for victims of circulatory disorders such as 'arteriosclerosis and atherosclerosis'. (Arteriosclerosis is the general term employed to encompass almost all disorders of the arterial and venous system which are considered to be due to "aging." More specifically, the term refers to "hardening" and "thickening" of the arteries, accompanied by loss of elasticity in the blood vessels, 'Atherosclerosis' is characterized by clogging of the arteries with fatty deposits on the walls. Once these deposits accumulate, they can break off and begin to clog and narrow arteries. This puts pressure on the heart which has to pump blood through increasingly narrowing arteries, just like a pump pumping water through a clogged hose. . If such a piece of material [a "clot" or "thrombus'] makes its way to the heart and/or blocks the flow of blood to the heart, then we have one of the common forms of "coronary thrombosis."

Still another benefit of Vitamin E is its anti-coagulant (anti-blood-clotting) power. Moreover, this anti-coagulant quality of the vitamin does not produce harmful side-effects as do the drugs heparin and dicumarol, which are now in common use in an attempt to treat and prevent the formation of clots - the clots (thrombi) being the leading cause of "coronaries" and "strokes", whether they be due to the formation of blood clots or to "flaking" away of the fatty deposits. The latter drugs must be used with extreme caution, for they tend to produce hemorrhages. There is great debate raging in the medical world as to whether these drugs should be used at 'all', as their action of artificially creating 'hemophillia' (bleeding which is extremely difficult to control) seems to outweigh their merit as anti-coagulants.

With Vitamin E, however, such is not the case no matter how massive the dosage employed. Further, Vitamin E has shown some tendency to 'dissolve' clots. Although Vitamin E is also a dependable, efficient anti-coagulant, its action stops when its anti-blood-clotting ability is no longer needed. Vitamin E can even help speed up wound healing and can even prevent scars from forming on the skin.

Still another recognized property of the amazing Vitamin E is its ability to maintain normal permeability of cellular membranes, notably the capillaries. You might recall that capillaries are tiny blood vessels which supply nourishment to individual cells. If the capillary walls become too impermeable (less penetrable), their function of feeding the cells is impaired; on the other hand, if the walls become too permeable, or sponge like, they leak out their precious cargo into the space in between cells where it does not belong, and, thus, the cells are deprived of nutrition.

Vitamin E is truly a wonder vitamin that treats heart disease as well as a host of other ailments and imbalances. The list of diseases vitamin E helps is endless; such as **diabetes** (many patients have been able to go off insulin entirely while others have had its use drastically reduced), it helps treat **menopause** (It has been dubbed "natures own tranquilizer," by various gynecologists, who have found that heavy doses of Vitamin E somewhat mirror the effects of estrogen - the female hormone - in relieving "hot flashes," nervousness, depression, anxiety, and irritability without the adverse side effects of the hormone), **eye disorders** in children (near-sightedness, crossed eyes, along with **mental retardation**, have been reported corrected or alleviated with extremely large doses of Vitamin E, up to 3000 international units a day for years), it has been shown to prevent and cure cirrhosis of the liver, it has been shown to have a great effect on treating **leprosy** (Hansen's disease), **lupus erythematosus** (a tuberculosis skin disease which is characterized by an intractable rash) and in the prevention of sickness due to x-ray therapy, it has been shown to improve **muscular dystrophy**(20%-50% of sufferers treated with massive doses of Vitamin E have been found to be helped dramatically), markedly improve in withdrawal symptoms from drug abuse, normalize blood pressure, it has even shown that in several series of experiments that childless couples when given massive treatments of Vitamin E (and this means both the man and the woman) can very often have children, when nothing else was effective.

These are some of the known benefits of Vitamin E. Vitamin E also treats various forms of **sexual dysfunction and lack of sex drive**. This property of Vitamin E - that of improving the quality of the sperm as well as the general health of both parents has been noted throughout the history of the vitamin. In fact, as we have mentioned previously, this ability to induce the production of healthy offspring caused it to be tagged as an "anti-sterility vitamin" and this is still considered by many medical authorities to be the vitamin's prime function.

There are plenty of other benefits which we don't know yet, but since Vitamin E cannot be patented and then sold by a big company, nobody wants to do more studies on it; so many other benefits of this vitamin will never be heard of.

A brief history of vitamin E

Dr. Evan V. Shute of London, Ontario, Canada, began to seriously investigate Vitamin E in the 1930s. His first patient was suffering from Purpura (a blockage of the smaller blood vessels) when doctors were considering removing his spleen in hopes that the condition would improve. But because the patient was suffering from severe heart failure the operation could not be performed - and lucky for him.

Researcher Skelton and Dr. Shute, using their findings from treating dogs of purpura, administered 200 IU of Vitamin E every day to their despairing patient. At the time, this dosage was much higher than had ever been used before to treat human beings. Today we know this dosage is extremely low, which helps to explain why back then many researchers could not obtain uniform or even satisfactory results - they weren't using enough Vitamin E to cause any significant changes.

Even so, their first patient's heart trouble quickly disappeared. Skelton and Dr. Shute's amazement in a simple vitamin grew and as did their curiosity. Their next patient was a barber who was dying from recurrent coronary thrombosis (this disease accounts for more than half of all deaths in men over 45). The barber was in the last stages of heart failure, complicated by a type of angina which was extremely painful and which nothing could relieve. Within three weeks of starting on Vitamin E he was freely playing drums in a local theatre. Their next patient was their own mother who suffered from severe angina pectoris, and again the vitamin worked, curing her pains and allowing her to resume her regular activities.

After these fantastic results, the gloomy picture of heart disease turned into a bright and clear glow of optimism. At the time of compiling their monumental work in 1954, Drs. Shute, et al., had treated more than 10,000 heart patients - with fantastic and credible results (now they have over 20,000 treated patients).

They thought their most careful scientific findings would be welcomed by the medical establishment, and then the whole world, that a cure for heart disease was finally found. But yet again they had to learn the hard way that the medical mafia is in no way interested in curing anybody, especially from such a profitable ailment like heart disease; and that is why you have never heard of Dr. Shute or his findings. Their work was rejected publication from journal after journal, yet in the name of truth they continued their research founding the Shute Foundation of Medical Research and successfully treating thousands of patients ever since.

Many other inventions that we currently use such as the encephalogram or x-rays had been ostracized and ridiculed when they first came out. Dr. Grubbe invented X-rays in 1896, yet the medical profession only recognized them as useful in 1951! He was asked what he thought was the reason for the authorities fighting the x-ray for so long, he replied bluntly: "The surgeons. They controlled medicine, and they regarded the X-ray as a threat to surgery. At that time surgery was the only approved method of treating cancer. They meant to keep it the 'only' approved method by ignoring or rejecting any new methods or ideas. This is why I was called a 'quack' and nearly ejected from hospitals where I had practiced for years." Nearly every single great invention of our time has gone through this process, and most are buried never to be heard from again. It's all about the money folks.

The Shute's scientific evidence clearly shows more than 10000 patients successfully cured of heart disease, yet he found the hard way that no matter how much evidence him and his researchers bring, the medical mafia would ignore and depreciate all evidence for as long as they can. However, as more researchers such as Dr. M.K Horwitt at the Elgin State Hospital in Elgin, Illinois, began to do studies on Vitamin E and proved conclusively that a deficiency of Vitamin E in the blood of the human being produces the destruction of red blood cells, the FDA was pretty much forced to admit that vitamin E was an essential nutrient (a small win after a long and hard battle). Yet despite all the evidence, the FDA still falsely claims that we receive adequate amounts of Vitamin E from food and do not need to supplement ourselves with it. So even though the government admits that you need Vitamin E, they still have the minimums set at a nearly useless level.

All sorts of studies made on Dutch and American diets indicate that the average of these diets provides no more than 12 IU a day and perhaps much closer to 6 IU. I don't know how this can be represented as "adequate." In fact, every scientist in the field would say that the average American exists in a chronic state of alpha tocopherol (vitamin E) starvation. The 30 IU per day minimum requirement is what prevents the destruction of red blood cells in our bodies, and that was known decades before the FDA decided to include vitamin E as an important vitamin. Can you believe this? As early as the 1940s scientists from all over the world brought overwhelming evidence that vitamin E was a cure for heart disease and sterility. This was known **IN THE 1940s**, yet we are still "looking for the cure" to heart disease!

"It was nearly impossible now for anyone who valued his future in Academe to espouse Vitamin E, prescribe it or advise its use. That would make a man a "quack" at once. This situation lasted for many years. In the United States, of course, the closure of the J.A.M.A. pages against us and tocopherol meant that it did not exist. It was either in the U.S. medical bible or it was worthless. No amount of documentation could budge medical men from this stance. Literature in the positive was ignored and left unread. Individual doctors often said: "If it is as good as you say, we would all be using it." But nothing could induce them as persons of scientific background to make the simplest trial on a burn or coronary."

The American Medical Association even **refused** to let the Shute's present their findings at national medical conventions. In the early 1960's, the United States Post Office successfully prevented even the *mailing* of vitamin E. Please re-read these sentences so they sink in.

Linus Pauling wrote, in the book's 1985 foreword:
"The failure of the medical establishment during the last forty years to recognize the value of Vitamin E in controlling heart disease is responsible for a tremendous amount of unnecessary suffering and for many early deaths. The interesting story of the efforts to suppress the Shute discoveries about Vitamin E illustrates the shocking bias of organized medicine against nutritional measures for achieving improved health."

Decades of Vitamin E research ignored:

1936: Vitamin E-rich wheat germ oil cures angina.
1940: Vitamin E suspected as preventive of fibroids and endometriosis, and curative of atherosclerosis.
1945: Vitamin E shown to cure hemorrhages in skin and mucous membranes, and to decrease the diabetic's need for insulin.
1946: Vitamin E greatly improves wound healing, including skin ulcers. Also demonstrated effective in cases of claudication, acute nephritis, thrombosis, cirrhosis and phlebitis. Vitamin E strengthens and regulates heartbeat.
1947: Vitamin E successfully used as therapy for gangrene, inflammation of blood vessels (Buerger's disease), retinitis and choroiditis.
1948: Vitamin E helps lupus erythematosus and shortness of breath.
1950: Vitamin E shown to be effective treatment for varicose veins, and in cases of severe body burns.
1954: The Shutes' medical textbook, *Alpha Tocopherol in Cardiovascular Disease*, is published.
1956: *The Heart and Vitamin E* is published.

The Shutes treated more than 30,000 cardiac patients over a period of more than 30 years. Their success cannot be easily dismissed. Today, the Shute Institute in London, Ontario, Canada, continues to see cardiac patients from all over the world, providing what is arguably the most thorough and successful vitamin E treatment for heart disease anywhere.

Knowing all this, people are still fed the rotten propaganda that "a cure is just around the corner" while we donate and donate in good faith to these corrupt organizations. You must realize that the only thing these pharmaceutical companies care about is their profits. They will discredit doctors and researchers trying to make a difference while lobbying politicians and the government into only approving their toxic drugs.

I hope that after reading this information you will be much more cautious in believing the baloney that is spewed from the medical establishment.

The Vitamin E Story, by Evan Shute, M.D. James C. M. Shute, editor. Forward by Linus Pauling. (Burlington, Ontario: Welch Publishing, 1985. 219 pages, softcover.) ISBN 0-920413-04-8 This book may be out of print so if you would like to acquire one you can try an internet bookseller search, or contact the Shute Institute, 367 Princess Ave., London, Ontario, Canada N6B 2A7. Email: shutemedical@lweb.net .

Natural Alpha Tocopherol (Vitamin E) in the treatment of Cardiovascular and Renal Diseases as suggested by Drs. Wilfrid and Evan Shute and the Shute Institute for Clinical and Laboratory Medicine, London, Ontario, Canada. Use only products labeled in terms of International Units (IU).

Acute coronary thrombosis: 450 to 1,600 IU a day started as soon as possible and maintained.
Older cases of coronary thrombosis: 450 to 1,600 IU if systolic pressure is under 160 Otherwise 450 IU for the first four weeks, particularly if a hypotensive agent is used concurrently.
Acute rheumatic fever: 450 to 600 IU daily.
Chronic rheumatic heart disease: give 90 IU daily first month, 120 IU daily second month and 150 IU daily for third month. 150 IU may be ideal dose. Occasionally more is necessary and advisable. Response will necessarily be slow.

Anginal Syndrome: 450 to 1,600 IU if systolic pressure is under 160. Otherwise start on 150 IU for four weeks then 300 IU for four weeks, particularly if hypotensive agent is used.
Hypertensive heart disease: 75 IU daily for four weeks, 150 IU daily for four weeks, then cautiously increase. Should be used with hypotensive agents. High doses of vitamin E have been shown to reduce high blood pressure in rats with chronic kidney failure. (Vaziri N. *Hypertension*, Jan 2002.)
Thrombophlebitis and Phlebothrombosis: 600 to 1,600 IU daily.
Thrombocytopaenic Purpura: 800 to 1,200 IU daily.
Diabetes Mellitus: Same schedule as for cardiacs.
Acute and Chronic Nephritis: Same schedule as for cardiacs.
Burns, Plastic Surgery, Mazoplasia: 600 to 1,600 IU daily, using vitamin E ointment or vitamin E spray as adjunct. (Editor's note: vitamin E may also be dripped from a thumbtack-punctured capsule.)

Among other things, vitamin E supplementation does the following:

* Reduces the oxygen requirement of tissues. Has an oxygen-sparing effect on the heart, enabling the heart can do more work on less oxygen. The benefit for recovering heart attack patients is considerable. 1,200 to 2,000 IU daily relieves angina very well.

* Gradually melts fresh clots, and prevents embolism. Vitamin E moderately prolongs prothrombin clotting time, decreases platelet adhesion, and has a limited "blood thinning" effect. This is the reason behind the Shutes' using vitamin E (1,000 - 2,000 IU/day) for thrombophlebitis and related conditions.

* Is a moderate vasodilator and improves collateral circulation and consequently offers great benefits to diabetes patients.

* Strengthens and regulates heartbeat, like digitalis and similar drugs, at a dose adjusted between 800 to 3,000 IU daily.

* Prevents scar contraction as wounds heal.

* Decreases the insulin requirement in about one-forth of diabetics.

* Stimulates muscle power.

* Preserves capillary walls.

* Reduces C-reactive protein and other markers of inflammation

* Epidemiological evidence also suggests that a daily supplement of vitamin E can reduce the risk of developing prostate cancer and Alzheimer's disease.

If everyone supplemented daily with a good quality multivitamin-multimineral, plus extra vitamins C and E, it could save **thousands** of lives a month.

CAUTIONS

The maintenance dose equals the therapeutic dose.

Do not take iron and vitamin E at same time. If iron is indicated, separate the doses by about nine hours.

The digitalis requirement is often reduced after vitamin E takes hold, so over-digitalization should be avoided. A patient receiving vitamin E should not be digitalized by the Eggleston massive dose technique nor any of its modifications. It is usually sufficient for full digitalization to give what is ordinarily a maintenance dose of 1 1/2 grains digitalis folia or 0.1 mg digitoxin per day. By the second day the patient is often digitalized.

Insulin dosages in diabetic cardiacs must be watched closely, for the insulin requirement may be considerably reduced very suddenly.

Estrogens should rarely be given at the same time as alpha tocopherol (vitamin E).

Safety of Vitamin E

The Shutes observed no evidence of harm with doses as high as 8,000 IU/day. In fact, "toxicity symptoms have not been reported even at intakes of 800 IU per kilogram of body weight daily for 5 months" according to the Food and Nutrition Board. This demonstrates a safe level would work out to be around 60,000 IU daily for an average adult, some 2,700 times the RDA! If anyone tells you Vitamin E may be toxic, they simply dont know what they are talking about.

External Uses of Vitamin E

Vitamin E is very effective on burns, first apply cold and then a vitamin E solution. You can drip the vitamin onto burned skin directly from a

Vitamin E capsule. This is sanitary, soothing and painless. Even third degree burns heal much more readily with twice-daily applications of vitamin E. Less scarring and greatly reduced inflammation are continually reported with its use. Absorption of the vitamin is best if the skin is dry before application.

For a large area of sunburned skin, mix a few 400 I.U. capsules with one or two tablespoons of olive oil. Gently rub this in as soon as possible after exposure. There will be little if any peeling if you apply this mixture promptly.

Individuals also report relief of hemorrhoids with topical use of vitamin E.

*As a side note to Vitamin E: since this vitamin is not water soluble and not able to effortlessly transfer the placental barrier as easily as other nutrients (such as B Vitamins because they are water soluble), mothers have a much higher amount of Vitamin E in their blood than do newborns. Breast milk provides the necessary method for not only a multitude of life saving nutrients but Vitamin E as well which is not found in necessary quantities in baby formulas. Breast feeding is one of the most important things a mother can do for her new born child.

Vitamin B6

"Pharmaceutical companies are very annoyed with niacin because their products have to compete with it. Some of their cholesterol-lowering drugs cost up to $150 a month while niacin costs about $10." -----Abram Hoffer, MD, PhD 1997 Interview by Peter Barry Chowka.

CLEVELAND, Nov. 14, 1995 -- People with low levels of the vitamin B6 have a greater chance of developing heart disease, a newly published study by a team of cardiologists and cell biologists at The Cleveland Clinic Foundation concludes.

Several recent studies have shown that high levels of homocysteine, an amino acid in the blood, is associated with coronary artery disease, often leading to heart attacks and strokes. Previous studies have focused on deficiency of the vitamin folic acid and its association with homocysteine. But the Clinic's study, published this week in "Circulation" magazine, indicates that the link between homocysteine and vitamin B6 is more profound.

"We have shown it is not just folic acid, but it's a vitamin B6 deficiency as well," said Killian Robinson, M.D., a cardiologist at The

Cleveland Clinic and principal investigator for the study. "It seems to be a very prevalent problem."

The study compared 304 patients (201 men and 103 women) being treated for coronary artery disease. The study found that vitamin B6 deficiency is as much a risk factor for coronary artery disease as smoking and high cholesterol. Deficiencies of folic acid and B12, which have been linked to homocysteine levels and vascular disease, were shown not to be as significant risk factors as B6 in coronary artery disease.

Magnesium deficiency http://www.execpc.com/~magnesum/index.html

"According to the U.S. National Academy of Sciences (1977) there have been more than 50 studies, in nine countries, that have indicated an inverse relationship between water hardness and mortality from cardiovascular disease. That is, people who drink water that is deficient in magnesium and calcium generally appear more susceptible to this disease. The U.S. National Academy of Sciences has estimated that a nation-wide initiative to add calcium and magnesium to soft water might reduce the annual cardiovascular death rate by 150,000 in the United States."--- Groundwater and Human Health, Groundwater Resources of British Columbia, British Columbia Ministry of the Environment.

Dr. Brian Leibovitz, Ph.D., editorialized in a recent issue of the Journal of Optimum Nutrition that magnesium: "is now recognized as a first-line medicine for the treatment of heart attacks. A study published in The Lancet, for example, reported the effects of a double-blind, randomized, placebo-controlled study in 2,316 patients with suspected myocardial infarction. The dose of magnesium was high (about 8.7 grams given intravenously over a 24 hour period), but the results were remarkable: magnesium reduced cardiovascular mortality by 25 percent. The author's conclusion: "
"Intravenous magnesium sulfate is a simple, safe, and widely applicable treatment. Its efficacy in reducing early mortality of myocardial infarction is comparable to, but independent of, that of thrombolytic or antiplatelet therapy..."

Green Smoothies

There is one food group that matches all nutritional needs of humans: **greens**. The truth is, most people do not consume even the bare minimum for green leafy vegetables. When was the last time you ate even a half cup of raw leafy greens?

I used to think that a few leaves that I put into my salad was good enough. Most people think that if they eat a small salad (usually a Greek salad with practically no dark green leaves) they are good for a few days. But we don't realize that dark leafy greens are the most important and beneficial living food that we have available. Dark greens are rich in almost all essential minerals and vitamins, as well as protein!

If you look at the composition of plants, you may notice that cellulose, the main constituent of plants, has one of the strongest molecular structures on the planet. Greens possess inside them more valuable nutrients than any other food group, but all these nutrients are stored inside the cells of the plant. These cells are very tough and are made to survive on the earth. In order for the nutrients to be released, the cell wall needs to be ruptured, which is not an easy task. If you eat plenty of greens, but you do not chew them thoroughly, you are not getting the full nutritional content of the plant. The plant needs to be swallowed in a creamy consistency to ensure full benefits.

After decades of eating mostly processed and cooked food, most modern people have lost their ability to chew normally. For some, their jaw has become too narrow or their jaw muscles have become too weak to chew through rough fiber. Not even to mention that our bodies have become so unaccustomed to eating leafy greens, that for most people they are very unpalatable. These obstacles make chewing and eating enough greens to satisfy the bodies' requirement not an easy task.

This is why blending greens in a high speed blender (especially in the high powered multi horsepower blenders) is the way to go. You can easily blend two bunches of greens with some fruits and sprouts and you have yourself a **delicious vitamin, mineral, protein, and nutrient packed drink**. Drinking 2-3 cups per day is enough to satisfy your body's requirement for most nutrients and is **one of the most important dietary additions you can add to your life**.

At first start off with a 60% fruit and 40% greens mixture, and as you get used to the taste and you body begins to actually crave greens, you can switch to a 40% fruit and 60% greens blend. Soon enough you will be drinking fully 100% green smoothies!

How to Make a Green Smoothie

The easiest way is if you acquire a small blender; they are usually around $50. The one i use was just $40, and is called "Magic Bullet" - where the cup you pour your ingredients in is what you will be mixing in and then drinking from. Makes cleanup a breeze.

1. Pour water halfway in the container.
2. Put in a handful of greens - spinach or kale.
3. Put in a banana, apples, or other fruits or berries.
4. Add your superfood or protein mix if you have it. Can also throw in some spirulina or chlorella and a teaspoon of bee pollen. A scoop of my green superfood powder has spirulina, chlorella, barley, wheatgrass, and more than 20 other superfoods.
5. Add raw coconut sugar, honey, coconut butter, or stevia for sweetness.
6. Mix all of this and drink. (If the blender doesn't mix well, just add more juice or water)

Start out by drinking one of these smoothies with your breakfast, or even as a breakfast replacement. Then start drinking 2 a day, and increase to even 3 a day.

Experiment with different combinations and varieties of fruits and veggies. But always try to include spinach, a green superfood powder, spirulina and chlorella as these have the highest amounts of nutrients, minerals, vitamins and proteins.

Benefits of Green Smoothies

- Spinach is considered a super food and one of the most nutritious live foods you can eat.
- Very easy to digest if blended well, ruptures the cell wall allowing for easy digestion and absorption.

- They are a complete food because unlike juices, they still have all the valuable fiber.
- Amongst the most palatable dishes for all people. Mixed with fruit, creates a wonderful, delicious sweet and zesty flavor. Most people are very surprised that something so green and healthy can taste so good!
- Green smoothies are chlorophyll rich. A molecule of chlorophyll closely resembles a molecule of human blood. According to Dr. Ann Wigmore, consuming chlorophyll is like receiving a healthy blood transfusion.
- They are very easy to make and cleaning up is a breeze. Consider this: spending 15 minutes making a bacon, egg and toast breakfast that has insignificant nutritional content, is full of nasty fats, and is terrible for your health, or spend 2 minutes making this amazing super-food.
- Enjoyed by people of all ages including children and babies six months or older.
- Consuming green smoothies forms a great habit for eating more greens. After a few weeks of drinking them, most people start craving and enjoying greens. Eating enough greens is often a problem for many people, and this provides a great alternative.
- Green smoothies can be consumed anywhere, just make some extra and take with you to work. They are much easier to make and much more efficient than a salad and can all fit in a small container.

Sprouts for Optimum Nutrition

Sprouts are considered as wonder foods. They rank as the freshest and most nutritious of all vegetables available to the human diet. By a process of natural transmutation, sprouted food acquires vastly improved digestibility and nutritional qualities when compared to non-sprouted embryo from which it derives. Sprouted foods have been part of the diet of many ancient races for thousands of years. Even to this day, the Chinese retain their fame for delicious mung bean sprouts. **Sprouts provide all the essential vitamins and minerals**, they are a natural multivitamin. They should form a vital component of our diet. Sprouting requires no constant care but only an occasional sprinkling of water.

All edible grains, seeds and legumes can be sprouted, if it is possible try to find ones that are organic and not genetically modified. Even if you are unable to acquire organic ones, they will still bring a ton of benefits.

Generally the following are used for sprouting :

Grains : Wheat, maize, ragi, bajra and barley.
Seeds : Alfalfa seeds, radish seeds, fenugreek seeds, carrot seeds, coriander seeds,
pumpkin seeds and muskmelon seeds.
Legumes : Mung, Bengal gram, groundnut and peas.

Alfalfa, as the name in Arabic signifies, is the king of all sprouts. Grown as a plant, its roots areknown to burrow as much as 12 meters into the subsoil to bring up valuable trace minerals of which manganese is especially important to health and digestion ; it is a vital component of human insulin. Apart from minerals, alfalfa is also a rich source of vitamins A,B,C,E and K and amino acids. Sesame seeds are another good source of nourishment. They contain all the essential amino acids in their 20 per cent protein content, and higher concentration of calcium than milk. They are high in letichin, unsaturated fats, vitamin E and vitamin B complex, besides other live nutrients.

How to Sprout

As a first step, a good variety of seeds should be used for sprouting. It should be ensured that the seeds, legumes or grains are of the sproutable type.

Soyabeans do not sprout well as they often become sour (soybeans should not be used at all in the diet, including soymilk). Wheat has to be grown in soil. It is advisable to use seeds which are not chemically treated as this slows down the germination rate. The seeds should be washed thoroughly and then soaked overnight in a jar of pure water. The jar should be covered with a cheesecloth or wire screening. The duration of soaking will depend upon the size of the seed.

You may place the seeds on a plate or in a jar with a little bit of water; the seeds must not be fully immersed in water. The seeds must not be in direct sunlight and must be covered. The seeds will expand about eight times their original size. It should also be ensured that the mouth of the jar is not completely covered so as to allow air in. The seeds should be rinsed and water replaced every day until fully sprouted.

Seeds are at their optimum level of flavour, tenderness, and nutritional value when a few millimetres has sprouted. To retain their freshness and nutritional value, they should be placed in a refrigerator, if they cannot be consumed immediately after reaching suitable maturity. It is best to eat sprouts fresh.

The main factors for sprouting are water, air, heat and darkness. There may be poor germination or no germination at all if any of these factors are not present such as insufficient water, or too much water, lack of sufficient heat, lack of fresh air, either too cold or too hot surroundings and too much light.

Benefits

There is an amazing increase in nutrients in sprouted foods when compared to their dried embryo. In the process of sprouting, the vitamins, minerals and protein increase substantially with corresponding decrease in calories and carbohydrate content. These comparisons are based on an equivalent water content in the foods measured. Analysis of dried seeds, grains and legumes shows a very low water content. But this increases up to tenfold when the same food is converted into sprouts. For accurate comparison each must be brought to a common denomination of equal water content to assess the exact change brought in nutritional value.

Sprouted mung beans, for instance, have a 8.3 increase of water content over dried beans. Hence the nutritional value of sprouted and dried mung beans can be compared by multiplying the analysed nutrients of sprouted mung beans by the factor of 8.3. Based on this criterion, the changes found in sprouted mung beans when compared with the figures for the beans in the dried state are as follows :

Energy content - calories Decrease 15 per cent.
Total carbohydrate content - Decrease 15 per cent
Protein availability - Increase 30 per cent
Calcium content - Increase 34 per cent
Potassium content - Increase 80 per cent
Sodium content - Increase 690 per cent
Iron content - Increase 40 per cent
Phosphorous content - Increase 56 per cent
Vitamin A content - Increase 285 per cent
Thiamine or Vitamin B1 content - Increase 208 per cent
Riboflavin or Vitamin B2 content - Increase 515 per cent
Niacin or Vitamin B3 content - Increase 256 per cent
Ascorbic acid or Vitamin C content - An infinite increase

The increase in protein availability is of great significance. It is a valuable indicator of the enhanced nutritional value of a food when sprouted. The simultaneous reduction in carbohydrate content indicates that many carbohydrate molecules are broken down during sprouting to allow absorption of atmospheric nitrogen and reforming into amino-acids.

The resultant protein is the most easily digestible of all proteins available in foods. Want a perfectly balanced and very inexpensive protein shake along with vitamins, nutrients, and minerals? Have some sprouts! There is also an increase in sodium content in sprouted seeds (not sodium chloride as in table salt). Sodium is essential to the digestive process within the gastro-intestinal tract and also to the elimination of carbon dioxide. Together with the remarkable increase in vitamins, sodium materially contributes to the easy digestibility of sprouts.

Dried seeds, grains and legumes do not contain discernible traces of ascorbic acid (vitamin C), yet when sprouted, they reveal quite significant quantities which are important in the body's ability to metabolise proteins. The infinite increase in ascorbic acid derives from their absorption of atmospheric elements during growth. Sprouts have several other benefits. They supply food in predigested form, that is, the food which has already been acted upon by the enzymes and made to digest easily. During sprouting, much of the starch is broken down into simple sugars such as glucose and sucrose by the action of the enzyme 'amylase'. Proteins are converted into amino acids and amides. Fats and oils are converted into more simple fatty acids by the action of the enzyme lipase.

During sprouting, the beans lose their objectionable gas producing quality. Research has shown that oligosaccharides are responsible for gas formation. For maintenance of health, some amount of gas production is necessary but it should be within safe limits. As the process of germination ends and sprouting begins, the percentage of oligosaccharides is reduced by 90%. Sprouts contain a lot of fibre and water and, therefore, are helpful in overcoming constipation.

Sprouts are an extremely inexpensive method of obtaining a concentration of vitamins, minerals and enzymes. They have in them all the constituent nutrients of fruits and vegetables and are 'live' foods. Eating sprouts is the safest and best way of getting the advantage of both fruits and vegetables without contamination and harmful insecticides.

It should, however, be ensured that seeds and dried beans are purchased from a store where they are fresh, unsprayed, not genetically modified, preferably organic, and packaged as food. Seeds that are packaged for planting purposes may contain mercury compounds or other toxic chemicals.

Health Fasting

Health fasting is the most beneficial cleansing routine you can do, not **one** of the most beneficial, **the most** beneficial. It is the quickest and strongest way to detoxify your body.

Fasting refers to complete abstinence from food and water for a short or long period for a specific purpose. The word is derived from the old English, 'feastan' which means to fast, observe, be strict. Fasting is nature's oldest, most effective and yet least expensive method of treating disease. It is recognised as the cornerstone of natural healing. Dr. Arnold Eheret, the originator of the muscusless diet healing system, describes it as "nature's only universal and omnipotent remedy of healing" and "nature's only fundamental law of all healing and curing. "

The practice of fasting is one of the most ancient customs. It is followed in almost every religion. The Mohammedan, the Buddhists, the Hindus and many others have their periods of strict fasting. The saints of medieval times laid great stress on this method.

Fasting during a state of disease was advocated by the school of natural philosopher, Asclepiades, more than two thousand years ago. Throughout medical history, it has been regarded as one of the most dependable curative methods. Hippocrates, Galen, Paracelsus and many other great authorities on medicine prescribed it. Many noted modern physicians have successfully employed this system of healing in the treatment of numerous diseases.

The common cause of all diseases is the accumulation of waste and poisonous matter in the body which results from eating cooked and dead food. Digestion and elimination become slow and the functional activity of the whole system gets disturbed. The onset of disease is merely the **process of ridding the system of these impurities, poisons, and toxins**.

Every disease can be healed by only one remedy - by doing just the opposite of what causes it, that is, by reducing the food intake or fasting. By depriving the body of food for a time, the organs of elimination such as the bowels, kidneys, skin and lungs are given opportunity to expel the overload of accumulated waste from the system. Thus, fasting is merely the process of purification and the most effective cure for almost all diseases and ailments. It assists nature in her continuous effort to expel foreign matter and disease producing waste from the body, thereby correcting the faults of improper diet and wrong living. It also leads to regeneration of the blood as well as the repair and regeneration of the various tissues of the body.

Duration

The duration of the fast depends upon the age of the patient, the nature of the disease and the amount and type of drugs previously used. The duration is important, because long periods of fasting can be dangerous if undertaken without being properly prepared. It is, therefore, advisable to undertake a series of short fasts of two to three days and gradually increase the duration of each succeeding fast by a few days. It is absolutely fine for most people to start with a 3 day dry or water fast, and increase each succeeding fast to 5, 7, 9, 14, 21 or more days.

This will enable the chronically sick body to gradually and slowly eliminate toxic waste matter without seriously affecting the natural functioning of the body. A correct mode of living and a raw food diet after the fast will restore your vigour and vitality. Fasting is highly beneficial in practically all kinds of stomach and intestinal disorders and in serious conditions of the kidneys and liver. It is a miracle cure for eczema and other skin diseases and offers the only hope of permanent cure in many cases. The various nervous disorders also respond favourably to this mode of treatment.

However, there are a few things you must know and take into account before doing a fast. The exit from a fast is as important as the fast itself, because if you exit the fast the wrong way, you can actually do more damage to your body than when you started.

The starting phase is not as important; you can either start right away without a transition stage, or you can choose a transition stage when you ease your body into the fast. The exit is the most important aspect to consider; **the exit transition must be at least as long as the fast itself.**

A precautionary measure which must be observed in all cases of fasting is the complete emptying of the bowels at the beginning of the fast by enema so that the patient is not bothered by gas or decomposing matter formed from the excrements remaining in the body. You can by an enema kit at most pharmacies. The proper way to do an enema is as follows; fill it with lukewarm water, lube the tip and insert. When there is no more water in the container you may stand up and walk around, you may also do a simple stomach massage by pressing with your hands all over your stomach to help fecal matter easily pass through. As you wait you may experience a few strong needs to expel, wait until the 3rd strong urge before you go.

During the fast it is strongly advised to get as much rest as possible because you will experience fatigue and drowsiness. The only time you may break a fast is when you experience severe headache or dizziness in which case you may drink some clean water or a small amount of a freshly squeezed juice. Sun and air baths should be taken frequently. During a dry fast (no liquids at all) do not take any showers or baths.

Benefits

There are several benefit of fasting. During a long fast, the body feeds upon its reserves. Being deprived of needed nutrients, particularly of protein and fats, it will burn and digest its own tissues by the process of autolysis or self-digestion. But it will not do so indiscriminately. The body will first decompose and burn those cells and tissues which are diseased, damaged, aged or dead, and it will starve all the bacteria and parasites in your body.

The essential tissues and vital organs, the glands, the nervous system and the brain are not damaged in fasting. Here lies the secret of the effectiveness of fasting as a curative and rejuvenating method. The capacity of the eliminative organs, that is, lungs, liver, kidneys and the skin is greatly increased as they are relieved of the usual burden of digesting food and eliminating the resultant wastes. They are, therefore, able to quickly expel old accumulated wastes and toxins. Fasting affords a physiological rest to the digestive, assimilative and protective organs. As a result, the digestion of food and the utilisation of nutrients is greatly improved after fasting.

The fast also exerts a normalising, stabilising and rejuvenating effect on all the vital physiological, nervous and mental functions. Fasting is the key to health and vitality, if you want to actually be younger, and not just look younger, then fasting is the answer.

Experiments showed that in cases of fasting or inadequate food intake, the small intestine begins producing melatonin which is well known to have anti-aging properties. With the intake of this hormone, tumours, fibromas, fibromyomas and cysts disappear, mastopathy and insomnia vanish. Animal experiments show this hormone to rejuvenate and defy aging. With age the quantity of melatonin in our bodies decreases. With a reduction below 20% of total normal levels, leukocytes are unable to recognize parasites and bacteria; oncology begins. This is why cleanses and periodic fasts are absolutely necessary for our bodies, they will literally make you younger.

During cleanses and fasting, the skin goes through an intense cleaning process. But there needs to be sweating for the excretion of many toxins out of the skin, which is why it is very important to sweat so the cells can easily excrete whatever toxins that might have accumulated. If you are unable to attend a sauna, and do not exercise, then you must take at least 2 showers in the morning and afternoon. It is very important to take a shower before 9am in the morning because during the night our bodies naturally detoxify, releasing toxins to the surface of the skin. If you do not take a shower before 9am, the skin will absorb all the toxins right back. If you are unable to take a shower then wipe yourself down with a damp towel.

The best health fasting rated by effectiveness are as follows; a dry fast, a water fast, a juice fast.

If you think you are ready, if you have done long fasts before, and you are healthy, then you can go on a 21 day dry fast followed by a 21 day water fast. This 42 day fast is the quickest way to totally clean up your physical body from all the bacteria, germs, and parasites, and totally rejuvenate every single organ and tissue to a baby like state. It is also the quickest way to clean your nadis (energy channels), and other metaphysical bodies such as your astral body.

3 Day Fast (with entry transition)

3 days before beginning – Eliminate all animal products from your diet, only grains, fruits, vegetables, oils, and nuts/seeds.

2 days before beginning – Eliminate all grains from your diet, only fruits, vegetables, oils, and nuts

1 day before beginning – Eliminate all oils and nuts from your diet, only fruits and vegetables

Start the 3 days of fasting, either dry or water, or a mix with 1 day dry, 1 day water, and 1 day dry.

After the 3 days of fasting, the first exit day is very important.

- Start with a 50 ml of water in the morning
- 30 minutes later drink 50 ml

- 30 minutes later drink 100 ml
- 1 hour later you can drink up to 250 ml
- 1 hour later you can drink as much water as you like throughout the day

Day 2 - You may drink freshly squeezed fruit/vegetable (do not mix fruits with vegetables) juices during the first half of the day and add fresh fruits or vegetables later

Day 3 – You may add nuts and oils

Day 4 – You may add cheeses, milk products, grains, and seeds

If you have already done dry fasting like this before then you can do a 5 or 7 day dry fast.

5 Day Fast

-3 – Eliminate all animal products from your diet, only grains, fruits, vegetables, oils, and nuts/seeds.

-2 – Eliminate all grains from your diet, only fruits, vegetables, oils, and nuts

-1 – Eliminate all oils and nuts from your diet, only fruits and vegetables

5 days of fasting, either dry or water, or a mix with 2 days dry, 1 day water, and 2 days dry.

+1 – The first exit day is very important.

- Start with a 50 ml of water in the morning
- 30 minutes later drink 50 ml
- 30 minutes later drink 50 ml
- 1 hour later drink 50 ml
- 1 hour later drink 100 ml
- 1 hour later you can drink up to 250 ml
- 1 hour later you can drink as much water as you like throughout the day

+2 – Drink only water or freshly squeezed fruit/vegetable (do not mix fruits with vegetables) juices

+3 – You may add fresh fruits and vegetables

+4 – You may add oils

+5 – You may add nuts

+6 – You may add grains/seeds

+7 – You may add cheeses and milk products

Beneficial and positive symptoms of fasting; headache, severe fatigue, blood pressure changes, heart arrhythmias, diarrhea, and others. There is a golden rule; the more fatigue you feel, the better your cleansing process is activated, so do not be alarmed when you feel severe fatigue, it means you body is working hard to detoxify.

Headaches, fatigue, and various pains do not occur because you are receiving inadequate amounts of energy, they happen because your body is detoxifying. This may take a while, and the symptoms may vary depending on what chronic illnesses you are carrying deep within your tissues. Some people feel weightless and full of energy, while others are lying in bed for weeks with high fever. It all depends on how much toxins your body will have to get rid of. The symptoms are different but everyone who switches can agree on the following; no disease, weight loss, energy levels are through the roof, a positive mood, skin becomes younger, and people constantly noticing the differences.

It is recommended that everyone do a 3 day fast once every month, that's unless you are on a 100% raw food diet for more than two-three years in which case you don't need to detoxify as your body is already clean.

Oil pulling

Oil pulling is a thousand year old Ayurvedic cleansing treatment that has been used by millions of people all around the world for amazing health benefits. It is so simple and so inexpensive anyone can perform this absolutely anywhere, all you need is a few spoonfuls of vegetable oil and 5 minutes a day. Dr. Bruce Fife, whose written an entire book on oil pulling, says the oil acts like a detox sponge.

"When you put it in your mouth and work it around your teeth and gums it "pulls" out bacteria and other debris. As simple as it is, oil pulling has a very powerful detoxifying effect. Our mouths are the home to billions of bacteria, viruses, fungi and other parasites and their toxins. Candida and Streptococcus are common residents in our mouths. It is these types of germs and their toxic waste products that cause gum disease and tooth decay and contribute to many other health problems including arthritis and heart disease. Our immune system is constantly fighting these troublemakers. If our immune system becomes overloaded or burdened by excessive stress, poor diet, environmental toxins and such, these organisms can spread throughout the body causing secondary infections and chronic inflammation, leading to any number of health problems."

The method consists of vigorously swishing vegetable oil (sunflower or sesame seed) in the mouth for 5-10 minutes. The movement of oil sucks up bacteria, germs, viruses, toxins, hormones, chemicals and heavy metals through the tissues, blood vessels, tongue, and mucous membranes in the mouth while the vitamins and minerals of the sunflower oil are absorbed.

Dr. F. Karach reports extraordinary success with the method of oil pulling on the following diseases: Headaches, bronchitis, thrombosis, asthma, cardiovascular diseases, chronic blood disorders, arthritis and other rheumatic diseases, eczema, stomach ulcers, chronic intestinal diseases, heart and Nierenbe complaints, gynecological illnesses, neurological diseases and liver diseases, and even **cancer**.

By reducing the toxic load through the elimination of toxins from our bodies our immune system is stimulated which allows all other systems and organs to work at optimal levels.

Oral Ecology

"It's amazing what you can see if you look carefully," says Mager, a fellow in oral medicine at the Forsyth Institute, an independent research institution in Boston. The view reveals hundreds of different kinds of bacteria, viruses, yeast, fungi, and other micro-organisms. Forsyth scientists, most of whom are on the faculty of the Harvard School of Dental Medicine, have found 615 different species of bacteria - and they're still counting.

It's a great place for micropests to dwell. Glistening white plateaus, dark crevices, and slimy surfaces boast steamy temperatures of 95 degrees Fahrenheit. The microbes bathe in a saliva-induced humidity of 100 percent, and eat a lavish diet of sugar and other carbohydrates. It's so lush and varied, Mager refers to it as a mini-jungle.
"In one mouth, the number of bacteria can easily exceed the number of people who live on Earth (more than 6 billion)," notes Sigmund Socransky, associate clinical professor of periodontology at Harvard. "These bugs don't colonize your mouth in a random way; rather, they form communities in a pattern that is dictated both by other bugs and by the environment. Bacteria affect their environment, and the environment affects them. Although they touch each other, the floor of the mouth is populated by different communities than the bottom of the tongue, and the top of the tongue hosts a biota unlike that on the roof of your mouth."

Years of detecting and identifying mouth tenants have revealed that those living in healthy mouths can be remarkably different from those living in diseased mouths. Some bacteria increase in number, while others decrease. By comparing communities of microbes in healthy people with those in the mouths of those with oral cancer, Mager has found a pattern that she expects will lead to the early diagnosis of oral cancers.

Bacteria and other microorganisms don't select our mouths, our mouths select them. The conditions in our mouths create an environment that favors certain types of organisms and allows them to grow and flourish. A healthy mouth (and healthy body) is filled with relatively benign bacteria for the most part. An unhealthy mouth attracts harmful bacteria. If you want to have a healthier mouth and body, you must change the environment in your mouth.

Researchers have tried various ways to alter the micro-populations in people's mouths. These populations can be altered *temporarily* by cleaning your teeth, using antiseptic mouthwashes, and even taking antibiotics. However, the ordinary inhabitants and their relative proportions to each other quickly reestablish themselves. Killing oral bacteria helps to reduce their numbers, but it does not change the types of organisms that thrive in the mouth.

By literally pulling out the germs and microbes from the mouth and toxins from the blood you are helping your body to detox while stimulating your immune system.

The Method

In the morning before breakfast on an empty stomach and after drinking a glass of clean filtered water, take one tablespoon in the mouth and begin to swish it around. Move the oil slowly and vigorously in the mouth as rinsing or swishing and Dr Karach puts it as "sip, suck and pull through the teeth" for fifteen to twenty minutes.

This process makes oil thoroughly mixed with saliva. Swishing activates the enzymes and the enzymes draw toxins out of the blood. The oil must not be swallowed, for it has become toxic. As the process continues, the oil gets thinner and white. If the oil is still yellow, it has not been pulled long enough. It is then spit from the mouth , the oral cavity must be thoroughly rinsed and mouth must be washed thoroughly. Just use normal tap water and good old fingers to clean.

Spit out in the trash, compost bin, or outside in the grass. The spittle contains harmful bacteria and toxic bodily waste. If one were to see one drop of this liquid magnified 600 times under a microscope, one would see microbes in their first stage of development.

Oil pulling intensifies your metabolism which leads to improved health. One of the most striking results of this process is the fastening of loose teeth, the elimination of bleeding gums and the visible whitening of the teeth.
The oil pulling /swishing is done best before breakfast. To accelerate the healing process, it can be repeated three times a day, but always before meals on an empty stomach.

Some people are not used to the strong texture and flavor of oil so if you have the gag reflex, don't fret, it will subside in a few days, just stick with it!

You can swish the oil while going about your regular morning routine. After you wake up and brush your teeth, put some oil in your mouth and begin to swish. Hold the oil as much as you can, the more the better, but if you can only do it for 5 minutes than it is better than nothing. You can use this method while at work, while walking your dog, watching TV, or doing something around the house.

For more information visit www.oilpulling.com

Enema and Colon Hydrotherapy

Colonic Hydrotherapy, also known as Colonic Irrigation, is a natural way to aid health and feel clean and balanced. Colon therapy has been used for centuries by European, Middle Eastern, and Far Eastern people for personal purification, health, and religious pursuits. Today, it is being used in alternative and naturopathic therapies for cancer treatment, candida and constipation, irritable bowel syndrome, and to ease labor and childbirth.

They are used for many conditions such as constipation, diarrhea, colitis, irritable bowel syndrome, painful menstruation, headaches, depression, toxicity, colds, parasitic infections, flu, sore throats, PMS, fever, dehydration, allergies, Candida, preparation for childbirth, and to stimulate the immune system to maximize health.

The colon is called the large intestine and is about 5-6 feet in length. The small intestine is wrapped around the colon and fits below the diaphragm (under the solar plexus all the way to the bladder) totalling about 30 feet. The colon cannot feel cold, heat, burning, or cutting, it can only sense stretching as with gas pains.

Benefits of Colon Hydrotherapy for Cancer

Colonic Hydrotherapy is especially useful in treating cancer patients. Colonics improve circulatory functions, stimulate the immune system, remove toxic waste, stimulate appetite, eliminate headaches, and boost energy.

When we eat a nutritionally deficient diet, the unused waste stagnates in the colon and the body absorbs these toxins. The organs in the body responsible for purification, such as the liver, kidneys, lungs, and skin, work overtime trying to purge the waste. This can result in a variety of illnesses.

Removing carcinogenic toxins from the body and boosting the immune system are paramount during illness, especially cancer. With cancer, large tumors can break and cause necrotic areas, formed of dead tissue. Since the body expels these toxic byproducts through the colon, it's vital to keep the colon flushed out with a cleansing colonic irrigation.

If a patient is weakened from the disease, frequent colonics help relieve the colon's toxic burden during the patient's healing process. But remember, colonic hydrotherapy is not a cure, nor should it be the only treatment for cancer. With a disease as serious as cancer, concurrent care under a physician is advisable.

Why Use Colonics for Cancer?

The American diet—full of processed foods, saturated fats, salt, bleached bread, additives, and artificial colors—leaves the colon clogged and stressed. Undigested food in the colon can ferment and putrefy, encouraging bacteria and toxins. Add to that a habitual lack of exercise and not drinking enough water and the result is constipation or diarrhea.

Colon Hydrotherapy releases congestion in the bowel, encourages beneficial intestinal flora, and detoxifies the body to improve overall health. After a colonic, people report feeling lighter in body and spirit, clean, clear headed, healthy, and even euphoric. Other benefits of colonics include less headaches, better mental clarity, better weight management, and relief from abdominal cramps, rheumatoid arthritis, and allergies.

The colonic procedure involves insertion of a disposable speculum connected to a hose into the rectum and the release of a solution, usually made of warm water or water and baking soda, to flush out the intestinal tract and upper bowel. The colon is flushed repeatedly to gently loosen fecal matter and flush away toxins.

Colonics for Cancer Prevention

Colonic Hydrotherapy can also be used as a preventative measure for cancers of the colon, liver, and digestive system, as well as for general health. When we normally move our bowels, we do not entirely empty the colon and material is left behind. A colonic flushes away what is left over, cleaning the body of waste and toxins that can build up and promote the growth of cancer cells.

Along with a healthy diet and exercise program, regular colonics are part of a proactive plan to ward off disease and promote well-being. A generally healthy person can undergo a colonic once every few months to maintain good health.

Q: How might I feel after the treatment?

How people feel after the treatment varies enormously. Some are ready to play for England, others would like to climb under the duvet for the rest of the day. You can feel a bit cold or shivery. Sometimes the treatment initiates emotional release as our feelings are often stored in the gut. You can then feel a bit vulnerable. After the first one or two treatments it becomes easier, and some fit it in their lunch break.

Q: How many sessions do I need?

It really depends on the condition of the bowel and how it responds to the treatment how many exactly are needed. It has taken a lifetime to build up the matter in the colon, so it is reasonable to expect that it will take a number of sessions to remove it. For healthy people 4 to 6 sessions will usually give a good clear out. Clients who take it further will always gain more! People with IBS sometimes respond quite well whereas others need more sessions. For any serious condition a treatment plan can be made in consultation with the therapist.

Q: Would enema's help me as well?

Yes, as an addition to colon hydrotherapy enema's can work quite well. Enema's cannot be compared to colon hydrotherapy though. Colon hydrotherapy inserts 20 or 30 gallons of water into the colon in one treatment and cleanses the bowel far better and far deeper. If you are unable to afford a colon hydrotherapy treatment an enema would be a great option (enema kits available at www.theictm.org)

Q: Will it make the bowel lazy?

No, it is an exercise for the bowel. Stimulation, contraction and relaxation will help tone and reshape the colon to aid incomplete elimination.

Q: Will it wash out all the good bacteria?

It will wash out some good bacteria as it will wash out lots of bad bacteria. In a healthy person the good bacteria will reproduce itself within 2-3 days especially now that the environment is cleaner. Probiotics or prebiotics may be recommended if it seems appropriate. In cases of candida or when antibiotics have recently been used a probiotic implant can be made and good bacteria placed directly into the clean bowel at the end of the treatment.

It is absolutely imperative that you conduct a **full bowel cleanse** before starting the cancer diet because your body will be going through a heavy detoxification process which will need a clean colon for proper toxin elimination. Dead cancer cells, chemicals, hormones, pollutants, and other waste will be leaving your body in very large amounts and a clean colon will make your cancer healing journey much easier.

If you can't afford a hydrotherapy treatment, I recommend an enema every few days for up to 8 treatments, then a month off and again 8 more treatments.

Home Enemas

Home enemas have been used for centuries as an inexpensive and effective treatment for a variety of diseases and illnesses due to its powerful cleansing and immune boosing effects.

Everyone has their own individual capacity, and it will change from one enema session to the next. However, the average amount of water one can usually comfortably retain is two quarts. This will vary depending on the amount of gas and waste in the colon. The most important thing to remember is never attempt to take in more water than is comfortable to retain. Initially, it may be difficult to retain the water for more than five minutes at a time. Later on, you will be able to work up to ten or fifteen minutes retention time.

Positions

Positions for taking an enema can vary with each individual's needs. Here are the three most common positions used.

Sims' Position
Lying on the left side, with right knee at about 90 degree angle, and left knee slightly bent.
POSITIVE: Less pressure on the abdomen.
NEGATIVE: Water remains mostly in the lower length of the colon (sigmoid and descending)

Knee-Chest Position
Body supported by the knees and the shoulders with chest nearly touching the floor.
POSITIVE: Gravity allows water to flow further along to the transverse colon and flexures. Allows air or gas to float up for ease of expulsion.
NEGATIVE: Not a comfortable position for an extended length of time.

Lying on the Back
Pillows under the head, knees raised or flat.

POSITIVE: The most comfortable position, allows you to massage the abdomen, water can reach the entire length of the colon.

NEGATIVE: Some pressure on the abdomen (can be relieved with gentle massage and by turning on either side).

Preparation and Procedures

Prepare the area where you will receive the enema — either bed or bathroom floor, or bathtub. Spread blankets or towels and a pillow or two for your head for comfort and warmth and cover with a vinyl sheet or large plastic garbage bag. Also, a blanket or extra large towel can be used to cover yourself. Keeping warm and comfortable is your first priority.

Prepare a pitcher with warm purified water Attach tubing to enema bag. Attach tip to tubing. (The larger tip will allow for filling without having to hold it in the rectum while lying on the back). Release valve on tubing over sink to release any trapped air.

Hang enema bag no higher than two feet above the rectum. Hanging it higher causes the fluid to flow out with too much pressure. Lubricate several inches of the tip.

Attempt to have a bowel movement and empty the bladder before the enema. A full bladder or colon makes taking an enema difficult and/or hard to fill.

Insert tip about two inches or so into the rectum in the direction toward the belly button. Do not use force; if there is any resistance, change the direction and re-insert. While in the Sims position, release the water very slowly into the rectum in this position, or roll onto the back position.

Attempt to take in as much fluid as tolerable and retain it for about five minutes. Gently massage the abdomen; rotate from back to left side and back, and onto right side and back throughout the process. Sit on the toilet and expel the enema and repeat the process until you have finished the first bag of water. Refill bag with pitcher of warm water and repeat the process, attempting to take in and retain more fluid for up to fifteen minutes. Repeat the process with the last pitcher of fluid, or use implant solutions.

Never try to forcibly hold in the enema. Expel the enema at any time you wish to do so. Nothing in this entire process should involve force or strain. This entire process should take approximately one half-hour per bag of water, or an hour and a half for a full three-bag session.

Changing positions can sometimes take the pressure off the urge to expel by moving the fluid around the entire length of the colon. You will be able to experiment with this as you become more comfortable with taking enemas.

Always thoroughly cleanse your equipment after each use and hang to dry before putting away.

Hydrogen Peroxide

Hydrogen peroxide is commonly used in an enema to kill parasites, germs, yeast infections (candida), and turbo boost the detox process. I always recommend hydrogen peroxide with an enema.

If you are going to use hydrogen peroxide (h2o2) in your enema regimen use only food grade hydrogen peroxide.

Using hydrogen peroxide in an enema is probably going to produce some gas in the large intestine. Causing some minor discomfort.

The 3% hydrogen peroxide (H2O2) available in grocery and drug stores on the shelf contain stabilizers (such as phenol, acetanilide, sodium stanate and Tetrasodium phosphate). This hydrogen peroxide is for external use only, not for internal use.

Three tablespoons of 3% food grade hydrogen peroxide mixed with a quart of filtered water makes a good enema or douche recipe.
Enema Recipe:
6 tbsp. 3% - H2O2
2 quarts (about 1.9 liters) warm filtered water (Mix well)

Enema solution Temperature 103° Fahrenheit at time of injection.
Dr. Kelley summarizes the effect,

> *"Essentially, the coffee enemas help the liver perform a task for which it was not designed — that of elimination in 1 or 2 years the accumulated wastes from many years of living in ignorance of the laws of nature."*

Coffee Enemas

There is some controversy over coffee enemas in the medical world. There are concerns over rectal infections, electrolyte imbalance, colitis, and possible heart failure. On Wikipedia, it says "The use of coffee enemas has led to several deaths as a result of severe electrolyte imbalance."

Dr. Gonzalez says he has researched the entire world's medical literature on coffee enemas and he found only 3 deaths attributed to this treatment. He also said in an interview that these 3 claims were quite dubious because the patients were already very sick from other complications, and 1 of the patients wildly overdid the coffee enema. If you compare this to the fact that literally hundreds of thousands of people have done coffee enemas through Dr. Gerson, Dr. Kelley, Dr. Gonzalez (these doctors are discussed in '*The Big Cancer Lie*'), and many others, with little to no problems, I would be skeptical to the motive behind the negative report on Wikipedia. Remember, very little money can be made off enemas, so as is pretty common with any successful alternative cancer technique, you find conventional websites like Wikipedia overemphasizing the problems, and underemphasizing the success.

Dr. Lawrence Wilson M.D. summarizes his use of coffee enemas,

"I have recommended coffee retention enemas to more than thirty thousand people. I have yet to hear about horrible side effects of any kind, although the procedure is somewhat inconvenient, especially at first. Most people get used to it quickly. The coffee retention enema is really quite simple, very safe when done properly, highly effective, able to be done in the privacy of your home, and inexpensive."

Inexpensive is not something cancer drug companies want to hear. Dr. Kelley also recommended a kidney cleanse, lung cleanse, skin cleanse, and nostril cleanse. See http://www.drkelley.com/CANLIVER55.html for details.

Heart Disease

Selenium

Selenium has been shown to be protective against heart disease by animal studies, epidemiological studies, lab animal studies, and human clinical studies. Selenium helps in maintaining the integrity of heart and artery tissue, regulation of blood pressure, regulation of blood clotting, and the reduction of plaque or cholestrol deposits in arteries.

Noninvasive heart centre http://www.heartprotect.com/

Angiograms

Dr. Wayne describes an important reason why bypass surgery and the use of stents may be considered obsolete. It is because of the heart's natural ability through angiogenesis to develop a network of new blood vessels around narrowed or occluded arteries. These tiny vessels are often referred to as collateral vessels, and are too small to be seen on an angiogram. Nevertheless, in spite of their small size, they are capable of delivering all the blood that is needed to the heart muscle. This is why although a coronary artery may appear to be blocked on an angiogram, there is no blockage of blood flow. In a sense the heart has put in its own bypasses allowing the heart muscle to function in a perfectly normal manner even if its main blood supply is is blocked. Yet the angiogram is unable to see these tiny collateral vessels because the technique cannot image blood vessels this small. It is also unable to image heart muscle because it is an x-ray, and x-rays cannot image muscle tissue. Thus, the coronary angiogram is unable to determine if the heart muscle supplied by an occluded coronary artery is functioning normally. It follows that this very dangerous and expensive test is useless as a diagnostic procedure. Yet it continues to be performed in over two million patients a year.

Dr. Wayne tells us that following these two million angiograms there are 5,000 heart attacks, 5,000 strokes, and 30,000 other vascular accidents. There are also 59,000 cases of kidney failure that require dialysis due to the toxic effect of the dye used in the angiogram on the kidney. The result is 7,000 needless deaths as a result of an unnecessary test. Yet, sadly, the only tests that are needed for the diagnosis and treatment of coronary artery disease can be obtained cheaply and safely with modern noninvasive imaging procedures, which cost only a small fraction of the cost of an angiogram, and without its dangers. Considering the fact that all cardiologists are required to perform 50-75 angiograms a year to maintain their hospital privileges, or they lose their privileges to perform this test and the income it provides ($10,000-$15,000), it is not hard to understand why most cardiologists urge all patients to have an immediate angiogram before they have a massive heart attack. Some have been known to schedule an angiogram even before seeing the patient.

None of Dr. Wayne's patients has undergone surgery in over 10 years, and none has had a major heart attack in 12 years!

"DO YOU REALLY NEED BYPASS SURGERY? A SECOND OPINION"
Howard H. Wayne, M.D., M. S., F.A.C.C., F.C.C.P., F.A.C.P.
Director, Noninvasive Heart Center
San Diego, California

In his book he clearly states that:

- The belief that bypass surgery is the only treatment for coronary artery disease is no longer true.
- That symptom relief after bypass surgery has nothing to do with the bypass procedure, and is due to numerous other factors.
- That the true frequency of complications after bypass surgery such as stroke and loss of cognitive function is as high as 30%.
- That the angiogram is the most inaccurate and dangerous test in cardiology, and frequently leads to unnecessary bypass surgery.
- That the heart can develop its own bypasses with proper medical treatment assuring a normal life span and life style.
- Despite new drugs and more sensitive diagnostic tests, patients with recent onset of chest pain who undergo stent insertion or bypass surgery have a 43% higher mortality compared to 25 years ago without these interventions.

Surgery, angiograms, stent insertions and other invasive procedures are big business for the medical mafia. There is no reason for them to tell you to take some vitamins which cost a few dollars, fix your diet which in most cases is free, when they can make thousands with surgery and toxic drugs.

Lower Your Cholesterol – Naturally!

What is a safe, inexpensive, nonprescription, convenient and effective way to reduce high cholesterol levels and reduce heart disease risk? Niacin (Vitamin B3)!

Niacin is a water-soluble B-complex vitamin, vitamin B-3. One of Niacin's unique properties is the ability to help you relax and fall asleep more quickly at night.

It is well known that niacin helps reduce the harmful cholesterol levels in the bloodstream since it is one of the best substances for elevating the "good" cholesterol HDL (high density lipoprotein). The finding that niacin indeed does lower cholesterol was confirmed by Parsons, Achor, Berge, McKenzie and Barker (1956) and Parsons (1961, 1961a, 1962) at the Mayo Clinic, which launched niacin on its way as a cholesterol lowering substance.

Since then it has been found to be a normalizing agent, meaning it elevates high density lipoprotein cholesterol, decreases low density and very low density lipoprotein cholesterol and lowers triglycerides. Grundy, Mok, Zechs and Berman (1981) found it lowered cholesterol by 22 percent and triglycerides by 52 percent and wrote, "**To our knowledge, no other single agent has such potential for lowering both cholesterol and triglycerides**." If the medical mafia actually wanted you to become healthy, this would have been on the front pages of the New York Times and Niacin would be taken all over the world to safely reduce cholesterol and help millions of people. But that would put them out of business, so you never hear anything about it.

It is well known that high cholesterol levels are associated with increased risk of developing heart disease. In addition to niacin, a typical diet to help keep cholesterol down as generally recommended by orthomolecular physicians can be described as a high fiber, sugar-free diet which is rich in complex carbohydrates such as vegetables and whole grains.

It is even possible to lower cholesterol levels with niacin without any changes to your diet. Boyle, then working with the National Institutes of Health in Washington, D.C., became very interested in niacin. He followed a series of patients taking 3 grams (3,000 milligrams) of niacin every day. He reported his findings in a document prepared for the physicians involved in Alcoholics Anonymous by Bill W (1968).

In his report, Boyle reported that he had kept 160 heart disease patients on niacin for ten years. Out of the 160, and against a statistical expectation that 62 would have died with conventional care, only six died. He stated, "From the strictly medical viewpoint I believe all patients taking niacin would survive longer and enjoy life much more." Continuous use of niacin will decrease mortality and prolong life.

Niacin Combined With Other Drugs Which Lower Cholesterol

Familial hypercholesterolemia is an inherited disease in which plasma cholesterol levels are very high. Illingworth, Phillipson, Rapp and Connor (1981) described a series of 13 patients with this disease whose cholesterol levels ranged from 345 to 524 and triglycerides from 70 to 232. When a drug plus diet did not decrease cholesterol levels below 270 mg/100 mL they were given niacin, starting with 250 mg three times daily and increasing it every two to four weeks until a final dose of 3 to 8 grams per day was reached. To reduce the niacin "flush," (a harmless blushing of the skin) patients took aspirin (niacin flush is known to be reduced with a vitamin C intake simultaneously) with each dose for four to six weeks. Even at such dosage of niacin, tests revealed no abnormal liver function. They concluded, "Long term use of such a regimen affords the potential for preventing, or even reversing, the premature development of atherosclerosis that occurs so frequently in this group of patients."

Fortunately, niacin does not decrease cholesterol to dangerously low levels. Cheraskin and Ringsdorf (1982) reviewed some of the evidence which links very low cholesterol levels to an increased incidence of cancer and greater mortality in general. Fortunately however, niacin keeps cholesterol at normal levels, which cannot be said about most other cholesterol lowering drugs. By treating symptoms for one disease, big pharma's drugs can cause you even more disease.

A niacin flush may be experienced with its use, and although it is completely normal and safe, the following steps may be taken:

If you are interested in the use of niacin you may go to a health food store and purchase a bottle of 100 mg niacin tablets and a bottle of 1000 mg vitamin C tablets.

One should expect to begin by taking 1000 mg of vitamin C and 50 mg of niacin three times a day, preferably after each meal. A niacin tablet may be broken apart and taken at 50 mg doses.

After three or four days, the niacin dosage is increased to 100 mg three times a day. One might continue increasing the niacin by 50 mg or 100 mg every three or four days until the dosage of 1000 mg of niacin and 1000 mg of vitamin C are taken three times a day.

It normally takes about three months on the higher dosage of niacin and vitamin C for cholesterol levels to stabilize at lower levels. It may cost about 50 cents per day for a regime of 3000 mg of niacin and vitamin C, which is hundreds less than some extortion priced medication, or should I say poisons.

Continuous use of niacin can be expected to reliably decrease mortality and prolong life.

Remember: So far, in all the years medicine while drugs continue to kill hundreds of thousands of people every year, there is not even one death per year from vitamins.

Pharmaceutical drugs, properly prescribed and taken as directed, kill over 100,000 Americans annually. And since many cases are not reported, that number in actuality might be doubled or even tripled.

Restoration of health needs to be done nutritionally, not pharmacologically. All cells in all persons are made exclusively from what we drink and eat. Not one cell is made out of drugs.
Source: http://orthomolecular.org

Diabetes, cholesterol, heart disease and other diseases are all linked! Our body is a very complicated machine and everything works together. Symptons are usually just hints of something big underneath, that's why just looking at symptoms as separate things can never work because treating disease must be done to the whole body.

Study: http://www.ajcn.org/content/89/5/1588S.abstract
In analyses before alterations in lipid-lowering medications, total cholesterol decreased by 20.4 and 6.8 mg/dL in the vegan and conventional diet groups, respectively (P = 0.01); LDL cholesterol decreased by 13.5 and 3.4 mg/dL in the vegan and conventional groups, respectively

A vegan diet is <u>3 times more effective</u> at lowering cholesterol than the diet recommended by the American Diabetes Association

Sterility/Infertility

Official American medicine will go to any lengths to prove whatever it wants, but it is astounding that it does not choose to validate the already existing European and Canadian studies concerning sterility in humans. The European studies are so conclusive to the value of Vitamin E in sterility that it is clear why there were not followed up here. Again, there is too much money at stake here and as barbaric as it sounds, healthy humans are not profitable.

There are hundreds of well-controlled studies which demonstrate the value of Vitamin E in producing healthy offspring in infertile couples. There are also hundreds of animal studies which support this fact in practically all mammals. As in the classic experiments of the Darlington-Chassels study of race horses, with regard to increasing the production of thoroughbreds, the same results are seen with people. This property of Vitamin E, that of improving the quality of the sperm as well as the general health of both parents, has been noted throughout the history of the vitamin. It has been tagged as an "anti-sterility vitamin" and this is still considered by many medical authorities to be the vitamin's prime function.

Throughout our extensive research on Vitamin E the phrase frequently appears, "There were 'no' anomalies with Vitamin E therapy, while there were the usual ones before treatment." It is logical to say that any condition that is caused by the deficiency of an agent can be cured by administering that agent. As in the action of Vitamin C in the prevention as well as the cure for scurvy; likewise Vitamin B-12 and pernicious anemia; niacin and pellegra; B-1 and beriberi; Vitamin D and rickets; and so on.

Now, can the sperm be qualitatively improved so that they can mate with the ova and produce healthy offspring? The answer is yes. Both males and females should take a course of Vitamin E therapy at least one to three months before conception, and then, after conception, should continue with Vitamin E - particularly the woman, if she wants to carry her offspring for the nine months with greater benefit.

One example of a study comes from West Germany, conducted by Dr. R. Bayer. Dr. Bayer treated 100 married couples. More than half of the group were victims of "primary infertility"; Although the couples were able to conceive, they lost 100 per cent of their conceptions. These couples had 144 pregnancies and had lost all of them prior to Vitamin E treatment. After Vitamin E treatment there were seventy-five pregnancies and only two women lost their babies, while most women had aborted almost all their babies before Vitamin E therapy. Dr. Bayer was, thus, able to reduce miscariage from 100 per cent to 2 and a half percent!

Dr. Bayer's second group had "secondary infertility" (the couples had some successful births rather than total failure). They were able to achieve a total of only 38 births out of 101 pregnancies. Yet with his standard dosage of 100 milligrams (1 IU is the biological equivalent of about 0.667 mg d-alpha-tocopherol, so 100 milligrams is 66.7 IU) daily for one month for the male and 200 milligrams daily for three months prior to conception for the female, Dr. Bayer observed '100 per cent' success rate. In other words, from forty-one pregnancies, there were forty-one births, and all of them healthy offspring.

But Dr. Bayer being a disciplined scientist, of a caliber rarely seen now days, carried his experiment even further. He wanted to prove it was Vitamin E and Vitamin E alone which produced such successful positive changes. In both groups he lowered the Vitamin E intake to one-third of what it was previous. The results were quite shocking. When the males in the first primary sterility group were lowered to 1/3 the full intake of Vitamin E, the miscarriage rate was 33% instead of the 2.5% with the heavier dosage.

In the second group ("secondary infertility") , when the amount of Vitamin E was reduced to 1/3 the full intake, miscarriage was reduced from 61 per cent (without Vitamin E) to 21 per cent, instead of 100 per cent successful births as with the heavy dosage.

Thus, we see that Dr. Bayer and his associates have not only proved that Vitamin E can be essential in human fertility and the health of the offspring but that the actual dosage of the vitamin must be therapeutic in order to achieve optimum results, i.e., a successful conception and a successful birth. Dr. Bayer's studies - particularly those concerned with sperm improvement - have been supported by many other experiments throughout the world. It is most interesting to note that not in a single experiment where the male and female were under intensive Vitamin E therapy has there ever been recorded the birth of any flawed child, either mentally or physically.

There were hundreds of men, women, and children involved in these experiments and, and by all laws of percentages, there should have been several deformations, and quite a few mentally retarded children, **but there were none**. Therefore, Vitamin E, in playing its many beneficial roles within the body, is able to improve the quality of the sperm in the human male; and, judging from the mass of evidence, both animal and human, Vitamin E is able to alter the female's reception of the sperm and to provide a good environment for the developing fetus. It is apparent that large amounts of Vitamin E given to the mother can, in turn, assist the rapidly-growing fetus.

Now, as we have stated, Dr. Bayer's essential findings have been supported by many researchers throughout the world, that Vitamin E therapy (oftentimes in conjunction with B-complex and other supplements) before conception decreases the chances of any unsuccessful birth.

Minimum vitamin E dosage should be 400 IU.

Influenza

Vitamin D

Vitamin D has known anti-viral properties and has been directly associated with fighting influenza in a recent scientific review. Extensive evidence shows vitamin D is an important factor in immune system regulation.

During a viral infection, the body can draw on vitamin D stored in the body to supply the increased needs of the immune system. The withdrawn supplies of vitamin D are quickly replenished with 4,000 to 10,000 IU/day doses for a few days. Due to biochemical individuality, we recommend vitamin D blood testing as a routine part of a yearly physical exam. Getting your daily dose of sunshine (even a 10-15 minute tan can give you a month's worth of vitamin D) is very important as well.

Niacin

Niacin has known anti-viral properties. The most convincing evidence comes from recent work with HIV patients. Niacin is required for cells to generate the energy they use to perform virtually all biological activity.

Niacin's effectiveness fighting viruses may have to do with accelerating wound healing as well as improving immunity. Accelerating tissue repair limits collateral damage and minimizes the risk of secondary infection. Niacin has been proven to promote healing of damaged skin in double-blind trials. Other recent findings show that niacin reduces injury to the brain after strokes and reduces inflammation in general.

Niacin, 500 to 2,000 mg/day in divided doses, is generally well tolerated during periods when the immune system is fighting viral infections. One takes such doses for several days starting at the onset of a viral infection. Dividing the dose reduces flushing (sudden redness and a sensation of warmth on the surface of the skin). Using "no-flush" form niacin (inositol hexaniacinate) eliminates the flushing side effect.

Vitamin C

Strong evidence shows that high doses of vitamin C prevent common colds and reduce a cold's severity and duration. Given the similarities between cold and influenza viruses, vitamin C has a tremendous positive effect on both. Fighting influenza with vitamin C has been tested in the clinical setting and reported to be effective at very high doses.

Extraordinary quantities of vitamin C, between 20,000 and 100,000 mg/day, are very well tolerated during periods when the immune system is fighting a viral infection. These large daily amounts are best taken divided up into as many doses per day as possible, beginning immediately at the first sign of a viral infection. To achieve maximum effect it is necessary to maintain high concentrations of vitamin C in the body. Large, very frequent oral intake of vitamin C can maintain much higher blood concentrations of vitamin C than is generally believed.

Thiamine (Vitamin B1)
Research has shown that the B-vitamin thiamine has anti-viral properties. Thiamine was also shown to be an effective treatment for chronic hepatitis B.

Prologue

If you have finished the book I want to again congratulate you on taking this giant step towards your bright, healthy, slim, and amazing future. What you have read might not be all that simple, and some of you might not know how to put all that information to use.

These next steps are what make winners, what make the success stories, and what will actually change your life. If what you learn doesn't get put into practice, then it's useless knowledge. So let's put some of the things we have just learned into practice. But remember, these things are a lot easier than what you might expect, and with a bit of patience will make your life happier and healthier!

The main thing to remember is that the more natural and raw food you eat, the faster and easier you will lower your risk of countless diseases and regain your health. There is nothing you need to "do," your body will do it all for you, you just have to turn the right key and the door will open by itself. Your "open sesame," your secret password, your master key is just eating and living the way your body was made to.

Most Important Steps:
Food additives are your TRUE enemy and are much more important to look out for rather than calories/fats/or carbs. Get rid of as many artificial food additives as you can.

Eat as much raw food and as little animal food as possible to regain your digestive function, stimulate toxin removal, increase your metabolic rate, improve all organ function, activate fat burning, and begin curing all your so called "incurable" diseases and ailments.
Drink a minimum 1.5-2 litres of clean filtered water EVERY DAY to guarantee a smooth and easy way for all your toxins to leave your body ensuring a lightning fast path towards weight loss and health.

Supplement with a good quality superfood green powder and a few vitamins so that your body has all the required nutrients to keep itself healthy (vitamin C, E, D, hydgrogen peroxide).

If your budget allows, try to get as much of your food organic - I know how expensive it can be, but sometimes organic is even cheaper than regular produce. For example in my local grocery store apples cost exactly the same, so I of course grab the organic ones, while some berries are nearly double the price, so I settle for regular non-organic ones. As long as you eat more raw fruits and veggies, be they organic or non-organic, you will have better health.

Open up your fridge and look at all of things that you now know are preventing you from achieving amazing health. If you want to keep popping prescription drugs, being fat, sick, or tired, then by all means leave everything as it is, but if you have decided to change your life, then I will recommend that you definitely change what's in your fridge and pantry.

Step 1 – Take a big garbage bag.
Step 2 – Go to your fridge and pantry.
Step 3 – Notice the Cookies? Cakes? Pastries? Chips? Chocolate bars? Frozen dinners? Take all that and place it gently in the garbage bag which you will later donate to someone or throw it all away.
Step 4 – Go to your favourite grocery store and begin your learning process! Go though the isles and begin studying the ingredients in every product that you usually buy. If you notice any of the following, you can safely place it back on the shelf knowing that you now have the power and freedom of educated choice!

Here is a list with identifying code numbers and names of the nasty food additives that we should avoid eating. These artificial food preservatives, food colors and flavour enhancers are dangerous chemicals added to our food and are known to be linked to Hyperactivity, Attention-Deficit Disorder (ADD), Asthma, Cancers and other medical conditions.

Where to look for food additives on a product label?

When buying groceries, these additives are listed on the food product's packaging under "INGREDIENTS:" or "CONTAINS:" section, usually next to "Nutrition Information" but the code numbers or names of these additives can be printed out in a small font.

Food additives give flavour to what otherwise might be flavour less, genetically modified, nutrition-less, useless food. Flavouring is added so that these meals are pleasing to the palate when they come out of the microwave oven or the oven.

Preservatives are added for shelf life. Most food without preservatives usually goes bad in days, but adding these horrible chemicals keeps the foods fresh for weeks and months.

In order to avoid chemicals food additives, I recommend you do most of your shopping in the fresh produce section. I know it will be hard to start eating a lot more fruits and veggies if you've been eating mostly processed food for most of your life, but you have to start somewhere. The best part is that you don't have to look at portions, count calories or carbs - you can literally eat as much fresh fruits and veggies as you want and you will never gain a pound.

You don't have to follow elaborate recipes or spend hours in the kitchen.

For example, in the morning I drink a large green smoothie, during the day I drink lots of water, for lunch I grab an avocado, scoop it out onto raw bread, sprinkle some salt and have myself a super healthy sandwich. For dinner I eat a very large bowl of salad with feta cheese. On the side I have regular cheese with whole wheat sprouted raw bread. The salad is just lettuce, tomatoes, cucumbers, and celery with olive oil and a dash of salt - takes around 10 minutes to prepare. For me salad isn't a side dish, but a main dish. You can make bowls of salad as large as you want and eat as much as you want, for snacks, for lunch/dinner, etc.

Of course it takes many months to get your body used to eating so much more green stuff, but it is possible and you won't even crave snacks or sweets. When your body gets the required nutrients, it doesn't stay hungry.

A good tip that works for me is that as soon as you start craving sweets or a snack, just drink a large glass of water - the craving just goes away. If the craving persists, eat an apple, orange, or any other fruit or veggie. When in the store, don't even go into the snack isle. If you don't have bad snacks in your house, you won't accidentally eat them.

I haven't included any recipes because there are countless free websites that you can get any recipes you like from. Here are some good ones:

http://www.living-foods.com/recipes/
http://www.welikeitraw.com/rawfood/recipes/index.html
http://allrecipes.com/Recipes/Everyday-Cooking/Vegetarian/Top.aspx
http://goneraw.com/

If you want to find more just type into the Google search bar "raw food recipes" or "vegetarian food recipes" or just "healthy food recipes" and get thousands of web pages. Remember each meal must be at least 50% raw (fresh vegetables, fruits, nuts, seeds, dried fruits, sprouted grains).

Now go into the isle that sells vitamins and start supplementing with what our current food can't provide us. Again, the most important daily dosages of vitamins are: 800IUof vitamin E, 4-10 grams of vitamin C (regular, **not** Ester-C), **4000** IU of vitamin D, marine grade Okinawan calcium, and B-complex vitamins.

If you don't have a water filter, I highly recommend you purchase one so you can have plenty of clean drinking water. Remember, 1.5-2 litres daily! Not juice or tea or coffee, plain old water. The best water filetrs are reverse-osmosis or distillation as they remove everything from the water leaving just plain H2O.

And that's pretty much it. Sounds simple? Well that's because it is!

Get rid of the things that are CAUSING your poor health, load up on the things that will stimulate your body to cure your diseases, drink plenty of water for energy and to ensure a smooth detoxification process, and supplement with vitamins to get everything your body needs that the food we eat does not provide us.

The more things that you do from the 7 Steps, the better and quicker you will see results, it's all up to you now, everything you dreamed of regarding your body and your health can be a reality if you put your mind to it! I know you can do it! Start slow, begin the changes, and you WILL see results, absolutely, without a doubt, I guarantee it!

Your 7 Steps to Health

What is written below is pretty much the absolute best that you can possibly do for a healthy, new you. If you decide to implement everything that is written, then you are a true warrior of your health, you will see the results quicker than anyone, and you will achieve a healthy glowing and beautiful body in no time. For some it may not be as easy so please remember to take it slow and do what you feel is best for you. Start slowly, see and feel the result, then continue to add further changes. Do what you can, as best you can, you don't have to overwhelm yourself.

This list provides your body with everything it needs to cure most diseases by itself, easily and absolutely side effect free. You will be alkalizing your body's PH level, you will be increasing the oxygen content in the blood, you will be providing your body with all the necessary nutrients, and you will be creating a perfect place for detox allowing your body to naturally get perfectly healthy! This is the "cure" for your diseases; alkalize you system, increase oxygen, decrease the foods that are causing stress and disease and increase the foods that are promoting health and wellbeing. That's it!

The number one most important thing that will lead to the best health restoration and disease elimination is to stop eating all meat products, pasteurized dairy, drastically reduce the intake of processed foods (basically anything that comes in a can, box, package, or fast food restaurant) and drastically increase your intake of fresh fruits and vegetables to a minimum of 50% of your entire diet.

Just these things alone will take you 90% of the way to perfect health.

Step By Step

1. Reduce and eliminate cooked food, meat, dairy (store bought pasteurized), alcohol, caffeine, tobacco, sugar as they are all very strong acidifiers among other negative effects they produce.

2. Detoxify and alkalize your system with raw foods, green smoothies (this is absolutely essential, drink 2-3 green smoothies daily), freshly squeezed juices, and health fasting a few times per month.

3. Supplement with whole food powders, superfoods, anti oxidants, sunshine, and fresh air.

4. Completely remove any food additive, colorant, flavor enhancer, artificial sweetener, or any artificial ingredients from your ration.

5. Drink at least 2 liters (half a gallon) of water per day.

6. Walk twice per day for at least 15 minutes each and/or attend fitness/yoga classes.

7. Reduce stress by spending time outdoors; meditating, listening to peaceful music, smiling, laughing, spending time with loved ones etc.

Bonus Tips– These steps will further increase you wellbeing and multiply the health benefits

Find an organic whole food superfood powder or one that has a high quantity of superfoods such as spirulina, chlorella, barley grass, wheat grass, etc. These are located in the supplements or natural food isle of your grocery store, or can be found in health food stores.

The reason I always recommend whole foods supplements instead of separately taking vitamins is because vitamins and minerals in foods are bound to natural food complexes with proteins, carbohydrates and lipids. The human body recognizes this entire complex and digests it much easier.

Most vitamins and supplements, however, are synthetic combinations of isolated USP vitamins and minerals. These are often formulated to claim 100% of the Daily Value (DV) on labels. But these vitamins and minerals are not bound to anything, and may have an entirely different chemical structure than those vitamins naturally found in foods.

This is why many opponents of vitamins claim that you are wasting your money, and they are - to an extent right. Most of the vitamin supplements sold in stores are synthetic, created in a lab, not tested and might not even be absorbed by your body, so instead you just end up urinating them out.

This is why it's important to supplement with whole foods, vegetables, fruits, nuts, seeds, and superfood green powders to assure proper absorption and assimilation of vitamins and minerals.

The synthetic man-made vitamins or extracts may ignore antagonistic and synergistic effects of vitamins and minerals both in regard to absorption and metabolic reactions once absorbed. Complex factors in whole foods that aid absorption, such as chelating agents, may be missing in laboratory formulated vitamins and minerals. It is well known that many man-made supplements, especially calcium and iron, are not well absorbed. Always choose whole foods rather than specific vitamins or nutrients if available or accessible to you.

Of course if you cannot acquire whole foods in the area where you live, it is better to go with store bought vitamin supplementation than nothing at all.

Protein - do not buy whey or milk derived protein, they are detrimental to your health and have a whole list of negative effects on your body. There are much more powerful alternatives in the form of vegetable sources. One of these is hemp seeds or hemp powder. These can be found in many grocery stores in the alternative foods or vegetarian section. If you can't find hemp protein, you can look for "vetetarian protein" powders which usually have protein sources like peas or beans. Or if you want to avoid powders, you can eat meals with protein rich veggies like sprouted grains, beans, lentils, peas, chick peas, spinach, asparagus, broccoli or cauliflower.

Take lentils for example, a cup has 18 grams of protein and 1 gram of healthy fat. While an 80 gram (3 ounce) steak has 20 grams of protein, 20 grams of fat, out of which 7 are saturated, unhealthy fats. In addition to potential growth hormones, antibiotics, and cancer causing chemicals that are produced when meat is prepared.

Another protein alternative is spirulina which has the highest protein content of any natural food (65%); far more than animal and fish meat (which only has 15-25%), soybeans (just 35%), dried milk (35%), peanuts (25%), eggs (12%), grains (8-14%) or whole milk (3%) and has tremendous amounts of vitamin B12, much higher than in beef!

Change Gradually

If you try to change everything about your diet all at once, you won't stick with it. Go slow. Change **one item at a time** and **get accustomed** to the healthier alternative before tackling another. Make sure to go at your own pace and remember that this is not a race or one of those useless "30 day diet programs," you didn't become sick overnight, and you won't get cured overnight.

Sample Health Schedule

The first few week are the most important where you want to see the results and begin to feel the changes in your body. The most important things you can do in the first few weeks are as follows. These are absolutely essential to begin your path to great health:

- Drink 500ml (16oz) of clean filtered water as soon as you wake up and get as close to 2 liters (half a gallon) as you can throughout the day
- Drink a large green smoothie with bee pollen before eating/drinking anything else
- Reduce your soda/fast food/junk foods/sweets to an absolute minimum
- Eat something raw with every meal, be it a fruit, vegetable or salad.
- Supplement your diet with a superfood powder, 800IU vitamin E, 5-10 grams of vitamin C, 6000 IU of vitamin D, marine grade Okinawan calcium, and B-complex vitamins
- Walk at least 15 minutes per day **outside**

Remember, you don't have to change everything; just whatever you feel is right for you. It is better to change a couple things and stick with them rather than change everything, get frustrated and just quit altogether.

The following is a sample monthly breakdown of what you may find yourself doing to achieve total health. Again, add things slowly, one at a time, get accustomed to the changes, and when you begin to see a brand new healthy body in the mirror your confidence in your new life will skyrocket!

Month 1-2:

- Drink 1-2 green smoothies every day, one in the morning and one in the afternoon/evening
- Increase your raw food intake by having some fresh vegetables with every meal (the quantity of raw food has to be as much as your other food 50-50). You may eat as much raw food as you like throughout the day.
- Remove **all** sodas, artificial sweeteners, fast food, and heavily processed food from your diet.
- Drink at least 2 liters of clean, purified water per day. Better if it is ozonated and/or ionized.
- Take a 15 minute walk every day **outside**, even if it is raining or snowing!
- Supplement your diet with a superfood powder, vitamins (Vitamin C – 5-10 grams, vitamin E - 800 IU, B complex), and minerals (marine grade Okinawan coral calcium, selenium – 100 micrograms, iodine, vitamin D minimum 5000 IU).
- You may pray or meditate every morning, or just sit quietly and concentrate on your breathing and try to stay in the present moment without any thoughts for 5-10 minutes each morning.

Months 3-6:

- Continue with everything in month 1.
- Eat only raw foods during breakfast and all snacks while maintaining 50% raw/cooked food ratio with your other meals. You may eat as much raw food as you like throughout the day.
- Slowly begin to phase out coffee, alcohol, dairy (if it is raw, unpasteurized dairy, then you may indulge in this wonder food as much as you like), remove sugar (you may sweeten with stevia, or unpasteurized honey), and keep removing meat from your diet by eating it only once per week.
- Drink at least 2 liters (half a gallon) of clean, purified water per day.
- Take 15 minute walks **twice a day, outside**, even if it is raining or snowing!

Months 6-12

- Continue with everything in the previous months.
- Drink 2-3 green smoothies daily
- Eat only raw food during breakfast and dinner while maintaining a 50% raw/cooked food ratio during lunch. You may eat as much raw food as you like throughout the day.
- Eliminate coffee, alcohol, dairy (unless they are raw, unprocessed, unpasteurized, and organic milk products), and sugar (you may sweeten with stevia, or high quality honey) from your diet.

Month 7-continued

- Slowly begin to phase out all cooked food from your diet, while eating as much raw foods throughout the day as you like. If you are not yet ready to take on this challenge, then it is fine if you allow yourself to eat one small cooked meal per day.
- Continue with everything in the previous months

Now remember, you don't have to do everything if you are unable to. The most important things are to eliminate all meat products, pasteurized dairy, sugar and processed foods and processed fats. Just removing these 4 things will bring you unbelievable health.

The most important aspect is to take it slow and change at your own pace. Set goals for yourself and write down what you need to do today. You may even create a simple checklist if it is easier for you. Do your best to avoid cheating but at the same time do not suffer or create unhappiness for yourself because of a lifestyle change. At first it might not be so easy to stick to your goals when you live around so many temptations, but as you progress and your lifestyle changes strengthen, it will become easier and easier day by day. If you happen to give in at some point, allow what happened, accept your action, but tell yourself that you will be stronger next time and do you absolute best to stick to your goals.

As you slowly start changing your diet and actions, you will naturally and easily take on the healthy lifestyle. You will begin to see the difference in yourself, your appearance, well being, and happiness levels will rise dramatically, and people will begin to notice. Take it slow, take it easy, but be consistent and believe in yourself!

Easy Dietary Additions

An easy way to start is with the following dietary additions.

If you get rid of all the junk and start your new diet with these items, you will see changes within your body within the first few days.

- ***50% of your meals have to be raw***. Meaning a salad with all meals and raw unprocessed nuts/fruits/dried fruits/raw food bars as snacks.
- Drink 2 green smoothies daily with hemp protein and a scoop of a whole food green powder.
- In the morning take a teaspoon of **bee pollen** under the tongue and let dissolve, then swallow. Or add it to your smoothies, shakes or salads.
- Drink at least 1.5-2 Litres of **clean filtered water daily** (drink 500 ml or 16oz of water as soon as you wake up).
- Supplement with **minimum** 5-10 grams of spirulina and chlorella each per day, as well as 5 grams of vitamin C (L-ascorbate), 800 IU of vitamin E, and 6000 IU of vitamin D.
- Take a 15 minute walk every day, rain or shine.

Final Thoughts

I would like to conclude this book with some final thoughts which will summarize what you have just read. The most important idea that I would like you to see and feel is that health and wellness comes from the inside out. The idea that there exists a miracle pill, remedy, cure, item, or anything else other than a holistic (physical, emotional, spiritual) approach to health, is simply a lie. If we do not eliminate the CAUSE of our problem, be it physical or emotional, no matter what we do, we will be treating the SYMPTOM of that problem, and never eliminate that one thing that is CAUSING it.

I will go back to my example of hitting your finger with the hammer. No matter how many prescription drugs, treatments, pills or creams you decide to use, if you do not stop hitting your finger with the hammer, you will be stuck in a closed loop, a situation without an exit, a problem that will continue to emerge no matter what you do.

All the "cures" I have listed are only but a sample of what is out there. There are literally hundreds of various cures for cancer, diabetes, heart disease etc. which most people have never heard of (we now know WHY we have never heard of them). I want to urge you to not get stuck on the treatments themselves, but understand **the big picture** of how and why they work. Because if you know the how's and why's, you are free to substitute various things to make up your own combinations.

The only thing, and I repeat the ONLY thing, that can make you lose weight, cure your diseases, and make you totally healthy is a holistic approach to your wellbeing. You need:

Real Food (raw alkalizing vegetables, fruits, nuts, grains, sprouts etc.)
Real Water (filtered, unchlorinated, unflouridated, alkaline, toxin free)
Real Air and Sun (get at least 15 minutes of sunshine and get out more; the air inside the home is usually more polluted than the air outside)
Real Rest (proper sleep as well as meditation/yoga/relaxation etc.)
Real Exercise (proper low impact, walking is enough to keep your health and weight in check)

Slowly but surely, begin to take these steps to a better you.

Additional Information

www.theicitm.org
www.mercola.com
www.naturalnews.com

Your Body's Many Cries for Water by F. Batmanghelidj

Fire Your Doctor! How to Be Independently Healthy by Andrew Saul

The Case Against Fluoride: How Hazardous Waste Ended Up in Our Drinking Water and the Bad Science and Powerful Politics That Keep It There by Paul Connett, James Beck, and H. Spedding Mickle

GMO Trilogy + Seeds of Deception (set): Why Genetically Modified Organisms Threaten Your Health, the Environment and Future Generations by Jeffrey M. Smith

12 Steps to Raw Foods: How to End Your Dependency on Cooked Food by Victoria Boutenko and Gabriel Cousens

Vitamin C: The Real Story: The Remarkable and Controversial Story of Vitamin C by Steve Hickey

The Gerson Therapy: The Proven Nutritional Program for Cancer and Other Illnesses
Cancer. Hepatitis. Migraines. Arthritis. Heart Disease. Emphysema. For years, the medical establishment has called these chronic or life- threatening diseases "incurable." But now, the Gerson Therapy offers hope for those seeking relief from hundreds of different diseases. Juice your way to wellness. One of the first alternative cancer therapies, the Gerson Therapy has successfully treated thousands of patients for over 60 years. Now, in this authoritative revised and updated edition, alternative medicine therapist Charlotte Gerson and medical journalist Morton Walker reveal even more on the powerful healing effects of fruits and vegetables. Not only can juicing reverse the effects of many degenerative illnesses-it can save lives. "The Gerson Therapy" shows you: How to beat cancer by changing your body chemistry; Special juicing techniques for maximum healing power; and, How to combat allergies, obesity, high blood pressure, AIDS, lupus, and other diseases. This unique resource will help and inspire anyone who has ever said, "I want to get well. Just show me how." "The Gerson Therapy" offers a powerful, time-tested healing option that has worked for others - and can work for you!

Psychodietetics by Emanuel Cheraskin

"Changing your diet can change your life. You don't have to take our word for it; you can prove it to yourself." (p 132) So say this team of medical doctor and dentist, in one of the most persuasive and readable books on megavitamin therapy for emotional illness. The authors put forward surprisingly effective cures for drug dependency, mental illness, senility, depression, anxiety, hyperactivity in children, alcoholism and other ailments, supported by case histories and 290 medical references. Self-diagnostic questionnaires and an Optimal Diet are included, plus a hypoglycemia diet and notes on how to administer large doses of niacin (vitamin B-3) without side effects. (225 pages, paper)

The Untold Story of Milk, Revised and Updated: The History, Politics and Science of Nature's Perfect Food: Raw Milk from Pasture-Fed Cows by Ron Schmid

The Myth of Mental Illness: Foundations of a Theory of Personal Conduct by Thomas Stephen Szasz
The most influential critique of psychiatry ever written, Thomas Szasz's classic book revolutionized thinking about the nature of the psychiatric profession and the moral implications of its practices. By diagnosing unwanted behavior as mental illness, psychiatrists, Szasz argues, absolve individuals of responsibility for their actions and instead blame their alleged illness. He also critiques Freudian psychology as a pseudoscience and warns against the dangerous overreach of psychiatry into all aspects of modern life.

The Big Diabetes Lie

Our Deadly Diabetes Deception

"Greed and dishonest science have promoted a lucrative worldwide epidemic of diabetes that honesty and good science can quickly reverse by naturally restoring the body's blood-sugar control mechanism"

Nexus Magazine, Volume 11, Number 4, 2004

Thomas Smith

Introduction

If you are an American diabetic, your physician will never tell you that most cases of diabetes are curable. In fact, if you even mention the "cure" word around him, he will likely become upset and irrational. His medical school training only allows him to respond to the word "treatment". For him, the "cure" word does not exist. Diabetes, in its modern epidemic form, is a curable disease and has been for at least 40 years. In 2001, the most recent year for which US figures are posted, 934,550 Americans died from out-of-control symptoms of this disease.

Your physician will also never tell you that, at one time, strokes, both ischaemic and haemorrhagic, heart failure due to neuropathy as well as both ischaemic and haemorrhagic coronary events, obesity, atherosclerosis, elevated blood pressure, elevated cholesterol, elevated triglycerides, impotence, retinopathy, renal failure, liver failure, polycystic ovary syndrome, elevated blood sugar, systemic candida, impaired carbohydrate metabolism, poor wound healing, impaired fat metabolism, peripheral neuropathy as well as many more of today's disgraceful epidemic disorders were once well understood often to be but symptoms of diabetes.

If you contract diabetes and depend upon mainstream medical treatment, sooner or later you will experience one or more of its symptoms as the disease rapidly worsens. It is now common practice to refer to these symptoms as if they were separable, independent diseases with separate, unrelated treatments provided by competing medical specialists.

It is true that many of these symptoms can and sometimes do result from other causes; however, it is also true that this fact has been used to disguise the causative role of diabetes and to justify expensive, ineffective treatments for these symptoms.

Epidemic Type II diabetes is curable. By the time you get to the end of this article, you are going to know that. You're going to know *why* it isn't routinely being cured. And, you're going to know *how* to cure it. You are also probably going to be angry at what a handful of greedy people have surreptitiously done to the entire medical community and to its trusting patients.

The Diabetes Industry

Today's diabetes industry is a massive community that has grown step by step from its dubious origins in the early 20th century. In the last 80 years it has become enormously successful at shutting out competitive voices that attempt to point out the fraud involved in modern diabetes treatment. It has matured into a religion. And, like all religions, it depends heavily upon the faith of the believer. So successful has it become that it verges on blasphemy to suggest that, the kind high priest with the stethoscope draped prominently around his neck is a charlatan and a fraud. In the large majority of cases, he has never cured a single case of diabetes in his entire medical career.

The financial and political influence of this medical community has almost totally subverted the original intent of our regulatory agencies. They routinely approve death-dealing, ineffective drugs with insufficient testing. Former commissioner of the FDA, Dr Herbert Ley, in testimony before a US Senate hearing, commented: "People think the FDA is protecting them. It isn't. What the FDA is doing and what the public thinks it's doing are as different as night and day." [2]

The financial and political influence of this medical community dominates our entire medical insurance industry. Although this is beginning to change, in America it is still difficult to find employer group medical insurance to cover effective alternative medical treatments. Mainstream coverage is standard in all states. Alternative medicine is not. For example, there are only 1,400 licensed naturopaths in 11 states compared to over 3.4 million doctor licensees in 50 states. [3]Generally, only approved treatments from licensed, credentialed practitioners are insurable. This, in effect, neatly creates a special kind of money that can only be spent within the mainstream medical and drug industry. No other industry in the world has been able to manage the politics of convincing people to accept so large a part of their pay in a form that often does not allow them to spend it as they see fit.

The financial and political influence of this medical community completely controls virtually every diabetes publication in the country. Many diabetes publications are subsidized by ads for diabetes supplies. No diabetes editor is going to allow the truth to be printed in his magazine. If a diabetes magazine starts putting up stories of how to cure your diabetes naturally, then what would be the point of having ads for drugs and supplies? Drug companies would stop sponsoring the magazine and it would go out of business. The only way the magazine can survive is by printing stories of how great the drugs are. This is why the diabetic only pays about one-quarter to one-third of the cost of printing the magazine he depends upon for accurate information. The rest is subsidized by diabetes manufacturers with a vested commercial interest in preventing diabetics from curing their diabetes. When looking for a magazine that tells the truth about diabetes, look first to see if it is full of ads for diabetes supplies.

And then there are the various associations that solicit annual donations to find a cure for their proprietary disease. Every year they promise that a cure is just around the corner—just send more money! Some of these very same associations have been clearly implicated in providing advice that promotes the progress of diabetes in their trusting supporters. For example, for years they heavily promoted exchange diets, [4] which are in fact scientifically worthless—as anyone who has ever tried to use them quickly finds out. They ridiculed the use of glycaemic tables, which are actually very helpful to the diabetic. They promoted the use of margarine as heart healthy, long after it was well understood that margarine causes diabetes and promotes heart failure. [5]

If people ever wake up to the cure for diabetes that has been suppressed for 40 years, these associations would soon be out of business. But until then, they nonetheless continue to need our support.

For 40 years, medical research has consistently shown with increasing clarity that diabetes is a degenerative disease directly caused by an engineered food supply that is focused on profit instead of health. Although the diligent can readily glean this information from a wealth of medical research literature, it is generally otherwise unavailable. Certainly this information has been, and remains, largely unavailable in the medical schools that train our retail doctors.

Prominent among the causative agents in our modern diabetes epidemic are the engineered fats and oils that are sold in today's supermarkets.

The first step to curing diabetes is to stop believing the lie that the disease is incurable.

Diabetes History

In 1922, three Canadian Nobel Prize winners, Banting, Best and Macleod, were successful in saving the life of a fourteen-year-old diabetic girl in Toronto General Hospital with injectable insulin. [6] Eli Lilly was licensed to manufacture this new wonder drug, and the medical community basked in the glory of a job well done.

It wasn't until 1933 that rumours about a new rogue form of diabetes surfaced. This was in a paper presented by Joslyn, Dublin and Marks and printed in the *American Journal of Medical Sciences*. This paper, "Studies on Diabetes Mellitus", [7]discussed the emergence of a major epidemic of a disease which looked very much like the diabetes of the early 1920s, only it did not respond to the wonder drug, insulin. Even worse, sometimes insulin treatment *killed* the patient.

This new disease became known as "insulin-resistant diabetes" because it had the elevated blood sugar symptom of diabetes but responded poorly to insulin therapy. Many physicians had great success in treating this disease through diet. A great deal was learned about the relationship between diet and diabetes in the 1930s and 1940s.

Diabetes, which had a per-capita incidence of 0.0028% at the turn of the century, had by 1933 exploded by 1,000% in the United States to become a disease seen by many doctors. [8] This disease, under a variety of aliases, was destined to go on to wreck the health of over half the American population and incapacitate almost 20% by the 1990s. [9]

In 1950, the medical community became able to perform serum insulin assays. These assays quickly revealed that this new disease wasn't classic diabetes; it was characterised by sufficient, often excessive, blood insulin levels.

The problem was that the insulin was ineffective; it did not reduce blood sugar. But since the disease had been known as diabetes for almost 20 years, it was renamed Type II diabetes. This was to distinguish it from the earlier Type I diabetes, caused by insufficient insulin production by the pancreas.

Had the dietary insights of the previous 20 years dominated the medical scene from that point and into the late 1960s, diabetes would have become widely recognized as curable instead of merely treatable. Instead, in 1950, a search was launched for another wonder drug to deal with the Type II diabetes problem.

Cure versus Treatment

This new, ideal wonder drug would be effective, like insulin, in remitting obvious adverse symptoms of the disease *but not effective in curing the underlying disease*. Thus it would need to be taken continually for the remaining life of the patient. It would have to be a patentable drug because natural medication is not patentable. Like insulin, it would have to be cheap to manufacture and distribute. Mandatory government approvals would be required to stimulate physicians to prescribe it as a prescription drug. Testing required for these approvals would have to be enormously expensive to prevent other new medications from becoming competitive.

Additionally, natural medications that actually *cure* disease would have to be suppressed. The more effective they were, the more they would need to be suppressed and their proponents jailed as quacks. After all, it wouldn't be very profitable for big pharma if diseases could be cured with cheap alternative methods.

This is the origin of the classic medical protocol of "treating the symptoms". By doing this, both the drug company and the doctor could prosper in business, and the patient, while not being cured of his disease, would just be temporarily relieved of some of his symptoms.

In many cases natural methods work better than most drugs prescribed by doctors. This is why the force of law has been and is being used to drive the natural, often superior, medicines from the marketplace, to remove the word "cure" from the medical vocabulary and to undermine the very concept of a free marketplace in the medical business.

Now it is clear why the "cure" word is so vigorously suppressed by law. The FDA has extensive Orwellian regulations that prohibit the use of the "cure" word to describe any competing medicine or natural substance. It is precisely because many natural substances do actually both cure and prevent disease that this word has become so frightening to the drug companies and mainstream medical community.

The Commercial Value of Symptoms

After the drug development policy was redesigned to focus on relieving symptoms rather than curing disease, it became necessary to reinvent the way drugs were marketed. This was done in 1949 in the midst of a major epidemic of insulin-resistant diabetes.

So in 1949, the US medical community reclassified the symptoms of diabetes [10]along with many other disease symptoms into diseases in their own right. With this reclassification as the new basis for diagnosis, competing medical specialty groups quickly seized upon related groups of symptoms as their own proprietary symptoms set.

Thus the heart specialist, endocrinologist, allergist, kidney specialist and many others started to treat the symptoms for which they felt responsible. As the underlying cause of the disease was widely ignored, all focus on actually curing anything was completely lost. Instead of treating the cause of all these problems, they were broken down and treated separately by themselves.

Heart failure, for example, which had previously been understood often to be but a symptom of diabetes, now became a disease not directly connected to diabetes. It became fashionable to think that diabetes "increased cardiovascular risk". The causal role of a failed blood-sugar control system in heart failure became obscured.

Consistent with the new medical paradigm, none of the treatments offered by the heart specialist actually cures, or is even intended to cure, their proprietary disease. For example, the three-year survival rate for bypass surgery is almost exactly the same as when no surgery is undertaken. [11]

Today, over half of the people in America suffer from one or more symptoms of this disease. In its beginnings, it became well known to physicians as Type II diabetes, insulin-resistant diabetes, insulin resistance, adult-onset diabetes or more rarely, hyperinsulinaemia.

According to the American Heart Association, almost 50% of Americans suffer from one or more symptoms of this disease. One third of the US population is morbidly obese; half of the population is overweight. Type II diabetes, also called adult-onset diabetes, now appears routinely in six-year-old children.

Many degenerative diseases can be traced to a massive failure of the endocrine system (the function of the hypothalamus, pituitary, thyroid, pancreas, adrenal, ovary/testes, and pineal glands which secrete various hormones and influences almost every cell, organ, and function of our bodies). This was well known to the physicians of the 1930s as insulin-resistant diabetes. This basic underlying disorder is known to be a derangement of the blood-sugar control system by badly engineered fats and oils. It is exacerbated and complicated by the widespread lack of other essential nutrition that the body needs to cope with the metabolic consequences of these poisons.

All fats and oils are not equal. Some are healthy and beneficial; many, commonly available in the supermarket, are poisonous. The health distinction is not between saturated and unsaturated, as the fats and oils industry would have us believe. Many saturated oils and fats are highly beneficial; many unsaturated oils are highly poisonous. The important health distinction is between *natural* and *engineered*.

There exists great dishonesty in advertising in the fats and oils industry. It is aimed at creating a market for cheap junk oils such as soy, cottonseed and rapeseed oils.

With an informed and aware public, these oils would have no market at all, and the USA—indeed, the world—would have far fewer cases of diabetes.

Epidemiological Lifestyle Link

As early as 1901, efforts had been made to manufacture and sell food products by the use of automated factory machinery because of the immense profits that were possible. Most of the early efforts failed because people were inherently suspicious of food that wasn't farm fresh and because the technology was poor. As long as people were prosperous, suspicious food products made little headway. Crisco, the artificial shortening, was once given away free in 2 1/2 lb cans in an unsuccessful effort to influence American housewives to trust and buy the product in preference to lard.

Margarine was introduced and was bitterly opposed by the dairy states in the USA. With the advent of the Depression of the 1930s, margarine, Crisco and a host of other refined and hydrogenated products began to make significant penetration into the food markets of America. Support for dairy opposition to margarine faded during World War II because there wasn't enough butter for the needs of both the civilian population and the military. At this point, the dairy industry, having lost much support, simply accepted a diluted market share and concentrated on supplying the military.

Flax oils and fish oils, which were common in the stores and considered dietary staples before the American population became diseased, have disappeared from the shelf. The last supplier of flax oil to the major distribution chains was Archer Daniels Midland, and it stopped producing and supplying the product in 1950.

More recently, one of the most important of the remaining, genuinely beneficial fats was subjected to a massive media disinformation campaign that portrayed it as a saturated fat that causes heart failure. As a result, it has virtually disappeared from the supermarket shelves. Thus was coconut oil removed from the food chain and replaced with soy oil, cottonseed oil and rapeseed oil. Our parents and grandparents would never have swapped a fine, healthy oil like coconut oil for these cheap, junk refined and processed oils. It was shortly after this successful media blitz that the US populace lost its war on fat. For many years, coconut oil had been our most effective dietary weight-control agent.

The history of the engineered adulteration of our once-clean food supply exactly parallels the rise of the epidemic of diabetes and hyperinsulinaemia now sweeping the United States as well as much of the rest of the world.

The second step to a cure for this disease epidemic is to stop believing the lie that our food supply is safe and nutritious.

The Nature of the Disease

Diabetes is classically diagnosed as a failure of the body to metabolise carbohydrates properly. Its defining symptom is a high blood-glucose level. Type I diabetes results from insufficient insulin production by the pancreas. Type II diabetes results from ineffective insulin. In both types, the blood-glucose level remains elevated. Neither insufficient insulin nor ineffective insulin can limit post-prandial (after-eating) blood sugar to the normal range. In established cases of Type II diabetes, these elevated blood sugar levels are often preceded and accompanied by chronically elevated insulin levels and by serious distortions of other endocrine hormonal markers.

The ineffective insulin is no different from effective insulin. Its ineffectiveness lies in the failure of the cell population to respond to it. It is not the result of any biochemical defect in the insulin itself. Therefore, it is appropriate to note that this is a disease that affects almost every cell in the 70 trillion or so cells of the body. All of these cells are dependent upon the food that we eat for the raw materials they need for self repair and maintenance.

The classification of diabetes as a failure to metabolise carbohydrates is a traditional classification that originated in the early 19th century when little was known about metabolic diseases or processes. Today, with our increased knowledge of these processes, it would appear quite appropriate to define Type II diabetes more fundamentally as a failure of the body to **metabolise fats and oils properly. This failure results in a loss of effectiveness of insulin and in the consequent failure to metabolise carbohydrates**. Unfortunately, much medical insight into this matter, except at the research level, remains hampered by its 19th-century legacy.

Thus Type II diabetes and its early hyperinsulinaemic symptoms are whole-body symptoms of this basic cellular failure to metabolise glucose properly. Each cell of the body, for reasons which are becoming clearer, finds itself unable to transport glucose from the bloodstream to its interior. The glucose then remains in the bloodstream, or is stored as body fat or as glycogen, or is otherwise disposed of in urine.

It appears that when insulin binds to a cell membrane receptor, it initiates a complex cascade of biochemical reactions inside the cell. This causes a class of glucose transporters known as GLUT4 molecules to leave their parking area inside the cell and travel to the inside surface of the plasma cell membrane.

When in the membrane, they migrate to special areas of the membrane called caveolae areas. [16] There, by another series of biochemical reactions, they identify and hook up with glucose molecules and transport them into the interior of the cell by a process called endocytosis. Within the cell's interior, this glucose is then burned as fuel by the mitochondria to produce energy to power cellular activity. Thus these GLUT4 transporters lower glucose in the bloodstream by transporting it out of the bloodstream into all the cells of the body.

Many of the molecules involved in these glucose- and insulin-mediated pathways are lipids; that is, they are fatty acids. A healthy plasma cell membrane, now known to be an active player in the glucose scenario, contains a complement of cis-type w=3 unsaturated fatty acids. This makes the membrane relatively fluid and slippery. When these cis- fatty acids are chronically unavailable because of our diet, trans- fatty acids and short- and medium-chain saturated fatty acids are substituted in the cell membrane. These substitutions make the cellular membrane stiffer and stickier, and inhibit the glucose transport mechanism.

In other words, the outer cell membrane, which is made from fat, is replaced by unhealthy fats when healthy fats are not present. These unhealthy fats like trans fats, modified fats, shortenings, fried fats, create a very sticky and stiff cell membrane which destroys the natural sugar intake process.

Thus, in the absence of sufficient cis omega 3 fatty acids in our diet (flax or hemp oil), these fatty acid substitutions take place, the mobility of the GLUT4 transporters is diminished, the interior biochemistry of the cell is changed and glucose remains elevated in the bloodstream.

Our diets in this country lack these highly unsaturated fatty acids and contain an excess of man-made oils known as trans fats (or partially hydrogenated oils). These oils are very much like cholesterol and our bodies cannot tell the difference. These oils get into our cell walls and destroy the electrical charge. Without the charge, our cells start to suffocate. Without the oxygen, the only way the cell can replicate is anaerobically.

They also are very tough oils and have a 20-year shelf life. They impede the process of cellular exchange, or letting nutrition in and letting wastes out. Trans fats are also responsible for Type II diabetes, since insulin is a very large molecule it has a difficult time passing through a cell wall created with man-made fats and not cholesterol.

It is absolutely critical to avoid ALL trans-fatty acids, ALL hydrogenated oils, ALL vegetable oils like canola or soy, ALL margarine and ALL other "bad fats" like the plague.

Elsewhere in the body, the pancreas secretes excess insulin, the liver manufactures fat from the excess sugar, the adipose cells store excess fat, the body goes into a high urinary mode, insufficient cellular energy is available for bodily activity and the entire endocrine system becomes distorted. Eventually, pancreatic failure occurs, body weight plummets and a diabetic crisis is precipitated.

Your diet must contain only the healthy fats which your cells can be made from. If you eat foods made out of bad fats its like building a home with cracked and broken bricks. You will never cure your diabetes if you eat bad fats. Its stunning that doctors don't tell their patients that the cause of diabetes is the man-made fats and trans fats found in almost all our foods.

Orthodox Medical Treatment

After the diagnosis of diabetes, modern orthodox medical treatment consists of either oral hypoglycaemic agents or insulin.

• **Oral hypoglycaemic agents**
In 1955, oral hypoglycaemic drugs were introduced. Currently available oral hypoglycaemic agents fall into five classifications according to their biophysical mode of action. [19] These classes are: biguanides; glucosidase inhibitors; meglitinides; sulphonylureas; and thiazolidinediones.

The *biguanides* lower blood sugar in three ways. They inhibit the liver's normal release of its glucose stores, they interfere with intestinal absorption of glucose from ingested carbohydrates, and they are said to increase peripheral uptake of glucose.

The *glucosidase inhibitors* are designed to inhibit the amylase enzymes produced by the pancreas and which are essential to the digestion of carbohydrates. The theory is that if the digestion of carbohydrates is inhibited, the blood sugar level cannot be elevated.

The *meglitinides* are designed to stimulate the pancreas to produce insulin in a patient that likely already has an elevated level of insulin in their bloodstream. Only rarely does the doctor even measure the insulin level. Indeed, these drugs are frequently prescribed without any knowledge of the pre-existing insulin level. The fact that an elevated insulin level is almost as damaging as an elevated glucose level is widely ignored.

The **sulphonylureas** are another pancreatic stimulant class designed to stimulate the production of insulin. Serum insulin determinations are rarely made by the doctor before he prescribes these drugs. They are often prescribed for Type II diabetics, many of whom already have elevated ineffective insulin. These drugs are notorious for causing hypoglycaemia as a side effect.

The *thiazolidinediones* are famous for causing liver cancer. One of them, Rezulin, was approved in the USA through devious political infighting, but failed to get approval in the UK because it was known to cause liver cancer.

The doctor who had responsibility to approve it at the FDA refused to do so. It was only after he was replaced by a more compliant official that Rezulin gained approval by the FDA. It went on to kill well over 100 diabetes patients and cripple many others before the fight to get it off the market was finally won. Rezulin was designed to stimulate the uptake of glucose from the bloodstream by the peripheral cells and to inhibit the normal secretion of glucose by the liver. The politics of why this drug ever came onto market, and then remained in the market for such an unexplainable length of time with regulatory agency approval, is not clear. As of April 2000, lawsuits commenced to clarify this situation.

• **Insulin**

Today, insulin is prescribed for both the Type I and Type II diabetics. Injectable insulin substitutes for the insulin that the body no longer produces. Of course, this treatment, while necessary for preserving the life of the Type I diabetic, is highly questionable when applied to the Type II diabetic.

It is important to note that neither insulin nor *any* of these oral hypoglycaemic agents exerts any curative action whatsoever on any type of diabetes. None of these medical strategies is designed to normalise the cellular uptake of glucose by the cells that need it to power their activity.
The prognosis with this treatment is increasing disability and early death from heart or kidney failure or the failure of some other vital organ.

Alternative Medical Treatment

The third step to a cure for this disease is to become informed and to apply an alternative methodology that is soundly based upon good science.

Effective alternative treatment that directly leads to a cure is available today for some Type I and for many Type II diabetics. About 5% of the diabetic population suffers from Type I diabetes; about 95% has Type II diabetes. Gestational diabetes is simply ordinary diabetes contracted by a woman who is pregnant.

For the Type I diabetic, an alternative methodology for the treatment of Type I diabetes is now available. It was developed in modern hospitals in Madras, India, and subjected to rigorous double-blind studies to prove its efficacy. It operates to restore normal pancreatic *beta* cell function so that the pancreas can again produce insulin as it should. This approach apparently was capable of curing Type I diabetes in over 60% of the patients on whom it was tested.

The major complication lies in whether the antigens that originally led to the autoimmune destruction of these beta cells have disappeared from or remain in the body. If they remain, a cure is less likely; if they have disappeared, the cure is more likely. For reasons already discussed, this methodology is not likely to appear in the United States any time soon, and certainly not in the American mainstream medical community.

The goal of any effective alternative program is to repair and restore the body's own blood-sugar control mechanism. It is the malfunctioning of this mechanism that, over time, directly causes all of the many debilitating symptoms that make regular treatment so financially rewarding for the diabetes industry. For Type II diabetes, the steps in the program are:

• **Repair the faulty blood sugar control system.** This is done simply by substituting the pristine looking but toxic trans-isomer mix of fats and oils found in attractive plastic containers on your supermarket shelves with clean, healthy, beneficial fats and oils. Consume only flax oil, hemp oil, coconut oil, fish oil and occasionally cod liver oil until blood sugar starts to stabilise. Then add back healthy oils such as olive oil. Read labels; refuse to consume cheap junk oils when they appear in processed food or on restaurant menus. Diabetics are chronically short of minerals; they need to add a good-quality, broad-spectrum mineral supplement to the diet.

• **Control blood sugar manually during the recovery cycle.** Under medical supervision, gradually discontinue all oral hypoglycaemic agents along with any additional drugs given to counteract their side effects. Develop natural blood-sugar control by the use of glycaemic tables, by consuming frequent small meals (including fibre-rich foods), by regular after-meal exercise such as a walk, and by the complete avoidance of all sugars along with the sensible use of only non-toxic sweeteners (such as stevia, raw coconut crystals, and no aspartame!). Avoid alcohol until blood sugar stabilises in the normal range. Keep score by using a pinprick-type glucose meter. Keep track of everything you do with a medical diary.

• **Restore a proper balance of healthy fats and oils when the blood sugar controller again works.** Permanently remove from the diet all cheap, toxic, junk fats and oils as well as the processed and restaurant foods that contain them. When the blood sugar controller again starts to work correctly, gradually introduce additional healthy foods to the diet. Test the effect of these added foods by monitoring blood sugar levels with the pinprick-type blood sugar monitor. Be sure to include the results of these tests in your diary also.

• **Continue the program until normal insulin values are also restored** after blood sugar levels begin to stabilise in the normal region. Once blood sugar levels fall into the normal range, the pancreas will gradually stop overproducing insulin. This process will typically take a little longer and can be tested by having your physician send a sample of your blood to a lab for a serum insulin determination. A good idea is to wait a couple of months after blood sugar control is restored and then have your physician check your insulin level. It's nice to have blood sugar in the normal range; it's even nicer to have this accomplished without excess insulin or harmful drugs in the bloodstream.

• **Separately repair the collateral damage done by the disease.** Vascular problems caused by a chronically elevated glucose level will normally reverse themselves without conscious effort. The effects of retinopathy and of peripheral neuropathy, for example, will usually self repair. However, when the fine capillaries in the basement membranes of the kidneys begin to leak due to chronic high blood glucose, the kidneys compensate by laying down scar tissue to prevent the leakage. This scar tissue remains even after the diabetes is cured, and is the reason why the kidney damage is not believed to self repair.

A word of warning... When retinopathy develops, there may be a temptation to have the damage repaired by laser surgery. This laser technique stops the retinal bleeding by creating scar tissue where the leaks have developed. This scar tissue will prevent normal healing of the fine capillaries in the eye when the diabetes is reversed. By reversing the diabetes instead of opting for laser surgery, there is an excellent chance that the eye will heal completely. However, if laser surgery is done, this healing will always be complicated by the scar tissue left by the laser.

The arterial and vascular damage done by years of elevated sugar and insulin and by the proliferation of systemic candida will slowly reverse due to improved diet. However, it takes many years to clean out the arteries by this form of oral chelation. Arterial damage can be reversed much more quickly by using intravenous chelation therapy. What would normally take many years through diet alone can often be done in six months with intravenous therapy. This is reputed to be effective over 80% of the time. For obvious reasons, don't expect your doctor to approve of this, particularly if he's a heart specialist.

Recovery Time

The prognosis is usually swift recovery from the disease and restoration of normal health and energy levels in a few months to a year or more. The length of time that it takes to effect a cure depends upon how long the disease was allowed to develop.

For those who work quickly to reverse the disease after early discovery, the time is usually a few months or less. For those who have had the disease for many years, this recovery time may lengthen to a year or more. Thus, there is good reason to get busy reversing this disease as soon as it becomes clearly identified.

By the time you get to this point in this article, and if we've done a good job of explaining our diabetes epidemic, you should know what causes it, what orthodox medical treatment is all about, and why diabetes has become a national and international disgrace.
Of even greater importance, you have become acquainted with a self-help program that has demonstrated great potential to actually cure this disease.

About the Author:
Thomas Smith is a reluctant medical investigator, having been forced into curing his own diabetes because it was obvious that his doctor would not or could not cure it.

He has published the results of his successful diabetes investigation in his self-help manual, *Insulin: Our Silent Killer*, written for the layperson but also widely valued by the medical practitioner. This manual details the steps required to reverse Type II diabetes and references the work being done with Type I diabetes. The book may be purchased from the author at PO Box 7685, Loveland, Colorado 80537, USA (North American residents send $US25.00; overseas residents should contact the author for payment and shipping instructions).

Thomas Smith has also posted a great deal of useful information about diabetes on his website, http://www.Healingmatters.com

Diabetes #1 Shame Of The "Orthodox" Doctors - Chromium & More

"DIABETES is the number one shame of the "orthodox" doctors in the 20th century. Diabetes is easy to prevent, easy to cure and treat (in laboratory animals and probably in humans) so you can avoid all of the terrible side effects (i.e. blindness, hypertension, amputations, early death, etc.). Since 1958, it has been known that supplemental chromium will prevent and treat diabetes as well as hypoglycemia. Just ask any health food store owner or N.D.! Walter Mertz (the director of the U.S.D.A. field services) published the facts associated with chromium and diabetes in the Federation Proceeding.

Here is the ultimate case of a whole specialty of medicine which could be wiped out by universal chromium supplementation Nevertheless these facts are kept secret and away from the public for purely economic reasons.. Additionally, in 1985, the medical school at the University of Vancouver, BC, Canada stated that "vanadium will replace insulin for adult onset diabetics." Chromium/vanadium and the diabetes story should be on the front page of the newspaper in the same bold print as VE DAY instead of announcing things like artificial heart pumps that will temporarily save one life for $250,000!"

There are many minerals that seem to have been systematically removed form our diets. I say systematically as the root causes for Diabetes, heart disease, AIDS, cancer are clearly known and many of these diseases have been resolved in animals already*. Clearly the current disease epidemic is not merely a "mistake" made by well intentioned, albeit misguided mad scientists. In addition to Chromium, Iodine that used be available in bread has been replaced with the toxic Bromine and now in some instances even removed from salt, when it is known that iodine is an essential element for the thyroid - on which our immune system literally depends! To further add insult to injury, the unsuspecting public yet again knowing subjected to water fluoridation to further depress the thyroid... It is a real testimonial to the creator given that with all these induced insults our bodies still continues to function. Sadly allowing continued abuse by the vested interests...

We also know from human and animal studies that essential minerals never occur in a uniform blanket around the crust of the Earth, they occur in veins like chocolate ripple ice cream. Whatever essential minerals might have been in the Earth's crust also have pretty much now pretty much depleted. An example of one such mineral is Selenium. See Harold Foster's (medical geographer) work that so clearly delineates diseases based on soil mineral geographies.

*Selenium deficiency causes infertility, miscarriages, cystic fibrosis of the pancreas, Sudden Infant Death Syndrome in animals, liver cirrhosis, stiff lamb disease, white muscle disease, muscular dystrophy, anemias, encephalomalacia (Alzheimer's disease), cardiomyopathy heart disease, and mulberry heart disease. In each case, selenium supplementation prevented the disease and in many cases reversed or cured existing diseases, which were all significant causes of animal losses to the livestock industry. (Page 33)

JAMA Dec. 25, 1996, Selenium Supplemented At 250 Mcg/Day Will Reduce Ones Risk Of Developing Prostate Cancer By 69 Percent.

This should have been and still be front page news! No drug, I repeat no drug, has, can or ever appraoch such a feat! Yet the thugs continue to clamour for these generally toxic solutions....
Athletes sweat out more minerals in five years than couch potatoes sweat out in 50 years. If you sweat out all of your copper and don't replace it you are at high risk of dying of a ruptured aneurysm. If you sweat out all of your selenium and don't replace it you're at high risk of developing a cardiomyopathy heart attack or cancer. If you sweat out all of your chromium and vanadium and don't replace it you're at high risk of developing adult onset or type 2 diabetes. If you sweat out all of your calcium, magnesium, and sulfur and don't replace them, you are at high risk of developing arthritis, osteoporosis, and kidney stones. (Page 141) QED

"....Almost 50 years ago the mineral chromium was established as an essential nutrient at the federal offices of the National Institutes of Health by Dr. Klaus Schwarz. It was precisely for its role in blood sugar metabolism that this trace element chromium was established as essential.
A molecule named Glucose Tolerance Factor (GTF) that corrected abnormal sugar metabolism was found to be composed primarily of the mineral chromium. Dr. Walter Mertz, then an assistant to **Dr. Schwarz, reportedly noted at that time in 1959 "Type II diabetes is not a disease. It is the lack of a natural ingredient, known as GTF Chromium."**....

....Chromium works together with insulin in providing sugar to the cells for energy. If chromium levels decrease then sugar delivery to the cells from insulin decrease accordingly.

Modern medical terms such as "insulin resistance" and "insulin sensitivity" should be replaced by "gross chromium deficiency". It is not that insulin is "resistant" or lacks "sensitivity," but rather that insulin is lacking a vital – in fact essential – component for sugar metabolism that is this mineral chromium.

Insulin is a transport mechanism. It is like a truck that transports glucose to the cell. At the cell destination there is an insulin receptor site that is comparable to a loading dock. This is where the glucose is unloaded and passed into the cell. Chromium rich GTF molecules are in essence dock workers that assist the sugar (glucose) from the insulin "truck" at the insulin receptor site "loading dock" into the cell. If there are less and less GTF chromium "dock workers" then the work of providing sugar to the cells for energy slows and becomes unproductive. A traffic jam of insulin "trucks" in the blood stream results in higher and higher levels of blood sugar as the problem of chromium deficiency increases with the passing of time.

Whole wheat and raw sugar from sugar cane are rich in chromium. **The refining of whole wheat into bleached, white flour removes 91 per cent of that chromium. The refining of raw sugar into white sugar removes 98 per cent of that chromium. [This is why raw foods, even some high in sugar content, are perfectly healthy due to the added minerals, vitamins, and enzymes which are perfectly balanced to that specific food, helping it digest and absorb flawlessly into your body. As soon as any food is refined or cooked it looses some, or all, of the required elements and thus becomes not as beneficial as it was before]**

The refined flour and refined sugar are quickly reduced in the body into simple sugars that require chromium to be efficiently metabolized – chromium that is substantially no longer there. The most important component for your body to use the refined flour and refined sugar is very nearly entirely removed. This turns foods wholly good for you into those which are essentially unholy foods to you.

Quite literally every time you consume a refined, white flour or refined, white sugar product your body loses chromium.

If we were to eat raw organic foods and sprouted grains that grew without pesticides or GMO on clean mineral rich natural soil, we would be eating so many natural vitamins, nutrients, enzymes, and minerals that there physically would be no disease in our bodies. It would be biologically impossible to get any disease (unless of course deliberately). There would also be no need for "natural cures" or "vaccines" or packaged vitamins since we would be getting them all from our food. Nature is perfect, and any meddling with perfection looses that perfection.

Dr. Henry Alfred Schroeder, M.D., Ph.D., graduate of Columbia and Yale, and professor at Dartmouth medical school wrote more than 30 years ago that "the typical American diet, with about 60 per cent of its calories from refined sugar, refined flour, and fat ... was apparently designed not only to provide as little chromium as feasible, but to cause depletion of body stores of chromium."

Dr. Schroeder compared tissue levels of chromium in teenagers and those 40 years of age in Americans to those of three other cultures that did not follow after Westernized dietary choices in Mideast, southeast Asian, and African communities. He discovered very little change in the non-American cultures but dramatic decreases in Americans. **Almost 25 per cent of Americans had no detectable levels of chromium at all by the age of 40!** <u>That was more than 30 years ago</u> and things have not gotten any better – if anything things are worse.

This is a significant part of the reason that the average age of adult onset (Type II) diabetes is continually decreasing. A hundred years ago diabetes was a disease primarily of old age. Now the average age is approaching 30.

There is a dramatic increase of children developing adult onset diabetes in the last ten years. Imagine that. Children are developing adult onset diabetes before they even become adults! The field of medicine is baffled but I am not baffled at all. This is only the logical end result of the SAD (Standard American Diet) choices of the past 80+ years.

Few, if any, scientific researchers of the last 100 years were more accredited and experienced researchers regarding cardiovascular health than the late Dr. Henry Alfred Schroeder, M.D., a long time Dartmouth University professor. Dr. Schroeder identified chromium deficiency as the primary cause of heart disease. I think that is a little overly simplistic, but chromium deficiency is most certainly a primary part of the problem with heart disease. Dr. Schroeder noted that **cholesterol increases were linked to sinking levels of the trace element chromium more than 30 years ago.**

Schroeder discovered that chromium was the factor that managed cholesterol as he wrote, "*We found that chromium in the aorta was not detected (too low to be found) in almost every person dying of coronary artery disease, one manifestation of atherosclerosis, and was present in almost every aorta of persons dying accidentally.*"

Cholesterol has been blamed for decades as a primary cause of heart disease. However, cholesterol problems are only an effect caused by a deficiency of chromium.

Schroeder wrote of "the typical American diet, with about 60 per cent of its calories from refined sugar, refined flour, and fat". He noted that this diet "was apparently designed not only to provide as little chromium as feasible, but to cause depletion of body stores of chromium."

"The result is a prevalent disease, in this case, atherosclerosis," concluded Schroeder, about chromium deficiency.

Schroeder noted chromium supplements that are grown rather than concocted by man in his laboratories to be "100 times more active". He expressed great hope for atherosclerosis and diabetes when these grown source chromium supplements became available. **It was not until after his death during the 1970s that these supplements became available. They have been tragically ignored ever since.**

My own personal observations with a great many individuals have confirmed the postulations from Dr. Schroeder and his research. Reductions of LDL and total cholesterol levels, and increases in HDL levels are consistently noted with use of chromium supplements from grown origins. Reductions of triglyceride levels have been noted as well.

It is the right form of chromium (that which is grown) in the right amount (100 micrograms three times daily) that has been consistently shown to help diabetics – and almost any and every other individual for their life and living.

I should note that I did not pull out of a hat 100 micrograms three times daily or through some extensive trial and error. Human studies 40 years ago determined that 200 to 290 micrograms of dietary chromium intake "maintained chromium equilibrium". In other words, that is how much chromium you need to take in so that you don't lose more than you use.

It was noted that chromium intake from SAD choices at that time varied from 50 to 200 micrograms daily with an average of about 60 micrograms daily. However, it was also noted that a diet considered adequate in all other nutrients could contain as little as 5 micrograms of chromium. This deficiency of chromium is a very serious one of very long standing. Today the average chromium intake is noted as much less than even 60 micrograms daily.
As for chromium and other diseases – that is a very long list. Chromium has great importance at the cellular level from before you are born until the day you die.

Briefly, there is gestational diabetes and prevention of birth defects regarding the beginning of new life. Then there is energy production. OK, that is not a disease matter UNLESS you want to get into hypoglycemia and Chronic Fatigue Syndrome. People have greater energy and also feel better due to mental health issues. You know, the brain uses more sugar than any other organ in the body.

Vision loss is another hallmark of chromium deficiency and that is why there is much more vision loss with diabetics than with non-diabetics.

Cancer is another condition in which chromium is of profound importance. A must read interview: Chromium: Your Body Needs It, You're Probably Not Getting Enough of It, and Without It, You Cannot Survive - *Chris Gupta*

"The diagnosis of diabetes is very easy to make and it should be considered in any disease where there is a chronic weight loss or weight gain. Frequent urination and chronic thirst are warning signs that should be explored. A six-hour Glucose Tolerance Test (GTT)** will show a steep rise of blood glucose at 30-60 minutes to over 275 mg % and may keep rising to over 350 and stay elevated after 4-6 hours. The urine should be tested for sugar with the "dipstick" test every time the blood is tested for sugar. A positive diabetic will always include a positive urine sugar during the six-hour GTT. A morning fasting urine sugar test is useless for the initial diagnosis of diabetes. Blood of the diabetic is also typical in that the lipids and cholesterol are elevated as well as the sugar.

Treatment of diabetes should include chromium and vanadium at 250 mcg/day in the initial stages to prevent "insulin shock" (sudden dropping of blood sugar because of a relative insulin overdose). **Keep checking urine blood sugar before and after meals, and as the blood sugar level drops you can adjust your insulin or pill medication just like you have been taught.**

You will also need to deal with food allergies that cause celiac-type intestinal lesions (i.e. wheat gluten, cow's milk, soy, etc.) and supplement with betaine HCl and digestive enzymes at 75-200 mg (three times a day) before meals. Have patience; the intestinal lesions take 60-90 days to heal.

Treatment of diabetes should also include zinc at 50 mg daily, B complex at 50 mg daily (be sure to include niacin which is part of the GTF "glucose tolerance factor"), essential fatty acids at 5 grams daily (flax/hemp oil), B12 at 1,000 mcg/day, bioflavonoids including quercetin at 150 mg/day, copper at 2-3 mg/day, lecithin at 2,500 mg (**not** soy derived), and glutathione at 100 mg/day.

High fiber, high complex carbohydrate diets are recommended. No natural or processed sugar and carbohydrates should be consumed.

Every time you eat processed carbohydrate (i.e. sugar, alcohol, mashed potatoes, etc.), you will loose 300 percent more chromium in your urine than when you consume complex carbohydrates!

Herbs are useful in treating diabetes and may include licorice (Glycyrrhiza glabra), jaborandi (Pilocarpus jaborandi), yarrow (Achillea Millefolium), Canadian fleabane (Erigeron canadense), and Jerusalem artichoke. Plant derived colloidal minerals are fantastic for diabetics!

**Six-hour GTT: A FASTING BLOOD SUGAR ALONE WILL NOT DIAGNOSE HYPOGLYCEMIA OR DIABETES IN 98 PERCENT OF THE CASES; THERE ARE NO SHORT CUTS TO THIS DIAGNOSIS!!! A finger prick is done in the morning while fasting and the fasting blood sugar level is recorded (normal is 75 mg % give or take 5 points). Then 100 gm of glucose (Glucola) is ingested and a finger prick blood glucose is taken 30 minutes after ingestion and the results recorded. A finger prick blood glucose is taken at 60 minutes after ingestion of the glucose and at hourly intervals thereafter for a total of eight finger sticks. It is of extreme importance to have an observer present during the entire test, not because the test is dangerous, rather because behavioral changes are best recognized by someone else. Having the "patient" write their name, draw pictures, etc. can be very useful, especially in children where they may have a difficult time describing how they feel. These tests and observations should be done every 30 minutes during the six-hour test. A chart is then developed using the numbers gathered to assess the patient's glucose status. Hypoglycemia exists when the low during the test drops below the level of the starting fasting blood sugar level. Elevated blood sugar can produce behavioral changes as the blood sugar rises after a meal much in the same way that alcohol or drugs do (in fact, many hypoglycemics are falsely accused of being intoxicated!). Diabetes can be diagnosed when the total of the results of the fasting, at the 30 minute, one hour, and the second hour blood sugar test exceeds 600 mg % and there is sugar in the urine during the test.
Extracted from pages 348-349

Citations from: <u>Dead Doctors Don't Lie</u> by Dr. Joel D Wallach, Dr. Ma Lan.

Vitamin E and Diabetes

We can say that almost no diabetic dies from the disease itself, per se, but it produces a constant degeneration of the circulatory system to which insulin has no clear effect. The disease also affects other areas of the body which have little or nothing to do with the insulin-sugar balance, particularly the circulatory system. The biggest effects were seen in the tiny capillaries and in the smaller blood vessels which have the huge task of supplying the individual cells with the elements needed for an effective metabolism; somehow this function of the capillaries was being disturbed. For one thing, the permeability of the capillaries was altered: that is, their walls were no longer able to give and take nutrients as they are supposed to.

The nutrients carried by the blood were leaking out of the capillary walls and not penetrating the tissue cells; also, waste products of the cells could not gain entrance to the blood cells to be transported back to the various organs for elimination or to be changed into neutral, harmless substances. Therefore, deprived of nutrients and unable to rid themselves of harmful materials, the cells died. If one cell dies it's not a big deal, but when millions of cells begin dying in the same place it becomes a serious matter; as in gangrene or leg ulcers.

Diabetics have a circulation problem and are dying from diseases which once were considered totally unrelated to diabetes.

Now because of Vitamin E's qualities as an oxygen conserver, vasodilator, regulator of the cell's permeability, and muscle stimulant, among other qualities, it should be able to assist the body in managing diabetes. Researchers discovered another interesting quality of Vitamin E; It actually decreases the blood stream sugar in a number of patients, just as it decreases high blood pressure in a number of hypertensives. It conducts a whole body operation, toward maintaining homeostasis, the tendency of the body toward the normal.

The Shutes, along with the previously mentioned Dr. Butturini, were among the first researchers to discover Vitamin E's role in treating diabetes. They have treated thousands of diabetics with partial to completely successful results in most of their cases - provided that damage has not been done that is irreversible. They also have found that a diabetic who is given large doses of Vitamin E can oftentimes completely stop taking insulin. In most cases, insulin can be eliminated entirely (usually with the early victims) or else cut to a fraction of the former dose. In 80 per cent of all diabetics, the need for insulin can be either eliminated or drastically reduced.

The Shutes are backed up in their findings on diabetes by no less than thirty-five studies all over the world, and all performed by reputable researchers who have published in leading foreign medical journals. Sadly enough, most of these positive reports on Vitamin E are kept from you but, even more sadly, are kept from your doctor as well.

Cinnamon

A 12-week London study was recently conducted involving 58 type 2 diabetics with hemoglobin A1c (HbA1c) levels over 7 percent. Hemoglobin A1c is a marker for long-term glycemic control in diabetics.

After 12 weeks on 2g of cinnamon per day, study subjects had significantly lower HbA1c levels, as well as significantly reduced blood pressures (systolic, SBP and diastolic, DBP).

The researchers' conclusion:
"Intake of 2g of cinnamon for 12 weeks significantly reduces the HbA1c, SBP and DBP among poorly controlled type 2 diabetes patients. Cinnamon supplementation could be considered as an additional dietary supplement option to regulate blood glucose and blood pressure levels along with conventional medications to treat type 2 diabetes mellitus."

Among this spice's most impressive health benefits is its impact on blood sugar and ability to improve glucose control.

For example, just half a teaspoon of cinnamon a day has previously been shown to significantly reduce blood sugar levels, triglycerides, LDL (bad) cholesterol, and total cholesterol levels in people with type 2 diabetes.

Another study found that the spice increased glucose metabolism by about 20 times, which would significantly improve your ability to regulate blood sugar. Cinnamon has even previously been indicated as a potential insulin substitute for those with type 2 diabetes due to a bioactive component with "insulin-like" effects.

Interestingly, cinnamon lowers your blood sugar by acting on several different levels.

It slows the emptying of your stomach to reduce sharp rises in blood sugar following meals, and improves the effectiveness, or sensitivity, of insulin.

It also enhances your antioxidant defenses. A study published last year stated that "polyphenols from cinnamon could be of special interest in people that are overweight with impaired fasting glucose since they might act both as insulin sensitizers and antioxidants."

Yet another bioflavanoid compound called proanthocyanidin may alter the activity of insulin signaling in your fat cells.

Researchers have suggested people with diabetes may see improvements by adding 1/4 - 1 teaspoon of cinnamon to their food, and I see no reason not to give this a try if you enjoy cinnamon.

Excerpts from scientific studies and articles

Study: http://spectrum.diabetesjournals.org/content/25/1/38.full
A 2009 study14 found that, among a range of diets from vegan to non-vegetarian, as consumption of animal products increased, so did diabetes prevalence, ranging from 2.9% in vegans to 7.8% among individuals with unlimited consumption of animal products.

- **Eating meat raises your risk of diabetes by 170%**

Data from the Harvard Women's Health Study, the Nurses' Health Study, the Health Professionals Follow-Up Study, and other trials were part of a systematic review15 of 12 cohort studies that found that men and women who ate the most meat had the highest risk of type 2 diabetes. Intake levels of red meat, processed meat, and fish were all associated with risk of type 2 diabetes.

Although medication changes were not a goal of the study, requirements for medication also dropped; 43% (21 of 49) of those following the vegan diet reduced their diabetes medications compared to 26% (13 of 50) in the conventional diet group. After 74 weeks, improvements in glycemia and plasma lipid concentrations remained greater in the vegan group.

- **A vegan diet is nearly 2 times more successful at eliminating the need for diabetes medication**

Ferdowsian et al.5 concluded that a plant-based eating pattern that includes nuts, soy, and/or soluble fiber can reduce LDL cholesterol by 25–30%, an amount comparable to what can be achieved with statin drugs.

- **Plant based diet works just as well as drugs at reducing cholesterol - but without you having to live with drug or disease side-effects or paying for drugs your entire life.**

Study: http://www.nejm.org/doi/full/10.1056/NEJMoa012512

The lifestyle intervention reduced the incidence by 58 percent and metformin by [only] 31 percent.

- **A vegan diet is nearly 2 times more successful at eliminating diabetes**

Study: http://www.pritikin.com/pritikin-center-explore-the-resort/your-experience/your-results.html

A meta-analysis of 864 diabetics found that fasting glucose fell on average 19% within three weeks. Of those on oral drugs, 74% left Pritikin free of these drugs, and the majority of the others had their dosages significantly reduced. Of those taking insulin shots, 44% left insulin-free.

Among children with the Metabolic Syndrome, 100% no longer had the clinical diagnosis of the syndrome within two weeks of starting ...

- **A vegetarian, raw diet completely eliminated diabetes in 74% of patients and eliminated Metabolic Syndrome in 100% of children.**

Article: http://www.dailymail.co.uk/health/article-461350/Could-change-diet-reverse-diabetes.html

Dr Fedon Lindberg, a Norwegian endocrinologist who has treated more than 18,000 diabetic patients in his four clinics in his home country: "My experience with type 2 diabetic patients is that a balanced low-glycemic diet coupled with a healthy lifestyle can reverse the disease,".

"We have had many patients coming to us who were injecting high doses of insulin, as many as 200 units daily, who have managed to quit insulin and come off medications for blood pressure and other conditions."

Another doctor also claiming dramatic success using diet to treat diabetes is Dr Neal Barnard, an American expert whose book, Reversing Diabetes, was published in the UK last week.

"We've run trials showing that a diet with zero animal fats can control blood sugar three times more effectively than the diet recommended by the American Diabetes Association,"

Study: Vegetarian diet: panacea for modern lifestyle diseases?
http://qjmed.oxfordjournals.org/content/92/9/531.full

Diets rich in fiber and complex carbohydrate, and restricted in fat, improve control of blood glucose concentration, lower insulin requirement and aid in weight control in diabetic patients. An inverse association has been reported between nut, fruit, vegetable and fiber consumption, and the risk of coronary heart disease. Patients eating a vegetarian diet, with comprehensive lifestyle changes, have had reduced frequency, duration and severity of angina as well as regression of coronary atherosclerosis and improved coronary perfusion.

People consuming more fruit and vegetables had fewer strokes. Consumption of fruits and vegetables, especially spinach and collard greens, was associated with a lower risk of age-related ocular macular degeneration. Consumption of dietary fiber intake was associated with a drop in incidences of colon and breast cancer as well as colonic diverticula and gallstones.

Diets rich in fiber and complex carbohydrate and restricted in fat improve control of blood glucose concentration, delay glucose absorption, lower insulin requirements, increase peripheral tissue insulin sensitivity, decrease serum cholesterol and triglyceride values, aid in weight control and lower blood pressure in diabetic patients. Studies using high-carbohydrate and high-fiber diets reported an average 40% reduction of insulin doses, a 6–27% reduction in fasting serum glucose values, and a 10–32% reduction in serum cholesterol values.
-Dr M. Segasothy, NT Clinical School of Medicine of Flinders University, Alice Springs Hospital

A meta-study from 2010, which included over 1.2 million individuals, concluded that eating just 50g of processed meat per day (which is only a fraction of what most people consume) was associated with **42% higher risk of heart disease and a 19% higher risk of type 2 diabetes.** Red meat seems to contain compounds that become carcinogenic during cooking. For example, one study found that eating grilled or well done red meat increases the risk of cancer by more than 50%.
-Micha, R; Wallace, S.K.; Mozaffarian, D. "*Red and Processed Meat Consumption and Risk of Incident Coronary Heart Disease, Stroke, and Diabetes Mellitus*". Circulation online journal

Study: Three-Week Diet-Exercise Study Shows 50 Percent Reversal In Metabolic Syndrome, Type 2 Diabetes
http://www.sciencedaily.com/releases/2006/01/060115182443.htm
"The study shows, contrary to common belief, that Type 2 diabetes and metabolic syndrome can be reversed solely through lifestyle changes," according to lead researcher Christian Roberts of University of California, Los Angeles.

"The results are all the more interesting because the changes occurred in the absence of major weight loss, challenging the commonly held belief that individuals must normalize their weight before achieving health benefits," Roberts said. Participants did lose two to three pounds per week, but they were still obese after the 3-week study.

"Aside from meat and dairy, the study participants could eat as much as they wanted," Roberts said. "Because the food was not as high calorie as a typical American diet, the participants ate less before feeling full. This is a departure from most diets, which usually leave the dieter feeling hungry," he said.

The men also exercised daily on a treadmill, including level and graded walking, for 45-60 minutes. The exercise program was tailored to ensure each individual reached 70-85% of maximum heart rate.
-Christian K. Roberts, Dean Won, Sandeep Pruthi, Silvia Kurtovic, and R. James Barnard, of the Department of Physiological Science at UCLA

Article: Diet with zero animal fats can control blood sugar three times more effectively than the diet recommended by the American Diabetes Association
http://www.dailymail.co.uk/health/article-461350/Could-change-diet-reverse-diabetes.html

Dr Fedon Lindberg, a Norwegian endocrinologist who has treated more than 18,000 diabetic patients in his four clinics in his home country.

"My experience with type 2 diabetic patients is that a balanced low-glycaemic diet coupled with a healthy lifestyle can reverse the disease," he says.

"We have had many patients coming to us who were injecting high doses of insulin, as many as 200 units daily, who have managed to quit insulin and come off medications for blood pressure and other conditions."

"We've run trials showing that a diet with zero animal fats can control blood sugar three times more effectively than the diet recommended by the American Diabetes Association,"

Article: Vegan diet reverses diabetes symptoms, study finds
http://abcnews.go.com/Health/Diabetes/wireStory?id=2244647#.UGsEJEbPZ8E

People who ate a low-fat vegan diet, cutting out all meat and dairy, lowered their blood sugar more and lost more weight than people on a standard American Diabetes Association diet, researchers said on Thursday.

The vegan dieters lost 14 pounds (6.5 kg) on average while the diabetes association dieters lost 6.8 pounds (3.1 kg).

An important level of glucose control called a1c fell by 1.23 points in the vegan group and by 0.38 in the group on the standard diet.

They lowered their cholesterol more and ended up with better kidney function, according to the report published in Diabetes Care, a journal published by the American Diabetes Association.

Participants said the vegan diet was easier to follow than most because they did not measure portions or count calories.

"I hope this study will rekindle interest in using diet changes first, rather than prescription drugs," Dr. Neal Barnard, president of the Physician's Committee for Responsible Medicine, which helped conduct the study, told a news conference.

Study: Physical Activity in the Prevention of Type 2 Diabetes
http://diabetes.diabetesjournals.org/content/54/1/158.short

Individuals who increased moderate-to-vigorous LTPA or strenuous, structured LTPA the most were 63–65% less likely to develop diabetes.

Thus increasing physical activity may substantially reduce the incidence of type 2 diabetes in high-risk individuals.

Healing Crisis or Herxheimer

As you begin your new nutrition routing and cleanses, your body will be dumping high amounts of toxins, chemicals, and billions of dead cells, microbes, and bacteria into your excretory organs, blood, and pathways. Many doctors do not recommend fasting or colon hydrotherapy or cleanses because they produce various symptoms like fevers, chills, fatigue, muscle aches, nausea, diarrhea, skin breakout and other conditions. Yet this is **solely** due to your body dumping trash from all the little corners and crevasses of your body in an attempt to cleanse and detoxify itself. Basically it means your body is releasing more toxins than you can safely dispose of. This is called a detoxification reaction or healing crisis.

The more toxins one's body, the more severe the healing crisis will be. Some feel worse and attribute it to the failing treatment, yet your attitudes should be completely the opposite. You should **welcome** these reactions with open arms, it means your body is finally becoming healthy and you are on the **right** track.

Such reactions are temporary and can occur immediately -- or within several days, or even several weeks, of a detox. Symptoms usually pass within 1-3 days, but on rare occasions can last several weeks. If you are suffering from a major illness, the symptoms you experience during the healing crisis may be identical to the disease itself. Sometimes discomfort during the healing crisis is of greater intensity than when you were developing the chronic disease.

This may explain why there may be a brief flare-up in one's condition. Often the crisis will come after you feel your very best. Most people feel somewhat ill during the first few days of a cleanse because it is at that point that your body dumps toxins into the blood stream for elimination. With a more serious condition there may be many small crises to go through before the final one is possible. In any case, a cleansing & purifying process is underway, and stored wastes are in a free-flowing state.

The symptoms can be absolutely anything, from new symptoms to old illnesses flaring up. Whatever symptoms begin after you start the protocol, it is a sign that everything is working.

You might also experience "brain fog" symptoms which feels like you can't think clearly or put thoughts together. This is also normal and is a result of dead microbes and waste matter being excreted.

Diabetes Eating Plan

If you bought this book as a package with "*7 Steps to Health*" then I highly recommend you read it as it goes into a lot more detail into each food group. Before I describe the plan, there are a few assumptions I make:

- You don't smoke or chew tobacco
- You don't drink soda/soft drinks or eat at fast food restaurants
- You don't use recreational drugs
- You don't drink alcohol
- You don't drink more than a cup of coffee a day

If you do any of these things you are creating the perfect environment for the development of diabetes, and thus I highly recommend you avoid them.

The list below is pretty much the **absolute best** that you can possibly do to destroy diabetes fast. If you decide to implement everything that is written, then you are a true warrior of your health, you will see the results quicker than anyone, and you will achieve a healthy glowing and beautiful body in no time. For some it may not be as easy so please remember to take it slow and do what you feel is best for you. Start slowly, see and feel the result, then continue to add further changes. Do what you can, as best you can, you don't have to overwhelm yourself.

For you to reap the full benefits of your health and wellbeing, never get sick or develop disease, the following list should become a lifestyle commitment and not just a temporary measure.

1. No junk fats. This is the main reason why diabetes occurs. You must never eat trans fats, hydrogenated fats, fried or heavily processed fats, canola oil, soy oil, margarine, crisco, etc.

2. No white foods. This includes sugar, white flour, white pasta, gluten containing grains, potatoes, as well as yeast. Many celebrities including Cameron Diaz and Oprah have endorsed this diet because of the toxic effects these ingredients have on our bodies. The only sweeteners that are actually good for you are raw coconut crystals, stevia, raw agave powder, and raw honey - you can eat as much of them as you like.

3. No animal protein. Animal protein has been linked in numerous world renowned international studies to directly promote cancer growth, diabetes, and heart disease like a switch. This is absolutely key to a successful diabetes treatment and one which is recommended by almost all the prominent holistic doctors and clinics. Beef, chicken, fish, eggs are all considered animal protein and should be completely avoided if you wish you cure your diabetes in a short period of time. For more information please refer to "*The China Study*" by Colin Campbell.

4. No processed foods. It's quite simple; "If it came from a plant, eat it. If it was made in a plant, don't!" This might be a little challenging at first, but it is crucial for your health. You have no idea how many toxic additives, chemicals, preservatives, and flavor enhancers are added to our foods which lead to nasty ailments and diseases. If it comes in a package, try to avoid it as much as possible. Also, if the label reads "spices" as an ingredient, this doesn't mean actual spices like basil, pepper, dill, or parsley, it can mean up to **10,000 different chemical additives** disguised under the word "spices." This also includes processed rancid and hydrogenated fats and oil which destroy your cell membrane. Get used to eating and cooking with fresh vegetables, fruits, nuts, seeds and combinations of them.

Most importantly for a diabetes patient, avoid processed and artificial oils and fats, margarine, Crisco, hydrogenated oils, fried oils, all fats used in store bought pastries, cookies and cakes. Consumption of these fats is creating a broken cell membrane and preventing you from ever achieving optimal sugar absorption and insulin balance thus preventing you from ever curing your diabetes.

5. No pasteurized dairy. Pasteurized dairy is directly linked to cancer, heart disease and diabetes. It is no surprise that countries that have the highest dairy consumption; Denmark, Norway, and Holland have the highest rates of breast cancer. Nations where cheese consumption has tripled in the last 30 years, like England and France and Canada and the United States, have tripling rates of asthma and breast cancers. Raw dairy is a completely different product if compared to pasteurized dairy. The heating process of pasteurization destroys virtually everything beneficial in the milk such as enzymes, vitamins, fats, immune supporting factors, and beneficial bacteria. If you can find a raw milk provider near you, I highly recommend all raw dairy products. Visit www.westonaprice.org or www.realmilk.com for more information on raw dairy.

6. Do not use microwaves (the microwave article should be included in your bonus material), **drink tap water** (chlorine and fluoride react with all supplements and oxygen making them inert as well as stealing oxygen from your own body which promotes an acidic environment=not good for anyone looking to get rid of their diabetes or stay healthy), **do not use non-natural air fresheners, body washes, soaps, deodorants with aluminum** (reduces electrical potential of your cells making them sick and cancerous), **and toxic household cleaners** (full of hormone disruptors, chemicals that are known and proven carcinogens, DNA inhibitors, and other very nasty effects that you do not want near you as you destroy your diabetes). I know this might sound a little over the top but every standard chemical puts and even greater toxic load on your system. Again, I'm just letting you know the facts, the choice is always up to you.

Yes Foods

The following foods are a diabetes fighting arsenal and you can eat them as much as you like.

1. Raw, whole, fresh fruits and vegetables. The easiest way to stay healthy is to pack your meals with at least 50% raw foods. Every meal should be at least half made of raw fruits or vegetables. Spinach, kale, broccoli, cauliflower, cucumbers, tomatoes, peppers, radishes, squash, carrots, leeks, sprouts etc. Buy them organic if you can.

2. Good Fats and Oils. The only oils that should go anywhere near your plate are flax oil, hemp oil, coconut oil, and some olive oil due to the fact that your cells walls are hard, rigid, and dont allow nutrients, insulin, or oxygen to flow in and out. If you want to get rid of diabetes and other diseases, you must never consume trans fats, hydrogenated fats, and regular vegetable oils like canola or soy. This includes all regular pastries, cakes, cookies, fast foods, pre-packaged foods, tv dinners, and mostly everything found in a grocery store. This is the reason the diabetes epidemic grows exponentially in our country, because there is simply no good fats found in our foods. **Good fats and oils are your main weapon against diabetes!**

3. Sprouted, gluten and yeast free breads. Ezekiel and Genesis brands have a great lineup of sprouted and gluten free breads. Find some raw butter and you have a delicious substitute for the standard diabetes causing white bread with sugar loaded jelly. Yeast is also cancer food; Japanese research links breast cancer with the ingestion of goods baked with yeast. The problem is mycotoxins, which are waste products of yeast. There are many health problems that can be directly attributed to yeast, including arteriosclerosis, obesity, and AIDS.

4. **Gluten free grains**. Amaranth, buckwheat, millet, montina, oats, quinoa, rice, sorghum, teff, wild rice are all great meat replacing meals that are packed with nutrition and health promoting factors. Sprouted grains are anywhere from 3 to 10 times more nutritious than unsprouted and I highly recommend the sprouted kind. Also do your best to get them organic if your finances permit.

5. **Raw, unpasteurized dairy products.** Milk, cottage cheese, sour cream, butter are all amazing potent and nutritious diabetes-busting foods. They provide your body with virtually everything.

6. **Green smoothies and shakes.** Water, spinach/Kale, and fruits/berries is all you need for a delicious alkaline promoting diabetes destroying meal packed with everything your body needs. You may make as many green smoothies as you like and mix them with various ingredients like bananas, apples,

7. **Raw nuts and seeds**. Any nut other than peanuts should be your friend. Loaded with healthy fats, vitamins, minerals, and healthy calories you may snack on nuts as often as you like. Just make sure they are unprocessed, not fried or baked, in their **raw** state.

8. **Salads**. Here you can be as creative as you like. Any combination of leafy greens, vegetables, spices, and oils like flax or hemp will be bursting with flavor. Try experimenting with different spices and vegetables to find a salad that is exciting and one you can eat every day.

9. **Cinnamon**. Within cinnamon, the key substance is called: methylhydroxychalcone polymer (MHCP).

Dr. Richard A. Anderson, at the Human Nutrition Research Center (USDA) discovered that MHCP can stimulate glucose uptake by our cells. It can even help in the synthesis of glycogen, a polymer of glucose that our bodies produce as a means of storing energy for later use, when it is depolymerized back to glucose. Most of our glycogen is found in the liver, but some is found in our muscles - a handy place to be when we start exercising and need quick energy. Producing adequate amounts of glycogen is a principal function of blood sugar metabolism, and MHCP can help.

Dr. Anderson says that MHCP has effects similar to those of insulin and works almost as well. Both of these substances work by chemically modifying our cells' insulin receptors in a manner that activates them to do their job, which is to allow glucose molecules to pass through the cell wall into the insulin cascade--the series of molecular events triggered by insulin's interaction with its receptor-is also triggered by MHCP. He also discovered that when MHCP and insulin act together, the effect is synergistic, i.e., the total effect is greater than the sum of its parts."

While this is published information, orthodox medicine does not encourage people to eat cinnamon as a prevention measure for type 2 diabetes. Nor do they mention that type 2 diabetes is caused by trans-fatty acids and other bad fats. Nor will they ever will, because diabetes is a very profitable disease.

Diabetes Protocol

Please note that everything outlined is a best-case scenario. The more of these foods you incorporate into your life, the healthier you will be and the easier your path to a diabetes-free future. I understand some people's financial situations might not allow them to purchase some of these foods, or they might not be available in every store, but try to do your best to get as many of these foods and follow as many steps as possible.

Food

50% Raw - Half of everything you eat must be raw fruits and vegetables. This will allow your body to detox, alkalize, fill up on enzymes and nutrients while destroying diabetes.

Baking Soda- Mix a teaspoon of regular baking soda with half a cup of boiling water until fizzing disappears. Pour half a cup of cool water, and drink first thing in the morning. Baking soda alkalizes the entire body improving the immune system, metabolism, mineral absorption, and eliminates yeast and fungal infections.

Bee Pollen - A tablespoon daily (3 teaspoons in a tablespoon). You may either take it directly or put it in shakes, smoothies, salads, and anything else that is not going to be heated or cooked.

Green Smoothies - At least one green smoothie daily. I usually have one in the morning as a breakfast. I put a teaspoon of bee pollen, a scoop of my green superfood powder (has spirulina, chlorella, barley, wheatgrass, and more than 20 other superfoods) and raw coconut sugar for taste. (Go to page 357 for more tips on green smoothies)

Water - **Minimum** 2 liters/68 oz of clean filtered water daily. **Try not to use tap water if you can** as it might have fluoride or chlorine it in which interferes with oxygen, nutrient absorption in the cell and slows your healing progress.

Alkalizing and immune stimulating herbs - Tansy, wormwood, cloves (seeds, which are used in cooking).
All components are ground into a powder and mixed in a ratio of 4: 1: 2 (by weight) - 4 parts tansy, 1 part wormwood and 2 parts clove. One serving is 2 grams (about one teaspoon, non heaping). Add to this one teaspoon of fennel seeds, cumin seeds, thyme, and half a tea spoon of knotweed.
Take one serving 30 minutes before a meal with a glass of water. Increase to 2 servings on the second day, 3 servings on the third day, and continue with 3 servings spread out to three times a day before meals (one serving in the morning, one at lunch, and one at dinnertime).
To clarify, one serving would be 2 grams of powder (tansy, wormwood, cloves), 1 teaspoon of fennel seeds, cumin seeds, thyme, and a half tea spoon of knotweed.

Healing Practices

Exercise - walk outside a minimum 15 minutes a day, rain or snow!

Oil Pulling - Detox doesn't have to be difficult! Do this every time you have 5-20 minutes free, and cleanse away.

Fasting - The most powerful way to detox is absolutely free. Do at least one water or freshly squeezed juice fast every month. (See page 364 for more info about fasting)

Sunshine - If you can, get at least 15 minutes of sunshine to at least 70% of uncovered skin. Make sure you are directly in the sunlight, not behind glass as glass stops most of the beneficial (in moderation) UV rays.

Sauna - Attend a sauna at least once a week to help your body sweat out toxins.

Supplements - Spread them evenly throughout the day

Green Superfood Powder - Add a scoop to your smoothies every day
Vitamin C - 5 grams of the regular ascorbic acid kind daily, **not** the Ester-C brand (l-Lysine and l-Proline have been found to stimulate the effects of vitamin C)
Vitamin E - 800 IU daily
Vitamin D3 - 6000 IU daily
Vitamin B12 - 1000 mcg daily
Chromium (ionic) - 250 mcg daily
Vanadium (ionic) - 250 mcg daily
Digestive Enzymes - Depends on brand, check bottle for guidelines
Zinc - 50 mg daily
B Complex - Depends on brand, check bottle for guidelines (minimum 50 mg daily)
Bioflavonoids including Quercetin - 150 mg daily
Borage oil - 1000mg capsules three times daily (perfect blend of omega 3 and 6, with GLA, LA, EA fats)
Iodine - 2 drops daily in a glass of water (choose an iodine supplement that has both iodine and iodide such as Lugol's or Iodoral), take with vitamin C and magnesium to enhance its effects
Cinnamon - 5 grams daily, may be mixed in shakes, green smoothies, salads, sprinkled on top of fruits or bought in pill form
MSM - 5-10 grams daily in capsule form, make sure the MSM has absolutely no additives (MSM helps the cell wall become more elastic)

30 Day Diabetes Protocol

Almost every single person who has dedicated 30 days to this protocol has seen their diabetes completely disappear. Take the 30 day challenge and watch your diabetes melt away. You must follow this protocol exactly as written if you want to get rid of your diabetes in 30 days, no exceptions. If you are unable to do everything, then your results might come a little slower, and it might take 2-6 months.

100% Raw

Everything you eat must be **100% raw**, uncooked, and unprocessed. Various salads, fruits, vegetables, green smoothies, fruit smoothies, raw nuts, sprouted grains, dehydrated fruits and vegetables, and anything that is in its raw form.

- No meat (beef, chicken, fish, eggs, etc.)
- No flour products (anything baked, cooked, or fried with flour products)
- No pasteurized dairy products (milk, cheese, yogurt, except the flax seed and cottage cheese mixture)
- No pre-packaged foods, nothing processed or cooked

Baking Soda- Mix a teaspoon of regular baking soda with half a cup of boiling water until fizzing disappears. Pour half a cup of cool water, and drink first thing in the morning. Baking soda alkalizes the entire body improving the immune system, metabolism, mineral absorption, and eliminates yeast and fungal infections.

Bee Pollen – At least a tablespoon daily (3 teaspoons in a tablespoon). You may either take it directly or put it in shakes, smoothies, salads, and anything else that is not going to be heated or cooked.

Exercise - at least 30 minutes of excursive, it can be a walk, a jog, a gym session, or a sporting event.

Green Smoothies - at least one green smoothie daily.

Fasting - The most powerful way to detox is absolutely free. Do at least one water or freshly squeezed juice fast every week. (See page 364 for more info about fasting)

Sunshine - If you can, get at least 15 minutes of sunshine to at least 70% of uncovered skin. Make sure you are directly in the sunlight, not behind glass as glass stops most of the beneficial UV rays.

Sauna - Attend a sauna at least twice a week to help your body sweat out toxins.

Rebounder - Buy a small trampoline rebounder and jump for 5-10 minutes a day. This gets the lymph flowing stimulating the immune system.

Colon hydrotherapy - A professional session at least twice a week until colon is clean, or weekly enemas done at home.

Supplements

Herb mixture - Tansy, wormwood, cloves, fennel seeds, cumin seeds, thyme, knotweed
Green Superfood Powder - Add a scoop to your smoothies every day
Vitamin C - 5 grams of the regular ascorbic acid kind daily, **not** the Ester-C brand (l-Lysine and l-Proline have been found to stimulate the effects of vitamin C)
Vitamin E - 800 IU daily
Vitamin D3 - 6000 IU daily
Vitamin B12 - 1000 mcg daily
Chromium - 250 mcg daily
Vanadium - 250 mcg daily
Digestive Enzymes - Depends on brand, check bottle for guidelines
Zinc - 50 mg daily
B Complex - Depends on brand, check bottle for guidelines (minimum 50 mg daily)
Bioflavonoids including Quercetin - 150 mg daily
Borage oil - 1000mg capsules three times daily (perfect blend of omega 3 and 6, with GLA, LA, EA fats)
Iodine - 2 drops daily in a glass of water
Cinnamon - 5 grams daily, may be mixed in shakes, green smoothies, salads, sprinkled on top of fruits or taken in pill form

Protocol

Morning

- Drink 500ml / 17 oz of warm water with baking soda on an empty stomach
- Have the herb mixture, with a green smoothie with a scoop of green superfood powder; take 3 grams of vitamin C, 400 IU vitamin E, 3000 IU vitamin D, B12, and 3 grams of cinnamon with the smoothie
- 1 hour later you make have a healthy breakfast, fruits, vegetables, nuts seeds, etc, and take your chromium, vanadium, and 2 grams of MSM in capsules
- You may eat as much raw fruits, vegetables, and raw nuts as you like

Lunch

- 2 grams of MSM, and 1000mg borage oil, and herb mix.
- You may have a big salad with your favourite vegetables and leafy greens, some olive/flax/hemp oil, spices, and sea salt for flavor; have your B-complex, Zinc, 3000 IU vitamin D, bioflavonoids, and digestive enzymes with the salad
- You may eat as much raw fruits, vegetables, and raw nuts as you like
- Take your two drops of iodine with a glass of water before the meal or a few hours after the meal and 3 grams of vitamin C along with it

Dinner

- You may have another herb mix, and 20 minutes laater a big salad or a green smoothie with 3000 IU vitamin D, 3 grams of vitamin C, 400 IU vitamin E, 1000mg borage oil

Snacks

- You may snack on any amount of fruits, vegetables, nuts, seeds, dried raw fruits, berries, or a combination of these throughout the day. Just make sure to leave an hour before and after the cottage cheese mix.

Suggestions

If you notice the healing crisis/Herxeimer reaction becoming very strong, this means you body is not handling the toxin release.

If you feel the symptoms getting very strong, which sometimes happens as a huge wave of toxins gets released into the system, fast for a day, drink green smoothies, herb mix, eat salads, at least 2-3 liters of water daily, vitamin C, D, E, attend a sauna every day, and nothing else. An enema always helps in such situations, even if you have a high fever and enema is known to reduce a fever (sauna also helps which will sweat out the toxins).

You may resume the protocol once the symptoms subside.

Highly recommended books on diabetes:

"The pH Miracle for Diabetes : The Revolutionary Diet Plan for Type 1 and Type 2 Diabetics" by Robert O. Young, PhD

"Infectious Diabetes" is by Doug Kaufmann and David Holland, M.D.

Banned in Europe

...for Causing 83,000 Heart Attacks - Are You Taking it?

A September 23, 2010 article in the *New England Journal of Medicine* announced that, finally, the FDA has stepped forward and decided on regulatory action for Avandia, a diabetes drug that last year claimed 1,354 lives as a result of cardiac-associated problems.

The FDA is restricting access to Avandia by requiring GSK to submit a Risk Evaluation and Mitigation Strategy, or REMS.

Under the ruling, the drug will be available to patients not already taking it only if they are unable to achieve glycemic control using other medications and, in consultation with their health care professional, decide not to take a different drug for medical reasons.

Current users of Avandia will be able to continue using the medication if they appear to be benefiting from it and they acknowledge that they understand these risks. Doctors will have to attest to and document their patients' eligibility; patients will have to review statements describing the cardiovascular safety concerns.

But did the FDA go far enough – could it be too little, too late?
Unlike the US FDA, British regulators have ruled that GlaxoSmithKline's diabetes drug Avandia could lead to heart attacks or strokes, and *benefits no longer outweigh the risks*.

And so last week, they told 90,000 British diabetes patients to stop taking it. Evidence linking Avandia to an increased risk of a heart attack or stroke has been building since 2007, and GSK has agreed to pay $460 million in damages to settle about 10,000 lawsuits in America linking its use to patients suffering serious medical injuries. But the US FDA has chosen only to monitor the drug, rather than ask for a recall.

The FDA is "monitoring" a toxic drug which caused tens of thousands of severe injries. Yet they spend millions pursuing and hounding natural home remedies and do everything they can to get them off the market. Go figure.

Endnotes

1. National Center for Health Statistics, "Fast Stats", Deaths/Mortality Preliminary 2001 data
2. Dr Herbert Ley, in response to a question from Senator Edward Long about the FDA during US Senate hearings in 1965
3. Eisenberg, David M., MD, "Credentialing complementary and alternative medical providers", *Annals of Internal Medicine* 137(12):968 (December 17, 2002)
4. American Diabetes Association and the American Dietetic Association, *The Official Pocket Guide to Diabetic Exchanges*, McGraw-Hill/Contemporary Distributed Products, newly updated March 1, 1998
5. American Heart Association, "How Do I Follow a Healthy Diet?", American Heart Association
National Center (7272 Greenville Avenue, Dallas, Texas 75231-4596, USA), http://www.americanheart.org
6. Brown., J.A.C., Pears Medical Encyclopedia Illustrated, 1971, p. 250
7. Joslyn, E.P., Dublin, L.I., Marks, H.H., "Studies on Diabetes Mellitus", American Journal of Medical Sciences 186:753-773 (1933)
8. "Diabetes Mellitus", Encyclopedia Americana, Library Edition, vol. 9, 1966, pp. 54-56
9. American Heart Association, "Stroke (Brain Attack)", August 28, 1998, http://www.amhrt.org/ScientificHStats98/05stroke.html;
American Heart Association, "Cardiovascular Disease Statistics", August 28, 1998, http://www.amhrt.org/Heart_and_Stroke_A_Z_Guide/cvds.html ;
"Statistics related to overweight and obesity",
http://niddk.nih.gov/health/nutrit/pubs/statobes.htm ;
http://www.winltdusa.com/about/infocenter/healthnews/articles/obesestats.htm
10. "Diabetes Mellitus", *Encyclopedia Americana*, ibid., pp. 54-55
11. The Veterans Administration Coronary Artery Bypass Co-operative Study Group, "Eleven-year survival in the Veterans Administration randomized trial of coronary bypass surgery for stable angina", *New Eng. J. Med.* 311:1333-1339 (1984); Coronary Artery Surgery Study (CASS), "A randomized trial of coronary artery bypass surgery: quality of life in patients randomly assigned to treatment groups", *Circulation* 68(5):951-960 (1983)
12. Trager, J., *The Food Chronology*, Henry Holt & Company, New York, 1995 (items listed by date)
13. "Margarine", *Encyclopedia Americana*, Library Edition, vol. 9, 1966, pp. 279-280
14. Fallon, S., Connolly, P., Enig, M.C., *Nourishing Traditions*, Promotion Publishing, 1995;
Enig, M.C., "*Coconut: In Support of Good Health in the 21st Century*",

http://www.livecoconutoil.com/maryenig.htm
15. Houssay, Bernardo, A., MD, et al., *Human Physiology*, McGraw-Hill Book Company, 1955, pp. 400-421
16. Gustavson, J., et al., "Insulin-stimulated glucose uptake involves the transition of glucose transporters to a caveolae-rich fraction within the plasma cell membrane: implications for type II diabetes", *Mol. Med.* 2(3):367-372 (May 1996)
17. Ganong, William F., MD, *Review of Medical Physiology*, 19th edition, 1999, p. 9, pp. 26-33
18. Pan, D.A. et al., "Skeletal muscle membrane lipid composition is related to adiposity and insulin action", *J. Clin. Invest.* 96(6):2802-2808 (December 1995)
19. *Physicians' Desk Reference*, 53rd edition, 1999
20. Smith, Thomas, Insulin: Our Silent Killer, Thomas Smith, Loveland, Colorado, revised 2nd
edition, July 2000, p. 20
21. Law Offices of Charles H. Johnson & Associates (telephone 1 800 535 5727, toll free in North America)
22. American Heart Association, "Diabetes Mellitus Statistics", http://www.amhrt.org
23. Shanmugasundaram, E.R.B. et al. (Dr Ambedkar Institute of Diabetes, Kilpauk Medical College Hospital, Madras, India), "Possible regeneration of the Islets of Langerhans in Streptozotocin-diabetic rats given Gymnema sylvestre leaf extract", *J. Ethnopharmacology* 30:265-279 (1990); Shanmugasundaram, E.R.B. et al., "Use of Gemnema sylvestre leaf extract in the control of blood glucose in insulin-dependent diabetes mellitus", *J. Ethnopharmacology* 30:281-294 (1990)
24. Smith, ibid., pp. 97-123
25. Many popular artificial sweeteners on sale in the supermarket are extremely poisonous and dangerous to the diabetic; indeed, many of them are worse than the sugar the diabetic is trying to avoid; see, for example, Smith, ibid., pp. 53-58.
26. Walker, Morton, MD, and Shah, Hitendra, MD, *Chelation Therapy*, Keats Publishing, Inc., New Canaan, Connecticut, 1997, ISBN 0-87983-730-6